Relational Psychoanalysis: Volume II
Innovation and Expansion

RELATIONAL PERSPECTIVES BOOK SERIES

Volume 28

Relational Psychoanalysis

Volume II
Innovation and Expansion

edited by
Lewis Aron
Adrienne Harris

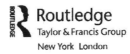

Routledge
Taylor & Francis Group
New York London

This edition published 2012 by Routledge

Routledge
Taylor & Francis Group
711 Third Avenue
New York, NY 10017

Routledge
Taylor & Francis Group
2 Park Square, Milton Park,
Abingdon,Oxfordshire OX14 4RN

Published by The Analytic Press, Inc.
101 West Street, Hillsdale, NJ 07642
www.analyticpress.com

ISBN - 9780881632705

Text set in Adobe Sabon 10/12 by Compudesign, Charlottesville, VA

To Steve and Mannie

Contributors

Neil Altman, Ph.D.—Coeditor of *Psychoanalytic Dialogues* and Associate Clinical Professor in the New York University Postdoctotal Program in Psychotherapy and Psychoanalysis. He is author of *The Analyst in the Inner City: Race, Class, and Culture through a Psychoanalytic Lens* (TAP, 1995) and coauthor of *Relational Child Psychotherapy*.

Lewis Aron, Ph.D., ABPP (Editor)—Director, New York University Postdoctoral Program in Psychotherapy and Psychoanalysis; President, Division of Psychologist-Psychoanalysts of the New York State Psychological Association (NYSPA); Editorial Board, *Studies in Gender and Sexuality*; Series Coeditor, Relational Perspectives Book Series. Dr. Aron is the author of *A Meeting of Minds: Mutuality in Psychoanalysis* (TAP, 1996) and coeditor of *Relational Psychoanalysis: The Emergence of a Tradition* (TAP, 1999).

Beatrice Beebe, Ph.D.—Clinical Professor of Psychology in Psychiatry, New York State Psychiatric Institute, Columbia University; Faculty, Columbia Psychoanalytic Center, the Institute for the Psychoanalytic Study of Subjectivity, and the New York University Postdoctoral Program in Psychotherapy and Psychoanalysis. She is coauthor of *Rhythms of Dialogue in Infancy* and *Infant Research and Adult Treatment: Co-constructing Interactions* (TAP, 2002).

Emanuel Berman, Ph.D.—Professor of Psychology, University of Haifa; Training Analyst, Israel Psychoanalytic Institute; Visiting Professor, New York University Postdoctoral Program in Psychotherapy and Psychoanalysis. He is editor of *Essential Papers in Literature and Psychoanalysis* and of Hebrew translations of Freud, Ferenczi, Winnicott, Hanna Segal, and Ogden; International Editor of *Psychoanalytic Dialogues*; and author of *Impossible Training: A Relational View of Psychoanalytic Education* (TAP, 2004).

Susan W. Coates, Ph.D.—Associate Clinical Professor of Medical Psychology in Psychiatry, Department of Psychiatry, College of Physicians and Surgeons of Columbia University; Teaching Faculty Member, Columbia Center for Psychoanalytic Training and Research. She is a coeditor of *September 11: Trauma and Human Bonds* (TAP, 2003).

Steven Cooper, Ph.D.—Training and Supervising Analyst, Boston Psychoanalytic Society and Institute; Faculty and Supervising Analyst, Massachusetts Institute for Psychoanalysis; Clinical Associate Professor of Psychology, Harvard Medical School; Consulting Editor, *Psychoanalytic Dialogues*; Corresponding Editor, *Contemporary Psychoanalysis*. He is the author of *Objects of Hope: Exploring Possibility and Limit in Psychoanalysis* (TAP, 2000).

Ken Corbett, Ph.D.—Editor, *Studies in Gender and Sexuality* and Associate Editor, *Psychoanalytic Dialogues*. He is a member of the Psychoanalytic Society of the New York University Postdoctoral Program in Psychotherapy and Psychoanalysis.

Muriel Dimen, Ph.D.—Professor and Supervisor, New York University Postdoctoral Program in Psychotherapy and Psychoanalysis; former Professor of anthropology, Lehman College (CUNY); Associate Editor, *Psychoanalytic Dialogues*; Incoming Editor (2006), *Studies in Gender and Sexuality*. She is the author of *Sexuality, Intimacy, Power* (TAP, 2003).

Darlene Bregman Ehrenberg, Ph.D.—Training and Supervising Analyst and teaching Faculty, William Alanson White Institute; Supervising Analyst, New York University Postdoctoral Program in Psychoanalysis and Psychotherapy; Teaching Faculty and Supervising Analyst, Northwest Center for Psychoanalysis (Seattle, WA and Portland, OR); Editorial Board, *Contemporary Psychoanalysis*; Consulting Editor, *Psychoanalytic Inquiry* and *International Forum of Psychoanalysis*; advisory board, International Association for Relational Psychoanalysis and Psychotherapy (IARPP).

Peter Fonagy, Ph.D., FBA—Freud Memorial Professor of Psychoanalysis, University College London; Chief Executive, the Anna Freud Centre, London.

Adrienne Harris, Ph.D. (Editor)—Clinical Associate Professor, New York University Postdoctoral Program in Psychotherapy and Psychoanalysis; Associate Editor, *Psychoanalytic Dialogues*. She is the author of *Gender as Soft Assembly* (TAP, 2005).

Theodore Jacobs, Ph.D.—Clinical Professor of Psychiatry, New York University School of Medicine; Training and Supervising Analyst, Psychoanalytic Institute, New York University and New York Psychoanalytic Institute; Supervising Child Analyst, Psychoanalytic Institute, New York University. He is the author of *The Use of the Self: Countertransference and Communication in the Analytic Process*, and coeditor of *On Beginning an Analysis*.

Daniel Kriegman, Ph.D.—Founding Member, Psychoanalytic Couple and Family Institute of New England; Faculty, Massachusetts Institute for Psychoanalysis; Former Chief Psychologist, Massachusetts Treatment Center for the Sexually Dangerous Offender.

Frank M. Lachmann, Ph.D.—Founding Faculty, Institute for the Psychoanalytic Study of Subjectivity; Clinical Assistant Professor, New York University Postdoctoral Program in Psychotherapy and Psychoanalysis; Editorial Board,

Psychoanalytic Inquiry. He is coauthor of *Infant Research and Adult Treatment: Co-constructing Interactions* (TAP, 2002); *Self and Motivational Systems: Toward a Theory of Psychoanalytic Technique* (TAP, 1999); *The Clinical Exchange: Techniques Derived from Self and Motivational Systems* (TAP, 1996); and *A Spirit of Inquiry: Communication in Psychoanalysis* (TAP, 2002).

Kimberlyn Leary, Ph.D.—Faculty, Boston Psychoanalytic Institute; Faculty, Psychoanalytic Institute of New England; Director of Psychology, Cambridge Health Alliance; Visiting Associate Professor of Psychology in Psychiatry, Harvard Medical School.

David Levit, Ph.D., ABPP—Diplomate in Psychoanalysis and Clinical Psychology; Faculty, Massachusetts Institute for Psychoanalysis; Assistant Clinical Professor of Psychiatry, Tufts Medical School; Adjunct Faculty, Smith College School for Social Work.

Karlen Lyons-Ruth, Ph.D.—Associate Professor, Department of Psychiatry, Harvard Medical School; Affiliate Scholar, Boston Psychoanalytic Society and Institute; Faculty, Massachusetts Institute for Psychoanalysis.

Karen J. Maroda, Ph.D.—Assistant Clinical Professor of Psychiatry, Medical College of Wisconsin; Advisory Board, IARPP; Board, Division 39 (Psychoanalysis) of American Psychological Association. She is the author of *The Power of Countertransference, 2nd ed.* (TAP, 2004) and *Seduction, Surrender, and Transformation: Emotional Engagement in the Analytic Process* (TAP, 1999).

Malcolm Owen Slavin, Ph.D.—Founder, Past-President, Faculty, and Supervising Analyst, Massachusetts Institute for Psychoanalysis (MIP); Advisory Board, IARPP; Contributing Editor, *Psychoanalytic Dialogues*; Editorial Boards, *Gender and Psychoanalysis, International Journal of the Psychology of the Self* (formerly *Progress in Self Psychology*), and *Self: Rivista Italiana Telematica di Psicologia Psicoanalitica del Sè e Intersoggettivita Psicoanalisi Relazionale.*

Joyce Slochower, Ph.D.—Professor of Psychology, Hunter College and the Graduate Center, C.U.N.Y.; Visiting Clinical Professor, New York Unviersity Postdoctoral Program in Psychtherapy and Psychoanalysis; Faculty, Psychoanalytic Insititute of Northern California; National Training Program, Object Relations Institute; Advisory Board, IARPP; Editorial Board, *Perspectives in Psychoanalysis.* She is the author of *Holding and Psychoanalysis: A Relational Perspective* (TAP, 1996).

Mary Target, Ph.D.—Reader in Psychoanalysis, University College London; Professional Director, the Anna Freud Centre, London.

Contents

Introduction

Lewis Aron
Adrienne Harris

▼   ▼   ▼   ▼   ▼

This volume was prepared and developed in a period of great promise and great loss within the relational and wider analytic community. Soon after the publication and welcome reception of Mitchell and Aron's (1999) *Relational Psychoanalysis: The Emergence of a Tradition* and shortly before Stephen Mitchell's untimely and completely unexpected death, Mitchell and Aron began to plan a sequel. Following Stephen's death, this plan was put on hold. When Adrienne Harris joined Lewis Aron as coeditor of the Relational Perspectives Book Series, the project was reenvisioned. Along with our colleagues and immediate community, now under the name the Stephen Mitchell Center for Relational Psychoanalysis, we began to imagine what relational psychoanalysis would look like without Stephen looking with us. Then, as we started to regain our strength to move forward and organize this collection, we sent Emmanuel Ghent the planned Table of Contents of Volume II and received his enthusiastic reply just days before his passing.

In the introductory essay to *Relational Psychoanalysis*, Mitchell and Aron (1999) referred to the relational tradition, rather than the relational school, to highlight that we were identifying a trend, a tendency within recent American psychoanalysis, not a more formally organized or coherent school or system of beliefs. Relational psychoanalysts share overlapping but not identical concerns, concepts, approaches, and sensibilities. While at times, and for specific purposes, Mitchell described these developments as revolutionary, rather than evolutionary, he recognized that this was not a simple depiction of social reality, but a construction designed to achieve certain ends in the architecture and aesthetics of theory building.

This volume has been undertaken in a much altered landscape. In the spirit of pluralism, we began with a guiding premise that there can be multiple pathways in the development of theories and that individuals in distinct and different communities work and interact and influence each other in ways that can only add to the health of our discipline and our practice.

Identities, including professional ones, are almost always more complex than single minded. Current theorizing in race studies (Lott, 1999) drawing on the seminal work of W. E. B. Dubois (1994), offers some instructive ideas. These postcolonial, postmodern thinkers reached back to a turn-of-the-century black social theorist to notice that multiplicity of racialized identity positions are not simply or solely problematic but also a brilliant and interesting set of solutions for living flexibly in multiple social/cultural worlds. Generic or single-valenced identities, however useful for certain political or strategic ends, miss the subtly nuanced multiplicity in all ethnic and cultural identities.

In this respect, our use of the term relational in this context is meant not so much to identify a particular school or a unified category but to signify a dimension of theory and practice that has become salient across the wide spectrum of contemporary psychoanalysis. Thinking of relational psychoanalysis along these lines encourages us to think about how the contributions of one school complement and compensate for the emphases of a different tradition. Following Mitchell (1988, 1997) by placing the centrality on the common relational dimension of these traditions, we attempt to structure and contain our work so that it does not disintegrate into a less than rigorous form of eclecticism.

Inevitably of course, despite the pleasure and commitments to process and trends and sensibilities, groups of people doing work together build structures. There is already a developing critical discourse about reifications, hegemonies, and revolutions that turn procrustean (Greenberg, 1995, 2001; Cushman, 1995; Spezzano, 2001; Botticelli, 2004).

This book and its earlier companion (Mitchell and Aron, 1999) attest to the practical and inevitable move toward structuring. People teach courses in relational psychoanalysis, form groups and associations, publish journals, hold conferences, and create their own terms and languages. All these developments may provide essential structure to further the elaboration of theory and practice, but they seem also to have the disadvantage of furthering the isolation and dissociation of one psychoanalytic school from another.

There are dangers and pleasures in "tradition." From friendly and amicable to contesting or antagonistic voices, the carapace of an emerging tradition deserves our attention. Shibboleths, new orders, new orthodoxies create difficulties internally and externally. (Any group founded in opposition to orthodoxy has to find its own vision beyond simple critique. Power inevitably snakes into the process.)

Irwin Hoffman (1998) described how analysts often feel that they have to "throw away the book" in an effort to maintain the dialectical tension between technique and the personally spontaneous. Of course, this tension implies that a new book becomes "the book." Our hope is that this book does and yet does not become "the book." Launching pad, progress report, a new clearing in the forest—these might be metaphors encompassing our hope for the usefulness and impact of this volume. Not a work of closure but an opening across schools and traditions. We can hope that there is some continuing influence from the spirits hovering over this particular book, Stephen Mitchell and Emmanuel Ghent, both deeply democratic and generative people. As ghosts and spirits, we hope they appear to us in the playful tradition of Puck or Ariel and not the Draconian voice of Hamlet's father. But this is decidedly a work undertaken at a moment when our generation feels newly empowered and newly bereft. A curious spot. Under these circumstances of mourning and melancholia, we want to be careful to turn ghosts into ancestors and resist any temptation toward rigid identifications or premature closure.

What Kind of Theory Is Relational Theory?

Let us go back to Mitchell's (1988) initial formulation of relational theory. In his first single-authored work, Mitchell, we believe, attempted two related but distinctive projects, both of which went beyond the delineation of the relational model that he had outlined with his colleague Jay Greenberg. In that earlier work, Greenberg and Mitchell (1983) distinguished the structural-conflict model from the relational model. There, relational theory was a description of a group of theorists who had neither defined themselves as relational nor seen their own work as related to that of others or to any movement or trend that would later be regarded as relational. It was only Greenberg and Mitchell, as historians and scholars of the development of psychoanalytic theory, who categorized them retrospectively as belonging to the relational turn in psychoanalysis.

According to Mitchell (1988), within the relational approach could be housed theorists who maintained a general allegiance to the drive model but who had developed perspectives that largely supplanted it. (Mitchell used Mahler as an example of this strategy.) The frame could also include authors who use drive-model language but redefine the key terms to express an essentially relational vision. (He used Winnicott and Loewald as examples of this strategy.) And the structure also could house authors who had explicitly broken with drive theory. (Here, Mitchell gave Sullivan, Fairbairn, and Kohut as examples.)

In his 1988 work, Mitchell extended his earlier collaborative work and moved beyond his position as a historian and scholar of psychoanalysis. Now he introduced two new innovations. First he developed a framework, a structure to contain, or a plan for how to elaborate, a relational theory. Then he began to develop his own particular integration of relational concepts into what he then called relational-conflict theory. This second project depended on the first but remained separate from and independent of it. We believe that this is a critical point to stress because it allows for the possibility that other thinkers will bring together the same or other relational concepts, in various combinations and with distinct emphases, and integrate these concepts in their own ways, forming their own different relational theories.

Let's examine the first innovation in greater detail. First, Mitchell established a framework or a schema, a plan of action, that allowed a thinker to integrate relational concepts from a wide variety of different psychoanalytic theories and formulate a unique relational integration. This framework includes three dimensions: a self pole, an object pole, and an interactional pole. This creative recognition allowed Mitchell to advocate that concepts be drawn from each of them and put together in new configurations thus allowing for the development of new theoretical integrations.

Mitchell proposed that, within this relational frame, a thinker could integrate a variety of relational concepts drawn from different psychoanalytic traditions and reorganize them into a new coherent theory. These three dimensions (self, other, and interaction), taken together, are what he called the relational matrix. This broad framework may be referred to as relational theory, but it is not itself actually a theory. It is, rather, a structure that holds together various concepts, thus allowing a theorist to integrate his or her own theory within it. We suggest that, rather than reifying it as a frame or structure, it is better thought of as a schema, a strategy, a plan of action that helps an analytic thinker take the action of bringing together diverse relational concepts and construct a new theory out of them. It is no accident that Mitchell (1988) titled his first book *Relational Concepts in Psychoanalysis*. He was working then on the level of bringing together concepts from many theories into his new framework. He was not thinking of any single relational theory that would dominate the field. In fact, he always eschewed such a project.

The second project that Mitchell began in his 1988 book and that he continued throughout the remainder of his life was to elaborate his own particular relational integration—his own theory (Mitchell, 1997, 2000). This theory evolved over the years, but it always tried to attend in some balanced way to issues of self-maintenance, self-regulation, identity, self-esteem, authenticity, and coherence as one dimension; issues of the other, internal objects and actual others, personifications, and mutual or field-regulation as a second dimension; and interactions, enactments, interpersonal behavior, and the who-did-what-to-whom as the third dimension. Moreover, Mitchell often placed a special focus on agency, on how we maintain and perpetuate the patterns of our relationships and the re-creation of our own psychic worlds. (Perhaps this idea may be subsumed under the self pole; perhaps it is better thought of as a separate dimension. Mitchell was not explicit in this regard.) Mitchell had his favorite authors and theorists (Sullivan, Fairbairn, Winnicott, and Loewald among others) and he drew upon them, more than on other writers, to construct his own relational integration.

Our key point is that what is often called relational theory can be thought of as two independent projects: one is a relational framework that can house numerous relational theories; the second refers to the multiple, specific relational theories constructed by different theorists. Mitchell's own relational-conflict theory is only one of these relational theories. Greenberg's (1991) development of his own dual-drive theory is another relational theory; Ogden's (1986, 1989, 1994, 1997) theory of intersubjectivity, Hoffman's (1998) social-constructivism, and Benjamin's (1988, 1995, 1998) intersubjectivity theory are yet other leading examples; and, of course, there are many more. Many theories are quite distinct from each other, but all draw on relational concepts, and all address, in one way or another, all three essential aspects of the relational matrix.

Indeed, both *Relational Psychoanalysis* and *Relational Psychoanalysis, Vol. II* contain articles that, when taken with the rest of the authors' works, reflect efforts to build individual relational theories along just these lines. Writers in this collection self-define in many ways. Relational psychoanalysis is a term that encompasses all these theories. It is not a theory in and of itself. To say that one is a relational theorist does not really describe which concepts in particular, and with what emphases, an analyst uses in his or her own clinical work or thinking. To do that, analysts need to think through the particular integration of relational concepts they draw on in their work. To say that relational theory is not a theory at all may be provocative even to our friends and close colleagues. It is certainly not a single theory. It lies on a level of abstraction different from any theory. It is, rather, a metatheory, a framework or schema that provides the necessary structure with which to go on building coherent and comprehensive relational psychoanalytic theories.

In crafting this introduction we have come up with a number of phrases or terms to describe relational work: a structure in which individual concepts are integrated; a plan, a schema, a framework, a metatheory; perspectives, points of view; a tradition. Probably this proliferation of terminology betrays both the enigma and anxiety in these claims. How do we design or describe a system of thought that is both powerful but flexible and malleable, generative rather than deductive, and not simply a new claimant on the theory food-chain ready to eat everybody in sight?

Probably the only way such a view can be developed and proposed is to situate relational theory in a set of overlapping, sometimes supportive, sometimes critical and contesting conversations. The only protection against reification, authoritarianism, hierarchy, and power moves is to be willing to engage, in good faith, in the kinds of conversations that make space for difference, for uniqueness, and for connection. Like all good pragmatist projects, relational theory is a "truth" to be made through talk and collaboration and conflict.

We believe that this view is consistent with the original platform on which the relational orientation was first institutionalized at the New York University Postdoctoral Program and put so well at that time by Emmanuel Ghent (1992):

> There is no such thing as a relational analyst; there are only analysts whose backgrounds may vary considerably, but who share a broad outlook in which human relations—specific, unique human relations—play a superordinate role in the genesis of character and of psychopathology, as well as in the practice of psychoanalytic therapeutics [p. xviii].

The Relational Tradition, Volume Two: Topics

The topics covered in this volume are continuous and discontinuous with the first volume. They reflect the vicissitudes in the wider field and the unique riverways that the writers in this collection have been following and, in some cases, building: Sexuality and gender development; the psychoanalysis of race and class; attachment; holding; intersubjectivity; mentalization; negotiation between and among selves; the inevitable conflict of interest between patient and analyst; emotional engagement; the fate of new and old objects; whose mind is it? whose body is it? whose analysis is it? the transpersonal experiences of representing self and self and other, of being mindful and minded; the play of countertransference and enactments.

Significantly, this volume includes four contributions drawn from the powerfully generative intersect of infancy research, attachment theory, and psychoanalysis. The linked papers of Fonagy and Coates, the theoretical innovation of Beebe and Lachmann, and the developmental and clinical challenges in the work of Lyons-Ruth cast a very interesting light on relational theory. The hybrid forms and cross-fertilizations in these essays are multiple and various. Sometimes relational psychoanalysis is in sight as an engaged interlocutor; sometimes common interests and perspectives seem to have arisen in parallel; and sometimes the work from this broad terrain of writers seems a necessary and useful challenge to relationalists to engage with questions of development. One of the trajectories developed in Mitchell's work might be seen to move from a place of critique of the "developmental tilt" (1984) or infantilization of patients (his interpersonal roots showing perhaps) to a new involvement (2000) with development questions and in particular with the challenge and contribution that attachment theory and developmental psychopathology can post to relational work.

In these developmentally inflected essays we can see influence and innovation, see the tremendous potential for careful integration of research traditions and cross-disciplinary conversations with psychoanalytic theory and practice. The writers might or might not define themselves primarily as relationalists. We include this work in the spirit of co-constructed conversations, not imperialism.

One of the themes that emerges repeatedly throughout the relational literature and is sounded in these papers is the "deconstruction" of misleading dichotomies and exaggerated polarization. Instead, the relational tradition has accentuated both/and over either/or thinking, even while recognizing that this very stand enacts a choice. The relational tradition places an emphasis on maintaining the tension between extremes, on ambiguity, on dialectic, on paradox, and on psychoanalytic dialogue. Deconstructing polarization, however, does not mean we avoid making careful distinctions or eschew differentiating among alternative approaches. Placing a value on maintaining tensions in the field does not mean that we should avoid making hard choices. Fluidity without sacrificing rigor.

This collection of essays was designed to display and continue that tension. Writers in this volume approach relationality, intersubjectivity, and the blend of interpersonal and intrapsychic with radically different agendas and theoretical preoccupations. Some are researchers whose writing is steeped in clinical process; some focus on the clinical experience; some are animatedly theoretical and metatheoretical preoccupations. Along with a breadth in methodology and modes of communication, the integrating impulse in these contributors takes many forms: literary-clinical, empirical-clinical, aesthetic-social, interpersonal-intrapsychic.

References

Benjamin, J. (1988), *The Bonds of Love: Psychoanalysis, Feminism and the Problem of Domination*. New York: Pantheon.

———— (1995), *Like Subjects, Love Objects: Recognition and Sexual Difference*. New Haven, CT: Yale University Press.

———— (1998), *Shadow of the Other: Intersubjectivity and Gender in Psychoanalysis*. New York: Routledge.

Botticelli, S. (2004), The politics of relational psychoanalysis. *Psychoanal. Dial.*, 14:635–651.

Cushman, P. (1995), *Constructing the Self, Constructing America: A Cultural History of Psychotherapy*. Boston, MA: Addison-Wesley.

Dubois, W. E. B. (1994), *The Souls of Black Folk*. New York: Dover.

Ghent, E. (1992), Foreword. In: *Relational Perspectives in Psychoanalysis*, ed. N. J. Skolnick & S. C. Warshaw. Hillsdale, NJ: The Analytic Press, pp. xiii–xxii.

Greenberg, J. (1991), *Oedipus and Beyond*. Harvard University Press.

———— (1995), Psychoanalytic technique and the interactive matrix. *Psychoanal. Quart.*, 64:1–22.

———— (2001), The analyst's participation: A new look—Reply. *J. Amer. Psychoanal. Assn.*, 49:417–426.

———— & Mitchell, S. A. (1983), *Object Relations in Psychoanalytic Theory*. Cambridge, MA: Harvard University Press.

Hoffman, I. Z. (1998), *Ritual and Spontaneity in the Psychoanalytic Process: A Dialectical-Constructivist View*. Hillsdale, NJ: The Analytic Press.

Lott, T. (1999), *The Invention of Race, Black Culture and the Politics of Representation*. New York: Blackwell.

Mitchell, S. (1984), Object relations theories and the developmental tilt. *Contemp. Psychoanal.*, 20:473–499.

———— (1988), *Relational Concepts in Psychoanalysis*. Cambridge, MA: Harvard University Press.

———— (1997), *Influence and Autonomy in Psychoanalysis*. Hillsdale, NJ: The Analytic Press.

———— (2000), *Relationality: From Attachment to Intersubjectivity*. Hillsdale, NJ: The Analytic Press.

———— & Aron, L., eds. (1999), *Relational Psychoanalysis: The Emergence of a Tradition*. Hillsdale, NJ: The Analytic Press.

Ogden, T. (1986), *The Matrix of the Mind: Object Relations in the Psychoanalytic Dialogue*. Northvale, NJ: Aronson.
—— (1989), *The Primitive Edge of Experience*. Northvale, NJ: Aronson.
—— (1994), *Subjects of Analysis*. Northvale, NJ: Aronson.
—— (1997), *Reverie and Interpretation: Sensing Something Human*. Northvale, NJ: Aronson.
Spezzano, C. (2001), How is the analyst supposed to know? Gathering evidence for interpretations. *Contemp. Psychoanal.*, 37:551–570.

Part I

Therapeutic Action

The relational turn has reverberated across multiple dimensions of psychoanalytic theory and technique and has left its mark on our theory of mind, our models of development, our understanding of psychopathology, and, perhaps most especially, on our theory of therapeutic action and its related implications for psychoanalytic technique. In this section we feature a collection of articles that have been influential in reframing questions of the analyst's role and the analytic process.

What kind of object is the analyst to be? What is the nature of analytic participation? How does our interest in the analyst's subjectivity and the patient's experience of the analyst's subjectivity lead to modifications in our views of analytic participation? How does relational theory change the way we think about conflict and resistance? What is the nature of the analyst's personal involvement in the work? What are the implications of the relational turn for contemporary psychoanalytic education and supervision?

Taken together, these articles highlight a significant shift in clinical psychoanalysis toward a greater appreciation of the analyst's personal responsiveness, spontaneity, and playfulness. There is now a greater emphasis on nonverbal communication and the affective link between patient and analyst and a new appreciation for the analyst's authenticity, vulnerability, personal openness and directness, as well as professional restraint and analytic discipline.

The Intimate Edge in Therapeutic Relatedness

(1974)

Darlene Bregman Ehrenberg

Editors' Introduction

While this book has largely drawn together contributions from the very recent psychoanalytic literature, this article by Darlene Ehrenberg is the notable exception, going back to an article first published in 1974. Ehrenberg has long been an innovator in psychoanalysis, and her work is often associated with a radically interpersonal approach to technique that features the analyst's use of self-disclosure. A careful examination of her work, however, reveals that she draws equally from both the interpersonal tradition and from Winnicott, Guntrip, and British object relations perspectives. We chose this article for inclusion because it set the tone for much of her future work, conveys the essential themes of Ehrenberg's writings, and highlights what we believe to be essential elements in a relational approach.

In a long series of publications, culminating in her 1992 book, *The Intimate Edge*, Ehrenberg demonstrated why, regardless of theoretical orientation, the recognition of the interactive nature of the analytic field has profound and radical implications for one's thinking about analytic technique. In this article, Ehrenberg begins by drawing on Martin Buber's philosophy of dialogue, which, much like Winnicott's psychoanalytic vision, relies on "the realm of the between." Ehrenberg sees patient and analyst as "observing-participants" who are engaged in a truly mutual, authentic, collaboration. Ehrenberg has gone on to show how working at the intimate edge of relatedness can extend the benefits of psychoanalysis to patients formerly considered unanalyzable and may be used to resolve clinical stalemates and situations of impasse.

In this article, Ehrenberg clearly states her radical position, namely, that the intimate edge is honed if analysts are willing to be open about their own reactions to the analytic field of mutual, shared experience. She elaborates a number of rationales for analyst self-disclosure including validating patients' perceptions, encouraging openness and directness, minimizing unnecessary hierarchy and authoritarianism, and avoiding an overreliance on idealization of the analyst. As always, Ehrenberg presents gripping clinical vignettes that illustrate her therapeutic principles.

Stephen Mitchell in 1997 pointed out that, whereas some analytic theorists and practitioners recognize the value of the analyst's disclosing carefully considered and highly processed reactions, Ehrenberg, by contrast, sees great value precisely in sharing her unprocessed, immediate reactions to her patients. For Ehrenberg, writes Mitchell, "We are what we do with others, and to withhold the analyst's reactions from the patient is to deprive the patient of precisely the insight she might find most helpful in understanding their experience" (p. 149).

Ehrenberg's work is characterized by several themes that have become identified with relational psychoanalysis across schools, including spontaneity; the unique value of playfulness; the role of authentic engagement in the process of working through; the therapeutic value of the analyst's openness, self-disclosure, and directness; and, perhaps most significant, the significance of mutuality and reciprocity between patient and analyst as they move toward the intimate edge of relatedness.

The Intimate Edge in
Therapeutic Relatedness*

▼ ▼ ▼ ▼ ▼

I

A clear conceptualization of the therapeutic process and of what in a relationship contributes to therapeutic outcome remains somewhat elusive and certainly controversial in the psychoanalytic literature. Despite Sullivan's note that interpersonal acts are "reciprocal" and "transformative" (Mullahy, 1945), Laing, Phillipson, and Lee (1966) remark that "psychoanalytic theory has no constructs for the dyad as such" and despite its importance, "the relationship *between* persons is undeveloped theoretically."

Though his main focus was not on the psychoanalytic situation, a notable effort to grapple with these questions is reflected in the work of Martin Buber (1957a, 1958), who wrote, "Distance provides the human situation, relation provides man's becoming in that situation." Buber believed that "Human life and humanity come into being in genuine meetings" and that the "inmost growth of the self" can be accomplished "between the one and the other, between men." For him the most profound growth and change in the treatment situation can only occur in the context of this kind of "personal relation." This involves what he labels an "I-Thou" relation in contrast to an "I-It" relation. It requires mutual confrontation, and he calls its unfolding the "dialogical," that condition of genuine dialogue which involves bringing oneself fully into it, without reduction or shifting ground and without holding back relevant thoughts or withdrawing. In Buber's framework the meaning of the interhuman is *"to be found neither in one of the two partners, nor in both together, but only in the dialogue itself, in this 'between' which they live together"* (italics added).

As in art, he states, it is the "realm of the between" which has become a form. Yet the processes of this "between," particularly as they must occur in the psychoanalytic situation, to facilitate the specific kinds of work that psychoanalysis requires, have never been clearly articulated.

The importance of this "between" and an effort to delineate its dimensions is also reflected in the seminal work of Winnicott. Winnicott (1971) writes of a "potential space" which is "at the interplay between

---

* Originally published in *Contemporary Psychoanalysis*, 10:423–437 © 1974 William Alanson White Society and Institute. Reprinted by permission.

there being nothing but me and there being objects and phenomena out-side omnipotent control."

He comments about the "place where it can be said that continuity is giving place to contiguity" in the potential space "which initially both joins and separates the baby and the mother." He states, further, "this potential space is a highly variable factor (from individual to individual), whereas the two other locations—personal or psychic reality and the actual world—are relatively constant, one being biologically determined and the other being common property" and adds that this potential space "depends on experience which leads to trust. It can be looked upon as sacred to the individual in that it is here that the individual experiences creative living."

Winnicott cautions that the psychoanalyst should not clutter up this space even as he helps enlarge or create it, by filling it with interpretations, which in effect are from the analyst's own creative imagination and *not* the patient's. He is less explicit about the processes that maximize the therapeutic possibilities of what goes on in this potential space.

In my own struggle to conceptualize the therapeutic *process*, and how the therapeutic relationship can be used to facilitate maximum growth, I have arrived at a concept which I call the "intimate edge" in relatedness. This paper is directed toward an elucidation of this concept and an elaboration of the therapeutic possibilities that I believe aiming for this "intimate edge" generates in the psychoanalytic situation.

By "intimate edge" I mean that *point of maximum and acknowledged contact at any given moment in a relationship without fusion, without violation of the separateness and integrity of each participant.* This point is not static, and may fluctuate from one moment to the next, so that being able to relate at this point requires ceaseless sensitivity to inner changes in oneself and in the other, and to changes at the interface of the interaction, as these occur in the context of the spiral of reciprocal impact. (My concept thus encompasses spatial as well as temporal dimensions.) More often than not this optimal point is over- or under-shot so that there is some kind of intrusion or else overcautiousness. In either case there is a failure on the part of psychoanalyst and patient to meet at the "intimate edge."

The concept is similar to what Winnicott (1971) refers to as the "continuity-contiguity moment" in relatedness. What distinguishes my conceptualization is the necessity for acknowledgment and explicitness since I believe the process of acknowledgment increases its dimensions, and changes the nature of one's experience of it. Ideally, the "intimate edge" thus becomes a point of maximum self-expression and maximum awareness of the individuality and boundaries of self and other for each participant. It is the point where each participant becomes acutely aware of his own active participation in a particular interaction, the choices he makes, and of where he ends and the other begins. The "intimate edge," over time, thus becomes the trace of a constantly moving locus, for each time this is identified it is also changed; as it is reidentified, it changes again. In a sense I am speaking of a kind of engagement in which both individuals are "observing participants" (in contrast to Sullivan's concept of the therapist as "participant observer") with a particular point of focus.

In the analytic situation studying moment-by-moment shifts in the quality of relatedness and experience between analyst and patient, permits exploration of individual patterns of reaction and particular sensitivities. Decisions to become increasingly involved or to withdraw can be studied in process. The feelings and associations surrounding these can be examined and can be used as the basis for fantasies and associations, and responded to by the analyst as he (or she) might respond to a patient's dream. The patient's associations to the immediate experience indeed become the metaphoric articulation of his unconscious hopes, fears, expectations, including the elucidation of the transference.

Actually even when the "intimate edge" is missed the *process* of aiming for it, the mutual focus on the difficulties involved in achieving a meeting, can facilitate such a meeting. The effort to study the quality of mutual experience in a relationship, the interlocking of both participants, as distinct from examining either participant separately, including a mutual focus on the failure to touch or on inauthenticity or collusion, can become the bridge to a more intimate encounter.

Such an engagement permits distortions in the perceptions of self and other, which result from false projections,[1] to be corrected through a dialectical interaction process in which clearer perceptions of the other force clearer perceptions of the self, and vice versa. Both percepts become more veridical. The necessity to engage in such distortions becomes available for analytic exploration once they cannot be successfully acted upon in the transference, and can be integrated into the self percept as one's own need to distort rather than accepted as an accurate view of reality. This kind of shift encourages clearer perception of the "interpersonal space" and simultaneously allows for clarification of the structure and dimensions of "inner space"; and for a shift form feeling victimized or helpless, stuck without any options, to the fresh experience of one's power and responsibility in relation to multiple choices. This also encourages the discovery of untapped individual potentialities, and the emergence of clearer self-definition in consciousness.

---

[1] Or false introjections.

Guntrip (1969) states that "what is therapeutic when it is achieved, is 'the moment of real meeting' of two persons as a new transforming experience for one of them" and that "transference analysis is the slow and painful experience of clearing the ground of left-overs from past experience, both in transference and countertransference, so that therapist and patient can at last meet 'mentally face to face' and know that they know each other as two human beings."

What I am suggesting is that Guntrip's idea of a "moment of real meeting" is not the end, but is itself an important starting point, and of continuing leverage in the analytic process.

Focusing on the interface of the analyst—patient interaction is not the same as focusing on the transference or countertransference. Rather, the focus is on the nature of the integration, the dialogue, and the quality of contact. Associations to the moments of contact are as useful as associations to the moments when this kind of meeting is not achieved. Analytic work does not stop when contact is made. It takes on new dimensions. I believe that an effort for a sustained and enduring, increasingly developing intimacy over time, not isolated somewhat discrete moments of meeting, ultimately becomes the condition for maximum growth; and that the "intimate edge" is the point from which such intimacy can develop. Guntrip remarks that "psychotherapy is a progress out of fantasy into reality, a process of transcending the transference" and "All this cannot go on unless the therapist is a 'real' person himself, giving the possibility of a 'real' relationship in the treatment situation, over and above the transference relations."

However, it is not simply a matter of enlarging, but also of analyzing this, so that ultimately each participant learns to know himself better through the immediate interactive experience. Focusing on this "real" interaction is analytically crucial, Wolstein (1959, 1971) stresses the importance of making this field of "shared experience" the focus of psychoanalytic inquiry. I am suggesting a particular way of focusing on this "shared experience."

In aiming toward the "intimate edge" instead of focusing on the content of distortions, projections, or transference, one must focus on the patterns of distorting. For example, if a patient drifts into a fantasy that figuratively takes him out of the room the content of the fantasy may indeed be meaningful, but the wish to be out of the room cannot be neglected. In fact, helping to identify what triggered the fantasy (and the content of the fantasy can provide useful clues) may be significant in helping the patient grasp the patterns of his own experience. Guntrip writes of the "sense of a gulf which the patient cannot cross but which perhaps the therapist can and does if he shows the patient that he knows about it" as being of the highest importance in treatment. I agree, and further suggest that the process of mutual and explicit focus on the very gulf between is exactly what transforms it into an "intimate edge." This involves a reversal of figure and ground, in which the space between becomes the focus, rather than the two individual participants or either of them or their fantasies separately. As in art, one can treat the "ground" or the "between" as a form that can be negotiated in its own right. The process of articulating this ground simultaneously defines more clearly the figures that shape it and makes vivid the fact that both participants in an interaction do *actively* shape the space between them. Winnicott (1971) refers to a conversation with Marion Milner in which she conveyed to him "the tremendous significance that there can be in the interplay of the edges of two curtains, or of the surface of a jug that is placed in front of another jug." In the case of two individuals, where each makes active choices at every moment, the situation becomes infinitely more complex.

The articulation of the "intimate edge," particularly when the quality of contact is minimal, validates the fact that each participant does make choices about how involved he wants to be. Winnicott (1965) points out that there are healthy uses of non-communication in the developing child. In his words, the development of the self may involve "a sophisticated game of hide and seek in which it is a joy to be hidden but a disaster not to be found." I believe that in the therapeutic situation it is important for the patient to consciously realize he is playing hide and seek if this is the case. Often the whole process is out of awareness. Making this explicit permits the recognition that one makes choices about what to hide and what to seek, and this helps define and sharpen the individual's sense of his own power and his own separateness in a relationship.

This approach is different from those of Greenson (1965), Greenson and Wexler (1969), Melanie Klein (1957), Myerson (1973) and others who have emphasized the importance of the "real relationship" between analyst and patient as a facilitating condition for successful analysis, but do not see it as the medium of the analytic work.

I believe the therapeutic potentiality of meeting at this "intimate edge" is heightened if the analyst is willing to be open about his own reactions to the mutual experience. Wolstein (1959) states, "If the method with the widest reach in the patient's experience is most desirable, then wider dimensions of the analyst's experience will also become involved in a therapeutic situation that is genuinely personal."

Levenson (1972) remarks that if the therapist uses himself as an instrument, examining his own anxieties about what the patient calls out in him, and presents these to the patient, he demonstrates most directly what it feels like to be engaged in the patient's world.

If the analyst is willing to be open about his own reactions these can be therapeutically useful in that they provide validation of the patient's impact, and serve to clarify exactly what this impact is, as Levenson suggests (1972). In addition, openness on the part of the analyst encourages the patient to deal with his reactions to the analyst's reactions explicitly, and to validate his own experience, as well as to draw his own conclusions in this regard. If the analyst openly acknowledges the limits of his capacities he generates a more intimate encounter so that studying explicitly the patient's reactions to the analyst's limitations is possible. As the patient is confronted with the analyst's fallibility he is also confronted with necessity for his own thoughtful participation in the analytic endeavor, which is also useful. At the same time this helps focus the common human dilemmas instead of leaving the patient with some vague sense that the analyst has reached some superior state of being that he, the patient, can never attain. Indeed, it can expose a patient's need to idealize the analyst, instead of perpetuate the idealization.

II

The following clinical examples highlight the process of working toward the "intimate edge":

At one point in the course of his treatment, a patient talked for a considerable length of time about how miserable he felt and how hopeless he believed he was. Despite the pain this might imply, it sounded to me like some kind of recording. And that it felt more as though he were trying to put me off rather than to communicate to me what his feelings were. I pointed this out to him. He reflected on it and came up with the realization that he preferred to keep a distance between us, and he formulated that what he had been involved in with me was actually a "pretense" of a relationship. I asked for his associations to his insights and he produced memories of experiences of humiliation as a child when he did allow others close to him, particularly his mother. When asked to elaborate, he said he did not see the point of all this but if it would make me "happy" he would try. I then asked what he meant by "if it would make you happy." He replied that he was willing to go along with my suggestion, even though it seemed a waste of time to him—"how could it help him with his current misery? It was all hopeless anyway"—to avoid a hassle and make things simpler for himself. He also stated that this was the way he usually "kept people off his back." I said it was more important he be honest than pretend and go through motions so as to "humor" me. He said he did not think it was a "big deal." I commented that I thought it was and suggested that he consider it. He then elaborated on some experiences with his mother that had been extremely painful. As he spoke about these experiences he began to show a degree of emotion he had never displayed before. I thought I had at this moment a better understanding of his pain and of his struggle than ever before and related this to him. He indicated that he was surprised and touched by this and responded by elaborating with a great deal of feeling how lonely and isolated he felt. Then, suddenly, he reverted to his former attitude, acting extremely indifferent and saying, *"What's the point of all this anyway, it's all hopeless."* I questioned the shift. He had no explanation and said it was not important anyway. I said I thought it was very important and suggested we try to pinpoint what triggered this sudden change. As we examined what had just gone on between us in minute detail, I realized that I had just glanced at the clock. I mentioned this to him, and we were able to unravel a sequence in which I had looked at the clock as he was talking, he had experienced this as evidence of my lack of interest, felt hurt, and automatically pulled back. It thus became exquisitely clear to both of us and we were able to make explicit the fact that his surface indifference really masked a deep sensitivity and a great deal of feeling. At this point he began to cry. This was followed by his concern that I would experience his tearfulness as childish and weak. I indicated that, on the contrary, I now experienced him as stronger and more human and that I now felt closer to him. His response to this was one of surprise and "feeling good."

In the next session he was considerably more open than usual and began to share some important details about his past and present life, details that he had been withholding. I stated that I was glad to learn about these, and thought it was important to our work together, but at the same time pointed out that although he had always questioned my trustworthiness in relation to him, I felt it was important for him to see that *he* had not been trustworthy in relation to me in the sense of being totally honest in his participation in our work. For example even if there were things he felt he could not discuss, he might have mentioned that this was the case and not pretended otherwise. He objected and said he had never actually lied but had simply withheld certain details. He also said that he had been more honest with me than with anyone in his life, and hastened to assure me not to take it personally. I questioned his "reassurance," whereupon he said he was only trying to be "nice." I said I thought it would be better if he would be honest. He became distressed and asked whether this meant I did not want to work with him anymore since he had lied. I questioned this expectation indicating that on the contrary it now seemed we had a sounder basis for working together than before. Nevertheless, I examined my own reaction to see what he might be responding to and realized I was becoming irritated with myself for having let myself be "taken in," for not being more perceptive about his withholding. I told him this. His response was to express a great deal of surprise that I should have any feelings about it at all, and to state that he suddenly saw me as more "human" than he ever had, and that he now felt "more equal" than he ever imagined he could feel.

The work that followed included the exploration of feelings that had not been accessible before, and by continuing to aim for the "intimate edge" it was possible to continue to intensify our relationship and deepen our understanding of his inner dynamics as well as for each of us to more sharply define ourselves. This permitted him to get more of a sense of his own maneuvers in the situation and served to highlight the issue of his responsibility in our relationship. Despite periods of doubt and ambivalence, and returns to his "affectless" posture, he began to speak of experiencing more "choices" and of feeling less "helpless" and began to take a more active role in relation to his own experience, in and out of the treatment situation.

Another patient had great difficulty defining her own boundaries and would repetitively set up situations in which she would try to get other people to make decisions for her. Then she would become angry at them for trying to control her. She was expert at setting up triangles where two people would be arguing over what she should do. She would take the aloof position of awaiting the decision of the "winner," assuming no responsibility herself. Invariably she would get angry at both parties and play them off against each other. She got them to express to each other her own negative feelings to each of them, which she then could innocently leave unacknowledged. This obscured the basic dilemma of her own inability to make her own decisions and be responsible for herself, and of her manipulativeness with regard to others as well as to herself. We had made some slight headway in facing this situation. Nevertheless, in one session even as she was talking about herself with some degree of awareness, she tried to set up an interaction in which I was to be the advocate of her taking responsibility for her own life, for making her own decisions, while she argued the case for not doing so. I told her that it was her conflict and thus it was her choice to make. I also pointed out that trying to structure this kind of debate between us was another example of how she managed to slip out of dealing with her own conflict, avoiding even recognizing it as her own conflict. She responded by becoming silent. Then she elaborated about her own awareness of this pattern, trying to develop some perspective on it on her own. I remained silent as she did this, only occasionally pointing out instances where she seemed to gloss over the emotional significance or seriousness of the dilemma, even as she described examples of the ways in which it recurred in her life. She then reported a dream in which her leg was shot, but, since people around her seemed to ignore it, she did too: corroborating the pattern of ignoring the seriousness to her of her own dilemma and not using her own resources to deal with it, as she let her responses be defined by the responses of others.

At the end of the session she tearfully expressed that the fact that I had listened and let her struggle with her own conflict made her feel "listened to" and closer to me. However, at the same time it was extremely painful for her and she resented me because it made her feel separate and aware of the boundaries between us, which made her feel lonely and lost. She said that if I had argued with her, even if it was her own inner conflict that was being projected and which became the basis for our argument, the act of arguing would permit her to feel involved and connected. She said this would be less difficult and painful for her to experience than the state of separateness with which my not arguing confronted her. I replied that the latter kind of relatedness had an illusory quality to it and that giving it up might suggest a more genuine kind of involvement. Her response to this was that a "deeper" involvement would be frightening because she feared she might "lose" herself. It was ironic because as the dream poignantly showed her line of "defense" was actually bringing about the state of affairs she seemed most to fear.

While this was not a totally new insight, the situation of having to confront the boundaries helped focus the issue and spell it out for analytic exploration. It helped shape our understanding of the functional structure of the pattern of her relatedness and its phenomenological dimensions and was a step towards working out the unconscious dynamics analytically instead of letting them be acted "in" our relationship.

III

In the preceding examples the analytic task seemed to be to identify the covert failures of contact, those that involved a false sense of more intimate connection than did in fact exist, or a relation to a projected part of the self rather than to the other. Farber (1966) alludes to this when he cautions that an illusory posture of intimacy is "a more deadly disability for the patient than any symptom that might have disappeared in the process," for to maintain this state of "pseudo-grace" no act may be admitted which challenges it and the possibility of genuine intimacy diminishes. In another context, Wynne, Ryckoff, Day and Hirsch (1958) discuss families that are characterized by "pseudo-mutuality," which is a phenomenon involving a "predominant absorption in fitting together at the expense of the differentiation of the identities of the persons in the relation."

They state that "what outside observers might regard as coercive or manipulative negative aspects are interpreted within the relation as simply part of the effort to dovetail more fully with one another."

This makes growth of the relation impossible. Schachtel (1959) goes even farther and suggests that such a mode of interaction, that involves a subtle kind of dehumanizing and distancing operation that avoids discovering the uniqueness of the other through a form of seeming familiarity and equality, is actually destructive. He suggests this form of "not venturing into the familiar," not allowing oneself to perceive the unknown in it, which involves the kind of perception that cuts off aspects of the object, becomes an act of subtle violation of the other. Others have focused on the operation of such processes in the specific context of psychoanalysis. Feiner (1970) in an attempt to define the inner experience of inauthenticity and its relationship to psychoanalysis, details inauthentic communication and relatedness and surveys the literature on the subject. Levenson (1972) describes the "reductio ad absurdum" of a false sense of understanding as an unproductive, growth inhibiting, symbiosis.

I believe that whenever such kinds of perceptual or communicative violation occur in relation to another, violation of the self is also involved. For example, to need to see oneself as controlled by another, requires seeing the other as having the power to control and seeing oneself as helpless to resist. I also believe that the pattern of "not venturing in the familiar" occurs in relation to the self as well as in relation to the other, so that one is often as out of touch with oneself as on might be with another, and can relate to oneself in violating ways just as one can to another. Feiner (1970) describes how the act of reification, relating the other as a thing, is ultimately turned on the self.

The process of aiming for the "intimate edge" in the therapeutic relation helps expose the false assumptions about both self and other and makes for the beginning of more veridical perception of self and other. Thus it facilitates the possibility or more intimate and more authentic therapeutic encounter.

As Buber (1957b) states, "The chief presupposition for the rise of genuine dialogue is that each should regard his partner as the very one he is." I believe this must also apply to the self, and that each must recognize and present himself as the very one he is himself in addition to recognizing who the other is, for such a "genuine dialogue" to occur, as Buber also suggests.

This process of focusing on the interface of the analyst-patient relationship both requires and makes it possible to identify what Laing calls "mystifications" (Laing, 1965), and permits them to be demystified in the immediate situation as the collusion involved in *both* mystifying (oneself or the other) and in the participation in being mystified is made apparent. The increasing illumination of the fact that each participant has an important role in the creation of what occurs between them stimulates each to see more clearly the nature of his own participation. This contributes to making the relationship a medium in which *both* participants expand and develop individually. Indeed the opportunity for the patient to experience the fact he can contribute to the analyst's growth and that treatment is not a one way process, itself can become a major stimulus for change (Wolstein, 1959, 1971; Singer, 1971). The possibility of a creative dialogue thus becomes a goal of treatment, and the medium in which it takes place as well.

Implicit in all of this is the conviction that the experience of intimacy must be *actively* created, and requires that both participants take responsibility for what goes on between them. It does not evolve simply through time spent together, but requires an active effort on the part of both participants to achieve. It is always the result of a collaborative[2] effort, a mutual willingness to adventure into the unknown. The mutual focus on the difficulties involved in this collaborative effort becomes the medium of the therapeutic process. And also implicit is the assumption that as the necessary shifts from a passive to an active involvement are made in the context of the analytic relationship, and through the medium of that relationship, corresponding shifts relating to an individual's view of himself and his role in all relationships become increasingly possible.

A meeting at the "intimate edge" is not simply intellectual, in which case either participant would be involved in an exercise of his or her own cleverness rather than in a more personally profound exchange. Nor is it simply affective, since it is quite possible for either participant to be emotional without ever being touched by the other. Nor is it simply personal,

---

[2] Sullivan (1956, *Clinical Studies in Psychiatry*. New York: W.W. Norton) distinguishes between collaboration and cooperation. He sees collaboration as involving a strong interest in a mutual achievement. In contrast he sees cooperation as more "juvenile," involving a strong interest in the other person's achieving as well as one's own, but easily subject to disruption and parting of the ways to avoid anxiety that either may arouse in the other. It seems therefore that in his framework collaboration involves a deep commitment to a mutual task, even if difficult, whereas cooperation is seen as a sympathetic side by side functioning that lasts only as long as it is comfortable.

since sharing intimate details about oneself might be no different from a recorded speech in which the words act as barriers rather than bridges. The essential qualities of the kind of engagement I am describing are *reciprocity* and *expanded awareness through authentic relation*.

Finding and making explicit the point of optimal closeness and distance in the relationship, a point which is constantly changing from moment to moment, provides the kind of experience in which the participants' awareness expands via the relationship as they clarify what they evoke and what they respond to in each other. This can only move in the direction of new experiences of mutuality and intimacy, and towards increasing self-knowledge and individuality.

It is commonly acknowledged that there is usually a discrepancy between how analysts work and how they think they work. I believe this is often a function of different levels of conceptualization, and that the level of the processes in the "between" is usually omitted from theoretical discussions of technique. I believe that more extensive articulation of the dimensions and processes that bridge interpersonal space is vital if a theory of psychoanalytic technique is to illuminate what it is in the therapeutic interaction that makes for growth and change.

References

Buber, M. (1957a), Distance and relation. *Psychiatry*, 20: (2).

Buber, M. (1957b), Elements of the interhuman. *Psychiatry*, 20: (2).

Buber, M. (1958), *I and Thou*. New York: Charles Scribner's Sons.

Farber, L. (1966), *The ways of the will*. New York: Basic Books.

Feiner, A. H. (1970), Toward an understanding of the experience of inauthenticity. *Contemporary Psychoanalysis* 7: No. 1.

Greenson, R. R. (1965), The working alliance and the transference neurosis, *Psychoanalytic Quarterly*, 34.

Greenson, R. R. & Wexler, M. (1969), The non-transference relationship in the psychoanalytic situation. *International Journal of Psychoanalysis*, 50.

Guntrip, H. (1969), *Schizoid phenomena, object relations and the self*. New York: International Universities Press.

Klein, M. (1957), *Envy and gratitude*. London: Tavistock.

Laing, R. D. (1965), Mystification, confusion and conflict. In: *Intensive family therapy*, ed. I. Boszormenyi-Nagi & J. L. Framo. New York: Harper & Row, Hoeber Medical Division.

Laing, R. D., Phillipson, H. & Lee, A. (1955), *Interpersonal perception*. New York: Springer.

Levenson, E. A. (1972), *The fallacy of understanding*. New York: Basic Books.

Mullahy, P. (1945), A theory of interpersonal relations and the evolution of personality. In: *Conceptions of modern psychiatry*, ed. Harry Stack Sullivan. New York: Norton.

Myerson, P. G. (1973). The establishment and disruption of the psychoanalytic modus vivendi. *International Journal of Psychoanalysis*, 54:(2).

Schachtel, E. G. (1959), *Metamorphosis*. Hillsdale, NJ: The Analytic Press, 2001.

Singer, E. (1972), The patient aids the analyst: some clinical and theoretical observations. In: *In the name of life*, Ed. B. Landis and E. S. Tauber. New York: Holt, Rinehart, Winston.

Winnicott, D. W. (1965), *The maturational processes and the facilitating environment*. New York: International Universities Press.

Winnicott, D. W. (1971), *Playing and reality*. New York: Basic Books.

Wolstein, B. (1959), *Countertransference*. New York: Grune and Stratton.

Wolstein, B. (1971), *Human psyche in psychoanalysis*. Springfield, Ill.: Charles C. Thomas.

Wynne, L. C., Ryckoff, I. M., Day, J., & Hirsch, S. I. (1958), Pseudo-mutuality in the family relations of schizophrenics. *Psychiatry*, 21.

Afterword

Although my thinking has evolved in many ways since my 1974 paper, I chose this first articulation of my conception of working at the "intimate edge" for this collection, and not a more recent articulation of my position, because I think it locates my thinking in historical context and because it remains fundamental to my position. My view was, and continues to be, that recognizing the interactive/ intersubjective nature of the analytic field requires us to re-conceptualize the data of psychoanalysis, the process of psychoanalysis, the analyst's role within this process, and the nature of therapeutic action.

As radical as this conception was considered to be at the time I first wrote about it in 1974, the irony is that this perspective takes an important aspect of Freud's thinking much more seriously than traditional theory has done. I am referring to Freud's (1915) observation, "It is a very remarkable thing that the *Ucs*. of one human being can react upon that of another, without passing through the *Cs*." (p. 194). Historically analysts seem to have assumed that, although this unconscious vulnerability applies to their patients, if they were "fully analyzed" themselves they could transcend it. They failed to realize that, as analysts, we are no less unconsciously vulnerable than our patients are, and that what we see in a patient may be responsive to some aspect of our own participation, of which we may be unaware.

When I say that the analytic field is interactive and that there is always much going on intersubjectively between patient and analyst, I am not talking about ways in which we may deliberately try to engage with our patients. I see this as a condition of analytic work, a given. It is not something we can avoid even if we try. The most classical analyst is interactively and intersubjectively involved, whether or not he or she realizes it. How we participate in this interaction, of course, will shape how the relationship will evolve, and what form it will take, for better or for worse; but the relationship remains "interactive" and "intersubjective" whether we are silent or we speak, and there is always an unconscious dimension to whatever transpires.

For this reason, however analytically sound our responses may seem on one level, and whatever we consciously intend, we may also be manipulative, seductive, or destructive, on another level, without even realizing it. Interpretation, even when "correct," for example, can be a form of harassment, impingement, competition, seduction, manipulation, or gratification, among other possibilities. The same is true for any other form of participation, including silence or disclosure. Silence is not necessarily "neutral." Often it is a response to interactive pulls we may not be aware of, and it can be integral to some kind of enactment between patient and analyst. Any kind of response can be authoritarian, assaultive, blaming, sadistic, collusive, gratifying, compliant, or some combination of these all at the same time, without our even being aware that this might be so. Even our efforts to monitor for unconscious enactment and collusion may involve enactment and collusion on another level. For these reasons, a so-called negative therapeutic reaction may not be a function of the patient's negative dynamic, as has often been assumed. Rather, it may be an iatrogenic reaction to an aspect of the analyst's participation of which the analyst may not be aware. We simply cannot ignore the power of unconscious communication, affective communication, and enactment in the analytic relationship. For the same reasons, even when things go well, we can never be sure whether it is despite our deliberate interventions or because of them (Ehrenberg, 1992).

Working at the "intimate edge" respects these constraints and actually embraces them. It involves an effort to expand the analytic dialogue to encompass in an explicit way the intersubjective dimension of the relationship and to generate specific kinds of movement within it. The analytic expanse is not only enlarged by this kind of effort, it is also transformed. The emphasis is on process, on engaging live experience, and on generating a new kind of live experience by so doing, in an ever-expanding way as the process of acknowledgment increases the intersubjective dimensions and changes the nature of the intersubjective experience. What is achieved is not simply a greater awareness of what is in play, but a new kind of experience.

What this requires is not a shift in focus from the internal to the interplay. It is much more complex. This is because what is intersubjective cannot be considered as "belonging" to either one or the other participant, nor can it be located as internal or external. It also is not simply "between." In addition, it is in constant flux.

My focus here is on some misunderstandings of how I define working at the "intimate edge" as well as on misunderstanding of my views about how and when "disclosure" might be used in this framework. My comments here, of course, also reflect some of the ways my thinking on these issues has evolved since 1974.

The editors, in their introductory comments, cite Mitchell's (1997) observation that my position is that "to withhold the analyst's reactions from the patient is to deprive the patient of precisely the insight she might find most helpful in understanding their experience" (p. 149). Though it is true that I believe that revealing our reactions can provide valuable feedback to patients about their effect on us, and about their ability to affect us, I also believe that how we decide what kinds of reactions we might want to reveal, and when and why, is not a simple matter. In addition, there is also the complex question of how we decide how to "frame" what we say. Certainly, also, there are times when revealing our "reactions" might not be useful or appropriate and when the best we can do is simply to listen and hear what a patient is trying to tell us. My view, therefore, is that disclosure is only one of many possible responses we can offer at any given moment. How to determine the kind of response that might be most analytically facilitating is the critical issue (see esp. Ehrenberg, 1995, 1996, 2003).

With regard to how we might "frame" our disclosures, I have found that contextualizing both our own and the patient's feelings, whatever they may be, as data to work with, and not to act on or simply react to them, is vital to establishing that all feelings are of analytic interest and can be explored safely. In so doing we also convey that our commitment is to the analytic work, no matter what feelings we or the patient may be experiencing. We also convey that we believe that a collaborative effort toward this end is possible, that no feelings are off limits, and that we are willing to engage with this patient in this way and are not frightened to do so (Ehrenberg, 1995, 1996, 2000, 2003).

Mitchell (1997) presented an example that I will use to clarify my position. Reflecting on what is meant by the "intimate edge," Mitchell asked us to consider the following scenario:

> A patient begins treatment. At the start of each session he lies down, exhales slowly, and sinks into what he experiences as a meditative mood conducive to free association and analytic self-reflection. After two or three minutes of silence, he begins to speak. The analyst finds himself with thoughts that seem important in those initial silences and begins to interrupt them with his own associations and reflections. The patient becomes angry; he feels interfered with and tells the analyst to be quiet, allowing the patient to create what he feels was the necessary analytic ambiance for himself. The analyst feels controlled by this ritualistic silence. He feels that to comply with it would be inauthentic on his part, destroying the necessary precondition for him to be engaged as an analyst. Eventually the patient quits [pp. 92–93].

Mitchell added in a footnote, "I am not at all suggesting that Ehrenberg would work in the way this analyst did. I am using this example to illustrate the perspectivistic nature of defining boundaries, edges and the 'here-and-now.'" (p. 93).

He then asked

> Where was the intimate edge between them? It depends on whom you ask. From the patient's point of view, there never was an intimate edge because the analyst never allowed the patient the preconditions necessary for him to be fully in the room. From the analyst's point of view, the edge was located at the point that the analyst felt constrained and told not to speak. Edges can be defined only within perspectives, and interactions, because they involve at least two parties, contain, by definition, more than one perspective. Therefore, any interaction can be described in more than one way. To place the central analytic focus on interaction is itself not enough, because what must be further considered is who is defining the interaction [p. 93].

I believe Mitchell's comments reflect a misunderstanding about what I conceive of as the intimate edge and about what is involved in working at the intimate edge. Let me try to explain how and why.

The intimate edge, as I conceive it, is an interactive creation that exists only intersubjectively. It is always unique to the moment. It is not "in the eye of the beholder," nor is the intimate edge something inherent in every moment. Sometimes analyst and patient are able to create and to engage at an intimate edge, and sometimes they may fail dismally, even when they try. Mitchell's question about where the intimate edge might be located in his example suggests that he assumed it is there to be found. I do *not* make that assumption, and

I do not see it as to be found in his example. Rather, what I see in this example is a very problematic enactment in play. What about Mitchell's concern about who is "defining the interaction"? Because each person inevitably will have a different experience of the same interaction, I believe it is *never* a matter of "definition." It is always a matter of personal experience and of *process*.

What about the process here? Mitchell commented that the analyst in his example felt that to comply with the patient's wish for him to be quiet "would be inauthentic on his part, destroying the necessary precondition for him to be engaged as an analyst." What exactly does this mean? And what exactly is that analyst's conception of what defines analysis? Although I think being authentic is vital, I also think responding in an analytic way requires more than simply being authentic; it is possible to be authentically destructive, authentically insensitive, authentically obtuse, and authentically nonanalytic. The question, therefore, is what would be most analytically useful here? In my view, if the analyst feels he is being asked to comply and that doing so would be a form of submission, then whatever power issues are being activated between his patient and him are precisely what should be clarified and engaged. Resisting would not be much better than complying. Neither choice would open to analytic scrutiny the issue of what is in play. If the pull is to become engaged in a power struggle, this is data to be curious about and attend to. Focusing on the interaction in this way is integral to how I conceive of working at the intimate edge and opens the analytic exploration in a uniquely important way. If such an effort failed, recognizing the failure would then be essential and would allow for exploring in minute detail what might be in play interactively.

These considerations apply not just when the interaction may be problematic in an obvious way. Sometimes the issues may be subtle. For example, when the pull from both sides is for the analyst to take a protective role, this too can be quite problematic. From my perspective, when this kind of enactment does occur, clarifying the collusion involved becomes crucial. In contrast, if the analyst assumes a protective role and does not attempt to explore what is in play, the patient may be robbed of a chance to see the ways in which she "gives herself over" to the other in this way or even pulls for it, and why. It also precludes a chance to clarify how each is responding to the other and in what ways. The idea is to clarify the interactive complexities so as to provide an opportunity for the patient to become aware of her vulnerabilities and be able to work these through, rather than to accommodate (or exploit) them, which would foreclose this kind of exploration. In effect, what is at issue here is the difference between providing fish and helping a person learn how to fish.

Deconstructing the pulls to enactment can be a means of helping a patient to access fantasies, wishes, and longings to be "taken over," or to be controlled, or to have all decisions made by another, or the reverse, and the extent to which a particular interactive structure may be eroticized in some way. Deconstruction can help illuminate the extent to which taking a helpless role may be a way to seduce the other into taking a helpful role, a way of asserting power or manipulating the other, or even humiliating the other in some form of sadomasochistic enactment without the other's knowing it,. To the extent that patient and analyst may be "colonizing" or "co-opting" each other internally in any way, clarifying this can be crucial. The same is true for varying forms of denial of boundaries that allow for maintaining an illusion of some kind of "oneness" or merger, for any number of reasons. Whatever the dynamics, opening to scrutiny what is in play in these enactments is critical if we are to help advance an analytic process.

Consider the process of projective identification from this perspective. Some analysts have described as "therapeutic" an interactive engagement in which the analyst receives the patient's projective identifications and returns them in some "processed" or "metabolized" form. My concern would be to clarify the collusion involved in this kind of enactment and the way in which it may allow for desire or agency, or both, to be located in the other, or surrendered to the other, or given over to the other, or taken over from the other. We might wonder if there is some desire to control the other or be controlled by the other from the inside? Is there a sexual fantasy at the heart of this way of relating, where one ends up inside the other or penetrated by the other psychically? Clarifying the pulls to collusion by both patient and analyst can allow for the exploration of the underlying fantasies and for understanding the extent to which this kind of engagement may be eroticized. I believe that deconstructing what is being enacted here is essential if the patient is to be helped to reclaim agency. In contrast, exploiting the dynamics involved or submitting to them, or colluding in any other way, can preclude a chance for the issues to be identified and worked through and can be undermining. To the extent that this may involve some form of reenactment, it can also be retraumatizing and can reinforce old assumptions without the patient or analyst realizing this.

With these matters in mind, let us consider a specific aspect of an interaction I have written about in great detail. It involves a moment when my patient Laura experienced her behavior as defensive.

Although I was well aware that her behavior was defensive, I also experienced it as aggressive (see Ehrenberg, 1985, 1992, 2003, for details of the process and earlier discussions of it). As we attempted to discuss the differences in our experience of the same interaction, she insisted I was "wrong" and that I was distorting her reality. I insisted that by accusing me of "distorting" her reality, she was challenging mine. The issue, as I saw it, was not whose perception was "right" or "wrong" or if it was possible for a response to be both aggressive and defensive at the same time. Rather, I was concerned about what was going on between us as we tried to discuss this issue. My position was that, if either of us tried to attack the other's right to have her own experience, this was a form of violation; it was possible and necessary for us to engage in a collaborative and mutually respectful way, even if we did not agree. What I tried to convey was that I was not invested in having her submit to my perception. Rather, I was interested in exploring the power issues that were in play between us and in questioning how we were each understanding what we were trying to do with each other. I also emphasized that I thought we had a right to disagree without its becoming cause for anger.

Much went on here beyond a simple exchange of words. It became an opportunity to discover that we could both survive the disagreement or difference in perception, and our reactions to it, and that being able to talk about it in this way could be interesting and constructive. Discovering that it was possible to engage constructively, even if we disagreed, and realizing that we now were actually engaging in a constructive discussion, challenged her assumptions about the relational possibilities. I believe that it was not just my words, but the actual experience of an intersubjective possibility that went beyond what she could have imagined as possible that had the greatest impact and was *mutative*.

Once her prior assumptions were thus challenged and she saw that they did not "hold," matters opened in a way they could not have been before. She spontaneously produced associations to experiences with her mother in which she now realized she had felt violated. In this context she reported realizing that what she had been doing with me was what her mother had done to her; the work began to move in many more directions and there were many more associations. The insight—the realization of a new intersubjective possibility—led to free(r) associations, not the reverse. It also allowed her to see the past through a new lens and with new degrees of freedom. Such questions as why she had felt she had to submit to her mother then, and to me now, and why she felt she had to fight to prove the other "wrong" so as to be able to feel she had a right to her own feelings could be engaged. So, too, could the question of why she ended up not knowing whether or not to trust her own experience in the face of conflict with mother and, later, with me. As she continued, she reported realizing that she was choosing to defer to mother, or to me, to get "approval" and feel "connected."

Realizing that deferring to the other to get "approval" and feel "connected" was her choice made clear that, despite her subjective experience to the contrary, she was actually not at the mercy of the other, as she had assumed; rather, she became aware that she was actually slave to her own need for the approval of the (m)other. Thus, even as she had assumed all along that it was the other who was trying to control her, now she realized that it was she who was trying to control the other and get the other to think and feel what she wanted the other to feel, no matter what the cost to herself. Then she would feel profoundly resentful of the other for the ways in which she felt "strangled." As this realization unraveled and she increasingly realized the extent to which she was the one doing this to herself, she was able to describe in detail moments when she had actually attacked people physically, without clearly understanding at the time what exactly had happened. She acknowledged that perhaps one of the reasons she had stormed out of our sessions in the past, when she was angry at me, was for fear that had she not done so at those moments of anger, she actually might have assaulted me. Although this admission was a bit shocking and difficult to integrate, the reclaiming (or the claiming) of agency that it allowed was liberating and empowering and allowed her to feel less threatened and "paranoid."

With an increasing sense of closeness and trust, she became aware of anxieties about our relationship, about how to know whether or not to trust her own judgment, and about her own vulnerability to influence. She noted with dread that she feared she would "lose herself" and not know whether she was feeling a certain way because of her own authentic wishes or because of her desire to please or to placate me. Even as she bemoaned how depressing it was that she still obviously had so much left to work on, she noted that this realization allowed her to feel whole and separate in a way she had never before felt. She experienced this change as a big step forward. Still, there were expressions of terror of needing or depending on anyone, and of fears that she would not be able to survive disappointment and hurt if she truly opened herself to anyone. Details of early experiences of having been victimized by others as a child, which had not been in awareness before, now became accessible.

Months later Laura spent a session telling me how much better she was feeling and that she was feeling "close" to me. She seemed to be risking a degree of vulnerability she had never dared allow herself to experience before. Then she expressed concern about how she would know when it was time to terminate. In the next session, however, she began with a challenge to me for all the times I had hurt her. I found myself feeling angry and defensive. She had obviously gotten to me. After some moments of silent reflection on how to respond, I finally said it was up to her whether she chose to negate all we had done together or to make use of it. She responded by pointing to my defensiveness and said that she was aware that what she had just done with me reflected her pattern of managing to "get" people by really figuring out their vulnerabilities and playing on them, even without necessarily being consciously aware of doing so at the time. She then gave me a list of examples and described how she felt her mother had done this to her. As we tried to determine what had prompted her to want to "get" me at that moment, it emerged that she felt I had hurt her in every session simply by telling her that we had to stop at its end. She continuously felt perplexed about how to deal with the pain of loss. The idea of termination, which she had raised in the prior session as a result of feeling better, had apparently triggered this particular reaction now. Becoming angry and negating the meaning of our relationship was a way to try to deal with these feelings. As this session ended, she playfully quipped, "I'll tame you yet." Then she smiled warmly. These sessions give a sense of how things continued to evolve, and they illustrate the progression of her growth and the kind of "freeing up" that working this way seemed to facilitate during this period of our work.

I think this example illustrates that taking apart the "seams" of the relationship in the way I have tried to describe here can free both parties to reengage in a different and more mutually satisfactory way. Instead of simply acting and reacting, patient and analyst can then begin to question, reflect, wonder, explore, and bounce off each other. When this occurs, being able to engage in this new kind of process and relationship is itself a measure of change, and the realization that change is possible is itself an insight. If both parties feel "strangled" in relation to each other, for example, experiencing that it is possible to engage in ways that are not "strangling" and that can be freeing, rather than crippling, and discovering that it is possible to talk about experiences of feeling oppressed in a constructive way, have dramatic impact. Each time experience opens, a new intersubjective possibility is achieved that, in turn, opens onto yet more new possibilities in a potentially endless progression.

Working at the intimate edge involves not only trying to study how things become "mixed" up between patient and analyst, but also a specific way of "mixing it up." This kind of process is different from an effort to focus on transference or countertransference because the latter effort implies that we can separate the two and that we think we can look from "outside" even when we are "inside." It is also different from focusing on the nature of the integration and the quality of contact in ways that assume an ability to "stand" in some "objective" place and take a "meta" view. What is required instead is something like turning our experience "inside out"— opening what I think of as the "internal boundary" of the relationship and explicating our experience from inside. In so doing, not only do we expand the analytic dialogue to include aspects of the intersubjective experience that normally are never explicitly acknowledged, we also allow new kinds of intersubjective experiences to evolve.

Even if the feelings between patient and analyst are antagonistic, the effort to engage collaboratively transforms the experience, generating a unique trajectory of evolving new experience in an ever-expanding way. The intimate edge, at any given moment, if it is achieved, thus becomes a point of new experience and also a point of entry to yet another possible kind of new experience. Each time we turn the moment "inside out," the experience changes and opens on itself and transforms yet again. This process is never linear. As the experience "opens," it opens in all directions simultaneously. The intimate edge thus is the "growing edge" of the relationship. It is the point from which intersubjective experience goes through ever-new transformations, as it moves forward from moment to moment in a specific and unique kind of way.

Blake's (1800–1803) image of finding "the world in the grain of sand" comes to mind. What I am after, however, is not a matter of simply finding what already exists and is there to be found. Rather, it is a matter of helping to generate something *intersubjectively* that did not exist before. If we can find a way to deconstruct what might have been toxic, or constrictive, it becomes possible to engage more freely and to bring the intersubjective moment alive so that what never might have been realized can be "born," and allowed to ripen and blossom. Such experiences are not "there to be found." They are intersubjective creations, wonders, and bits of magic. When they are achieved, they are never static, and there is no way to "hold" them, for they are in constant flux.

Working this way requires something akin to the idea of "Negative Capability" (Keats, 1817, p. 43), on the part of both patient and analyst. Keats defined this as "when man is capable of being in uncertainties, Mysteries, doubts, without any irritable reaching after fact and reason." What I have in mind involves a tolerance for and respect for "not knowing" not just cognitively, but also *affectively*. If we are willing to be emotionally available and accessible and open *to finding out where the experience might take us if we dare to let it*, we allow for the unexpected, sometimes the unimaginable in the immediate interaction. Insight then comes precisely in the form of the new experience that is generated as we work and engage in this way. From this perspective we must consider that the need to "know" where the work is going at any given moment may be a defense against the anxiety of "not knowing" and that presuming we can and should "know" limits what is possible analytically and experientially. If we could know beforehand what will happen, it would be more like plugging someone into our own script than really allowing ourselves to engage with and be touched by another. This would allow no room for surprise and for experiencing the real mystery and wonder of another or for exploring the limits of relational possibility.

Working this way allows for arriving at the unexpected, sometimes the unimaginable, in the immediate interaction. To the extent that this becomes transformative for both participants, the work is truly alive and can help to liberate creative and imaginative capabilities not only for the patient but also for the analyst.

Though *the intersubjective exists only intersubjectively*, and changes from moment to moment across time, each time a new intersubjective possibility is realized, specific as it may be to the particular dyad and to the specific moment between them, something internal also changes, and consciousness is expanded in a way that leaves neither person the same. Something rearranges internally for each, so that each participant actually then does "own" something not "owned" before. The insight that one is capable of an experience of a kind one did not even know was possible is something we keep, even after the experience may be over, and it becomes a kind of "private property." For example, one patient, in response to a dramatic kind of internal "opening" that occurred as we engaged this way, described his experience very eloquently. He reported that it felt as if "the ceiling was lifting on his imagination."

However critical "new experience" is here, what I am describing is never simply a matter of facilitating a "new experience" or "working in the moment." *There are many kinds of "new experience" and many ways of "working in the moment."* I am interested in the unique new experience that is generated if we work in the moment in the particular way I describe as working at the intimate edge.

It is striking to me that many of the points I argued in the 1974 paper and my later publications, which were so controversial then, have now come to be widely accepted. Nevertheless, that it has been and still may be difficult to apprehend my position, even in its most recent articulations, may be in part because, as I noted at the outset, this way of working, which is based on an appreciation of the interactive/intersubjective nature of the analytic field, and of the power of what goes on unconsciously between patient and analyst, may be difficult to grasp. I believe that where this is the case, it is precisely because it challenges traditional ideas about the data of analysis, about the process of analysis, and about how we use ourselves as analytic instruments. It also requires a radical shift in how we think about the change-process and about the nature of therapeutic action.

References

Blake, W. (1800–1803), Auguries of innocence. In: *The Complete Poetry of William Blake*, ed. D. V. Erdman.. New York: Doubleday, 1998.

Ehrenberg, D. B. (1992), *The Intimate Edge: Extending the Reach of Psychoanalytic Interaction*. New York: Norton.

_____ (1995), Countertransference disclosure. Panel discussion on "Self Disclosure: Therapeutic Tool or Self Indulgence." *Contemp. Psychoanal.*, 31:213–228.

_____ (1996), On the analyst's emotional availability and vulnerability. *Contemp. Psychoanal*, 32: 275–286.

_____ (2000), Potential impasse as analytic opportunity: Interactive considerations. *Contemp. Psychoanal.*, 36:. 573–586.

_____ (2003), A radical shift in thinking about the change-process: Commentary. *Psychoanal. Dial.*, 13:581–586

Freud, S. (1915), The unconscious. *Standard Edition*, 14:159–215. London: Hogarth Press, 1957.

Keats, J. (1817), Letter to his brothers, George and Tom Keats, December, 1817 In: *Letters of John Keats : A Selection*, ed. R. Gittings. Oxford: Oxford University Press, 1970.

Mitchell, S. A. (1997), *Influence and Autonomy in Psychoanalysis*. Hillsdale, NJ: The Analytic Press.

Holding:
Something Old and Something New*

(1996)

Joyce Slochower

▼ ▼ ▼ ▼ ▼

Editors' Introduction

When is the analyst's subjectivity a useful clinical resource to be brought to the foreground of an analysis, and when should it be kept in the background, carefully monitored and restrained? Among the most significant contributions of relational psychoanalysis is its focus on the inevitability of the psychoanalyst's participation, the therapeutic value of enactment, the ubiquity of interaction, and the importance of the analyst's subjectivity and of the clinical exploration of the patient's experience of the analyst's subjectivity. Joyce Slochower has consistently made important contributions by pointing to the excesses and one-sidedness of this focus, but, basing her thinking on the seminal contributions of D. W. Winnicott, she has done so from within the very center of relational theory.

In her 1996 book *Holding and Psychoanalysis* and throughout her body of work, Slochower explores the limitations of an overly interactive analytic style. There are times, she proposes, when certain

---

* An earlier version of this chapter appears in Joyce Slochower, *Holding and Psychoanalysis*. © 1996 The Analytic Press, Inc.

patients simply cannot tolerate the intrusion or impingement of the analyst's separate subjective presence. Building on and expanding Winnicott's notion of the analytic holding environment, Slochower provides an important corrective to other relational authors by highlighting the analyst's capacity for restraint in the service of protecting the patient from the analyst's "otherness." Slochower points to the necessity, at certain choice clinical points, for the analyst to suspend active investigatory and interpretive work. During moments of holding, patient and analyst together co-construct an illusion of analytic attunement that permits the analyst to be subjectively, rather than objectively, perceived.

Framing the question as holding and interpretation is polarizing. Placing containment and restraint on one side versus engagement and interaction on the other sets up a clash of models that is simplistic and reduces the complexity of all psychoanalytic schools. Slochower's work is rich and complex in that she views both of these models as necessary and interrelated strands, thus integrating the holding metaphor within a relational framework. Slochower addresses holding in a variety of clinical contexts—with severely regressed patients, in relation to issues of dependence, self-involvement, hate, mourning, religious ritual, and contemporary feminism. In the sample to follow, as in all her work, Slochower presents an illuminating clinical vignette that highlights the mutual and intersubjective aspects of the holding process.

Holding:
Something Old and Something New

▼　▼　▼　▼　▼

The Holding Metaphor in a Relational Context

It has always been easy to frame the practice of psychoanalysis and psychotherapy in terms of how we can best communicate with our patients about dynamic process. After all, much of psychoanalysis is focused on clarifying *meaning*: the meaning of transference, of early experience, of unconscious process. When we actively engage with our patients dialogically or work to deepen and make self-experience more complex, we use ourselves and what we know, and we tend to feel at our professional best. It is more difficult to feel comfortable in those moments when our activity—whether interpretative or interactive—is anything but helpful to our patient. We may be slower to recognize how clinical movement is sometimes effected not by our capacity to make meaning, but by our ability to create an emotional space within which inner experience can be articulated rather than challenged.

The Evolution of the Holding Metaphor

In his use of the holding metaphor, Winnicott (1960b)[1] sought to evoke the parallel between the developmental function of maternal care in infant development and the analyst–patient relationship. The Winnicottian mother/analyst protected the very vulnerable baby/patient from noxious environmental impingements in order to support access to previously hidden true self-experience. That idea generated a powerful response. If the analyst symbolically can become the mother, the possibility of reworking early trauma is enormously increased; what cannot be remembered can be reexperienced and then repaired; the patient can, in fact, be a baby again but with a better, more responsive mother.

This romantic portrait of the nurturing function, however, is dissonant with contemporary understandings of motherhood. Feminist (Chodorow, 1978; Dimen, 1991; Harris, 1991; Bassin, Honey, and Kaplan, 1994) and psychoanalytic perspectives (Benjamin, 1988; 1994; Kraemer, 1996) alike argue persuasively for a more complex view of mothering that explicitly includes the mother's subjectivity. The contemporary mother struggles intensely because she *cannot* be fully identified with her baby. Rather than spontaneously offering a holding experience from a position of pure identification with her baby's needs, she sometimes offers maternal care with a bit of reluctance. By making room for the ubiquity of maternal subjectivity, we offer the mother much more emotional breathing room than was accorded the idealized mother of the past, and we deepen our understanding of that primary relationship (Slochower, 1996a).

There is an evident clash between Winnicott's holding metaphor and relational/feminist thinking. The holding metaphor ignores, even implicitly *deletes*, the reality of the mother's subjectivity while placing the baby in a relatively passive position vis-à-vis good-enough maternal care (see Little; 1959; Loewald, 1960; Sandler, 1960; Balint, 1968). There is

---

[1] Although Winnicott is most frequently associated with work on the holding process, many others have also contributed to the concept of holding or containment. They include Bion (1959, 1962, 1963), Little (1959), Loewald (1960), Sandler (1960), Khan (1963), Balint (1968), Kohut, (1971), Bollas (1978), and Sandback (1993).

little room in this model for those aspects of a mother's experience that are not congruent with the needs of her baby.

In a similar way, the traditional holding analyst does not appear to contend with the analyst's[2] own incongruent subjectivity. The analyst seems to attend to the patient's needs (deficits) from a position of identification and caring concern, and it is as difficult to locate evidence of the analyst's noncongruent subjectivity in this vision as it is in the idealized mother–infant relationship. The analyst's capacity to evaluate and then meet her patient's needs places her in an emotionally certain, remarkably unflappable, and omniscient position vis-à-vis the passive patient/baby. And the patient, like a baby, is thereby rendered *unknowing*, unable to recognize the analyst as a subject. How can this patient/baby access adult-level self-experience within the holding metaphor?

It is not surprising that contemporary relational thinking takes issue with the maternal metaphor. It argues cogently that a patient is very much an adult, capable of a reciprocal, adult relationship with the analyst (see, e.g., Mitchell, 1988, 1991b; Aron, 1991; Hoffman, 1991, 1992; Burke, 1992; Stern, 1992; Tansey, 1992; Shabad, 1993).[3] From these perspectives, holding represents a near charade, an "as if" analytic position that ignores the complex subjectivities of both analyst and patient, rendering both parties idealized and one dimensional.

---

[2] Throughout this text, I use the feminine pronoun to refer both to female and to male patients and analysts.

[3] Mitchell (1988a, 1991b) questioned the idealized position in which the analyst/mother is placed by "developmental tilt" models and noted that the patient is consequently infantalized. He further suggested that these models sidestep the question of whether a patient's *wishes* (conflicts) or her *needs* (deficits) are the central therapeutic issue. Aron (1991) believes that the "analyst as holder" deprives the patient of a complex and adult type of intimacy. Stern (1992) points out that the analyst-as-mother has limited freedom and that her patient will be similarly restricted. He notes that the patient/baby metaphor implies that the patient is relatively unable to "see" the analyst in ways that are inconsistent with the empathic, mothering position. The baby/patient cannot easily communicate such perceptions to the analyst, and the resulting therapeutic interchange would thus be one that addresses only a rather circumscribed area of exchange between the two. Hoffman (1991, 1992) underscores the centrality of the analyst's *uncertainty* and her inability to "know," in any absolute sense, what the patient needs. He argues against the analyst's ability to engage in anything like an objective assessment of the patient's need for a holding process.

A Relational Holding Model

It is my aim to address this clash between relational and holding models and to propose a perspective on holding that is integrated within a relational framework. For, although I agree that the vision of patient-as-adult engaged in subject-to-subject relatedness with the analyst (Benjamin, 1994) enormously enriches the analytic interaction, this vision is often more a goal than a given in our psychoanalytic work.

Can all our patients tolerate and make use of explicitly intersubjective analytic process? It is my thesis that the intersubjective analytic relationship is a hard-won therapeutic achievement that often does not emerge until well into the treatment process. Many patients find it close to impossible to work with and integrate the marked contrasts between their subjective process and the analyst's separate perspective.

When mutuality is experienced as noxious rather than enriching, it becomes necessary, at least temporarily, that the analyst *not* be known; and in these moments, holding becomes a central therapeutic theme. Most patients need this experience at certain critical moments; some may need it for longer periods. A protected holding space can crucially support the expression and exploration of heretofore dissociated or denied aspects of affective life that are difficult to access or articulate in more ordinary analytic interchange.

In this book, I expand the meaning of the holding theme and explore its place within a relational perspective. I address the impact of holding on both patient and analyst and construct a more complex and shaded view of the analyst's struggle to be affectively "with" a patient. Holding becomes crucial at those moments when the analyst's separate input feels highly emotionally dysjunctive, that is, "out of sync" with a patient's affective state.

Holding has historically been associated with the needs of dependent patients in a state of regression. This view of holding is based on a maternal metaphor, wherein the analyst meets the patient's needs in an idealized way. Holding, however, can also be critical to working with difficult emotional states that may evoke anything *but* a synchronous, maternal response from the analyst. It is my intention to unpack the tight link between holding and dependence by exploring how we use holding in work around issues of rage, ruthlessness, and self-preoccupation wherein the analyst's role is far from idealized. As I take up these emotional themes, I consider the therapeutic function of a holding stance, the impact of holding on both patient and analyst, the clinical risks associated with the holding position, and the limits of work within the holding metaphor.

The holding theme is ubiquitous in analytic work, at times explicit and at other moments implicit. In "ordinary" therapeutic moments, the holding function remains in the background; we use both our affectively resonant responses and our more separate ways of understanding patients' processes quite explicitly by way of a complex of interventions, including, but not limited to, interpretations. In treatment situations with very difficult patients, however, interpretation or intersubjective exploration can be disruptive rather than facilitative, and the analyst may eventually turn to a holding position with the sense that her patient cannot tolerate anything other than this protected process.

When the reality of my separate subjectivity consistently disrupts inner process and cannot be worked with or worked through, I turn to the holding process. I use holding in a metaphoric sense to allude *to the coconstructed creation, by patient and analyst, of an illusion of analytic reliability and attunement.* That illusion has many affective colorings but always involves the analyst's struggle to establish a contained emotional space within which a range of difficult experiences can safely be experienced and expressed (Slochower 1991, 1992, 1994, 1996a, b). The illusion of attunement supports the patient's exploration of inner states in an analytic process that involves a minimum of potentially disturbing input on the analyst's part. Within this highly protected space, especially vulnerable patients may first be able to fully experience, work with, and integrate painful affective states.

When an analyst attempts to work within a holding process, she actively struggles to *bracket*, that is, *neither ignore nor introduce her dysjunctive subjectivity into the therapeutic interaction.* The analyst's struggle to hold herself crucially supports the dual capacity for affective containment and aliveness. This struggle is essential if the analyst is to sustain the holding metaphor without abandoning a two-person psychoanalytic model; if she altogether loses contact with her inner experience, holding will cease to represent a metaphor. The analyst is stripped of her subjecthood. Unaware that the more complex dimensions of her own experience and relationship to her patient have been lost, she "becomes" an idealized container for the patient.

Because the holding analyst attempts to contain her own subjectivity, she tends to feel constrained in her ability to make full use of her ideas and affective responses to her patient in these moments. The analyst often experiences enormous pressure actually to feel what her patient needs her to feel, whether that be, for example, empathic understanding, firm resolve, or anger. She may struggle quite a bit to contain those subjective responses that do not "fit" with her patient's emotional experience. It may even be difficult for the analyst to be absolutely certain that her subjective response to her patient is, in fact, her own; the possibility exists of a shared subjectivity, that is, of an area of confusion between the patient's and analyst's affective response.[4]

To explicate the holding theme, I focus on work with patients who are highly reactive to the analyst's separate input and who cannot easily move in and out of a holding experience. However, holding and interpretation can rarely be cleanly parsed. These separate, yet interpenetrating, themes in analytic work tend to alternate quite rapidly. The holding experience supports the analyst's interpretive or confrontative intervention, and the holding analyst sometimes *does* interpret, but with special awareness of her patient's vulnerability to disruption. At moments, interpretations themselves function as a container (holding) for affective experience. On yet another level, the therapeutic holding function carries its own symbolic communication, representing an implicit interpretation in its own right (Winnicott, 1954; Pine, 1984).

Illusion and the Coconstructed Holding Metaphor

The analytic process requires that we tolerate paradox and illusion as the treatment space is transformed into the particular affective arena needed by the patient (Ghent, 1992; Pizer, 1992). Despite their problematic edge, illusions enhance a capacity for play and creativity within and outside of the psychoanalytic situation (Mitchell, 1988; Slochower, 1998). Winnicott (1951) called this arena transitional space.

Within the holding situation, transitional space takes on a particular quality. Whatever its affective ambience, holding involves the mutual establishment, by patient and analyst, of a temporary *illusion of analytic attunement*. The analyst seems to remain evenly and consistently present, intact, and available to the patient. While the analyst may represent a maternal, nurturing figure, it is also possible that an illusion of attunement will organize around the patient's experience of the analyst as nonretaliatory, alive, and firm, consistently able to recognize and tolerate her patient's intense and toxic affect states.

---

[4] With patients who make extensive use of projective identification, this is particularly likely (see Klein, 1955; Bion, 1959; Ogden, 1994). To the degree that a patient has split off or disowned aspects of her own experience (e.g., an unconscious sadistic attack on the dependent self), the analyst may experience these attacking feelings as internally generated. In such a situation, the analyst may be uncertain whether her ambivalence about bracketing her subjectivity reflects her questions about the process or an identification with the patient's self-attack.

The holding process transforms the separate subjectivities of patient and analyst in the direction of increased synchrony. This leaves the analyst with the task of retaining, largely unexpressed, an image of the wider area created by their shared yet separate experience. This overarching analytic third (Ogden, 1994), a space within which patient and analyst can negotiate around two separate sets of subjectivities), must be sustained in the mind of the analyst. If that idea is altogether lost, then holding ceases to be a metaphor; analyst and patient lose contact with the illusory quality of the holding experience. The analyst "becomes" the parental holding figure and the patient becomes the baby in an enactment that is more literal than symbolic. The absence of metaphor will, in all likelihood, destroy the symbolic function of holding and ultimately disrupt the therapeutic function of the holding frame.

Holding and the Analyst's Subjectivity

In my experience, when patients are involved in an "ordinary" psychoanalytic interchange, my emotional variability will, unless extreme, either go nearly unnoticed or be directly responded to so that it can be explicitly addressed. As Aron (1992) and others have clearly elaborated, dialogue that directly addresses the analyst's subjectivity deepens the treatment relationship and patients' experience of themselves. While patients may have a variety of reactions to evidence of our subjectivity (including anger, pleasure, frustration), their struggle with it and with us is most often strengthening and results in a freer and deeper level of therapeutic interchange.

However, if my patient reacts violently to evidence of my separate personhood, to indications that my emotional experience, my ideas about her experience, are discrepant from hers, I will begin to explore the nature of our interaction. It is possible that my patient's reaction reflects her own *conflicts* around recognizing some aspect of our mutual interaction. Alternatively, my patient may have reacted to what, or the *way* that, I intervened. I am likely to keep trying to work with my patient around these issues unless it becomes inescapable that my separateness and emotional "misses" have a consistently toxic effect both on our work and on my patient's outside life. Only then will I move toward a holding position.

Holding involves an ongoing attempt on my part to contain my subjectivity. However, my success is likely to be approximate rather than absolute. Even during moments of holding, my patient may well be peripherally aware that I have more complex feelings about our relationship (and that I am a more complex person) than she is prepared to assimilate or deal with directly. To sustain the holding experience, my patient thus brackets (usually unconsciously) those aspects of my personhood or behavior that would disrupt the experience of being held. This bracketing stands in stark contrast to those moments when the patient is able directly to take up the question of our differences, whether affective or cognitive.

The holding space is not established by the analyst alone; patients unconsciously participate in sustaining the holding experience by excluding aspects of the analyst's presence that threaten to disrupt it. In this sense, the holding experience requires the patient's implicit participation. On one level, patient and analyst implicitly agree not to question the analyst's intactness, reliability, or holding capacity. Yet a tacit, unarticulated negotiation between analyst and patient maintains the boundaries of the holding experience. The patient makes clear, through both conscious and unconscious communications, what is essential for *her* during the holding process, and the analyst also (sometimes unwittingly) asserts the limits of her capacity to sustain the holding stance. These tacit negotiations stand in marked contrast to the very explicit negotiations that take place with patients engaged in a more mutual analytic interchange.

Holding as Enactment

There is increasing consensus among theorists across the psychoanalytic continuum that enactments are an inevitable part of the treatment process (Mitchell; 1991a, b; Burke 1992; Tansey, 1992; Bromberg, 1993). These moments carry important historical meaning for patient (and analyst) and are thus pivotal analytic "grist" that embodies potential for change. Simultaneously, however, enactments reflect the analyst's partial *failure*— to understand and articulate before acting. And some enactments are anything but useful; these so powerfully recapitulate early parental failures in form or content or both that they have a retraumatizing effect, reinforcing defensive style, creating a therapeutic stalemate, or precipitating a traumatic collapse. When the analyst's misunderstandings, interpretive errors, failures, and the like freeze rather than move the treatment process, holding represents a crucial treatment stance.

Is holding itself an enactment? Does the analytic holding function arise spontaneously out of the relational matrix? Or does the analyst decide to hold on the basis of an objective assessment of her patient's emotional state? In a relational context, is it not impossible ever to be certain that a patient *needs* a holding experience?

The shift toward a holding stance emerges out of an inherently sub-jective, negotiated interaction between patient and analyst that reflects the interweaving of apparently objective and subjective elements in the psychoanalytic situation. On one level, I assess what is going on with my patient, within me, and between us, and I move toward a holding posi-tion based on a clinical judgment informed by all those factors. Yet, despite the objective elements that inform my choice, the shift to a hold-ing stance inevitably emerges out of the subjective, mutual pulls of our relationship. My sense of a patient's relative vulnerability, of the force of her need, her anger, her reactivity to impingement, are all informed by my emotional experience of her. Do I feel like mothering her (i.e., have I identified with the parental metaphor)? Is my move toward a holding stance in part a reaction to feeling "shut out" of the analytic interaction? Do I need to insulate myself from my patient's anger? Have I responded to unconscious communications on my patient's part by moving into a holding position? Alternatively, do I struggle against the obverse pull, resisting abandoning my subjectivity and insisting that I be known?

The Limits of the Holding Metaphor

The very idea of a relational "holding" analyst is a paradoxical one. For while the analyst's capacity to hold the patient is real and powerful, the patient is not a baby and the analyst not the mother. The vision of ana-lyst as maternal provider clashes with the reality that the patient is an adult, capable of complex levels of awareness and conflict as well as need. The analyst is vulnerable to her own and her patient's subjective process; the analyst's holding capacity is significantly limited by her inevitably idiosyncratic reactions to her patient and by the treatment setup itself. Additionally, the analyst's ability to know *just what* her patient needs is open to question. What the analyst perceives to be an affectively conjunctive response may not always feel conjunctive to her patient; similarly, what feels dysjunctive to the analyst may at times actu-ally "fit" a patient's process far more closely than the analyst imagines. Even the most empathic, attuned analyst experiences a multiplicity of responses to her patient that may limit her ability to work within the holding metaphor.

How, then, can holding occur at all? It seems clear that the holding process requires that both patient and analyst bracket their awareness of the illusory nature of absolute analytic attunement for a time. The illusion of attunement—an illusion that patient and analyst share—reflects their confidence in the analyst's reparative powers. The patient (and sometimes the analyst as well) to some extent suspends, reframes, or temporarily sets aside her awareness of those elements that would put this emotional reliability into question. These may include the analyst's absences, her inevitable emotional variability, her affective "misses" or misunderstandings. That awareness, however, hovers at the edges of the analytic experience and occasionally breaks into process. Yet it is simultaneously clear that disruptions of the holding frame, whether expressed through unconsciously motivated enactments or the inevitable unreliability of the setting itself (e.g., vacations and other disruptions), are sometimes not only temporarily derailing but also are actually traumatizing, representing a repetitive parental failure that cannot be worked with or integrated. It is for this reason that the holding frame largely excludes the ordinary ways in which the analyst's subjectivity and emotional variability enter the treatment setting. The patient's extreme emotional reactivity underscores the temporary *reality* of her need for an unusually high degree of adaptation on the analyst's part.

Of course, it is only the deluded analyst who enters any kind of holding situation with absolute confidence about its therapeutic efficacy. To the extent that the holding process is functioning in a therapeutic way, the analyst must remain peripherally aware that she is indeed, *not* the mother. If the analyst too fully enters the holding fantasy, the element of enactment intrinsic to the holding experience will lose its metaphoric edge and take over in a more complete way. That enactment will ultimately have disastrous consequences when the holding fantasy collides with the reality of the analyst's incongruent subjectivity. It is thus essential that the analyst (and, at moments, the patient as well) acknowledge the paradoxical nature of the holding metaphor even while it is experienced as simply real.

So the analyst is *there* as a holding presence and also is *not there*. Her holding capacity, even if good enough, inevitably will fail, for the nature and boundaries of the analytic relationship are such that patients ultimately come up against the limits of the analyst's availability, reliability, or intactness. Further, by virtue of her ability to bracket her subjectivity, the analyst inevitably reveals something of herself to her patient—if only her emotional resilience and willingness to struggle with her experience.

Holding and Collaborative Psychoanalytic Work

Holding is, of course, not enough. When my patient and I live within the illusion of analytic attunement, my patient's self-experience remains relatively unchallenged and I remain a subjective, rather than an objective, object, inevitably *unknown*. The holding experience protects my patient from the reality of my externality as an object and a subject. A high price is paid for this degree of protection, for it leaves my patient at the mercy of my affective evenness, without much resilience vis à vis my inevitable variability. Ultimately, my patient needs to be less reactive to my (inevitably uneven) presence at any particular moment. If we are to work together to deepen and complicate a narrowed range of experience with objects—internal and external—my patient must be able to respond to and to integrate my subjectivity. Only if the analyst's separateness is experienced as potentially enriching can the work proceed outside the holding frame.

When analytic process begins to shift away from holding toward collaborative interchange, patient and analyst are better able to work with explicit evidence of the analyst's separate (if sometimes unwelcome) understanding of the patient's process and their interchange. As a capacity for collaborative investigation is deepened, the holding theme will ordinarily evolve into a more momentary or transient aspect of the work. The evolution of collaborative process involves mutual movement by patient and by analyst as well. At times, the analyst unconsciously responds to subtle cues on the patient's part indicating that some tolerance for difference may now be possible by introducing her subjectivity. Alternatively, the patient may make the first move toward collaboration, and the analyst may responsively shift toward a more separate position. Although an increased capacity for collaborative analytic work represents a treatment goal, I do not view this evolution to be unidirectional. The need for holding experiences pervades both the life span (Slochower, 1993) and the analytic process. It reemerges at times of emotional crisis and remains a crucial dimension of analytic and human experience.

It is, of course, inevitably risky for the patient fully to acknowledge the external reality of the analyst while simultaneously living with the very powerful loving and destructive feelings that are evoked in this work. In this sense, the achievement of a capacity for collaboration implies that we, as analysts, have allowed our patients to know us (both objectively and subjectively) as *people*—capable of doing and receiving real and projected harm as well as good. Our patients, of course, struggle with the dangers inherent in this awareness.

Illusion and the Holding Metaphor

If we recognize, but keep silent about our awareness that the holding experience is, in part, illusory, are we colluding with our patients?

Certainly, we fail to disabuse our patients of this somewhat "distorted" view of us; we might even be accused of emotional inauthenticity. Yet the illusion of analyst-as-ideal-parent may sometimes be critical for our patients *and for ourselves*. Are such partial illusions not, in fact, intrinsic to all intimate relationships? When my five-year-old son said to me, "You are the best mommy in the whole world," was it necessary that I present a more complex view of myself and disabuse him of his feeling? Should I have reminded him that I wasn't always so great, that he didn't always feel that way about me? Or was it instead essential *not* to question his feeling but, rather, to appreciate and even share it for that moment? Do we not permit such illusions to pervade romantic love relationships? If we feel wedded to absolute truthfulness, it becomes necessary to continually remind the other of the limits of our capacity to meet her needs, thereby leaching the relationship of any element of idealization.

Despite the narrow ways in which an analyst can "become" the holding object, the illusion of a protected space and of a highly resilient, attuned, steady analyst can crucially support therapeutic process and create a powerful background for the elaboration of painful, often dissociated aspects of internal process. Illusions can facilitate analytic experience and are especially central to the holding process. Yet illusions also carry considerable risk, particularly when they are held so tightly that their rupture feels toxic, if not catastrophic. To illustrate both the therapeutic and problematic dimensions of the holding experience and the illusion of attunement, let me describe a recent treatment in which intense moments of holding alternated with profound states of disillusionment and repetitive breakdowns of the holding space.

A successful academic, Anne entered analysis with eagerness and hope despite her pervasive depression. Anne seemed open, affectively alive, and extremely sensitive. She made intense eye contact, appearing hungrily to take in my physical presence in a careful way. When I inquired about this, Anne said that she was not accustomed to having anyone's full attention and found the treatment process extremely powerful. Anne had experienced her parents to be utterly caught up in their own concerns and emotionally detached; there was no sense of safety at home. During her first year she had had a very early positive relationship with a nanny who then left abruptly, never to be satisfactorily replaced. We suspected that therein lay an important source of her sensitivity to loss and tendency carefully to track my emotional responses.

After some months of work, Anne shyly expressed strong feelings for me. She said that she felt understood for the first time. She longed for me to be as close as possible, literally and symbolically, and I responded to her with warmth and caring. Anne slowly seemed to relax and open up, and our work deepened. I felt like the best of analysts—alive, connected, empathic, insightful, and we both responded with pleasure to the rich relationship that was unfolding between us.

During this relatively brief period of our work, Anne and I together bracketed dysjunctive aspects of our relationship; my holding stance and Anne's illusion of near-perfect analytic attunement supported a rich and unfolding process. Anne needed, and seemed to find, a sense of affective resonance, and the holding function allowed us to work deeply and well together. She experienced me as attuned, responsive, present; and, within this protected space, she contacted and worked with disturbing inner states.

Some months later, I became aware that there was something unusual about the holding frame within which we worked. Whereas many patients involved in a holding experience tend to exclude or bracket potentially disturbing aspects of the analyst's presence in order to preserve the holding experience, Anne did not. The illusion of attunement that supported Anne's holding experience was actually quite tenuous, and, after the initial honeymoon period, Anne became increasingly anxious, wary, and vigilant. I came to realize that Anne was, half consciously, testing out the reliability of my holding function, tracking me for confirmation that I was affectively present and for any indication that I was not. Her vulnerability to disruption was not, in itself, surprising; many patients are highly reactive to evidence of analytic ruptures. What was especially difficult here, however, was the simultaneous reality of the holding experience and Anne's conviction that the holding illusion was potentially toxic. Its toxicity resided in its vulnerability to collapse.

As Anne exposed more of her vulnerability to me, she scanned me with increasing intensity for evidence that I was repulsed by her. Eventually she found that evidence. A new pattern took hold: moments of holding that intensified Anne's longings were followed by renewed vigilance as she scanned for disruptions of that experience. Inevitably, disruptions occurred, leaving her feeling exposed and hurt. It became increasingly clear that our early and easy connection has been based on a precarious illusion. For any affective miss, no matter how predictable or minor, broke into the holding experience and disrupted the analytic space, which Anne now found false and devoid of feeling. And so, when I ended the session, if I failed to smile or to smile warmly enough, Anne felt devastated, unable to recover or to hold on to other dimensions of our relationship. In those moments, our connection was destroyed. I was merely a professional doing my job, there was nothing personal between us, and Anne reminded herself to guard against her own need for me. Neither resonating with her experience nor attempting to link her reaction historically helped Anne to shift or complicate her experience; the illusion of analytic attunement had utterly collapsed and we entered a period during which a narrowly defined emotional space gave me very little breathing room.

This pattern of holding, followed by disruption and very gradual, painful, repair, came to dominate our work. In one session, for example, Anne described her very conflicted relationship with a new boyfriend. As we spoke, Anne turned her face toward me from the couch, her face softened, and she cried softly, saying how good it felt to have me understand. This deep and connected work felt good to me as well, but, as the session moved toward its close, I felt a growing tension. I was aware that, by stopping Anne, I would again rupture things in a major way. Trying to find a way to shift what had become a predictable pattern, I gently said that I knew that when things felt close between us, our ending felt like a betrayal. I added that I knew that, no matter how tactfully I were to stop her now, there was a risk that we would repeat that old pattern of closeness followed by abandonment. I said (probably wistfully) that I wished we could find a way out of the box we were in. Anne, nodding with recognition, said sadly that she didn't think that she'd ever be able to feel differently. Our mutual recognition of this reenactment, however, did not seem to help Anne, who came into our next session depressed; despite all we had said, she felt again that our connection wasn't real, that she was "just a patient." Anne responded to the disrupted illusion by closing down emotionally, becoming wary and bitter, convinced that nothing could help her experience her life differently.

Anne repeatedly reexperienced this cycle of intimate holding followed by abandonment—when she felt that she "had" me, the certainty of abandonment increased and Anne guarded against that possibility by vigilantly scanning me. Over time, I felt increasingly frustrated, oppressed by Anne's scrutiny, helpless to do more than articulate the bind in which we found ourselves. Anne sought both to disconfirm and to confirm her grim certainty that I, like her parents, did not really care about her. As Anne's experience of repair was shattered, so was my sense of being a good analyst.

For Anne, the question of whether our relationship was real rendered its boundaries intolerable. Any breach in the reality of my emotional attunement and holding capacity destroyed the illusion of attunement that she seemed desperately to need. There was no element of play here; I either did or did not care enough about her; nothing bridged the doubleness of the treatment relationship. Without a capacity to sustain paradox and illusion, Anne could not bracket potentially disturbing aspects of my presence, and my holding function was regularly and powerfully breeched.

Anne and I lived in this excruciating treatment space for years. I struggled with intense frustration and sometimes despair as Anne and I reworked the reenactment of repair and rupture to no apparent avail. Anne usually felt enormous relief at my understanding and pain at the smallest of ruptures; we spoke often about the cycle and its antecedents. But inevitably, it seemed, the pattern recurred. When I gently let Anne know what I was feeling, she became devastated. She could not integrate the idea that I could have caring *and* frustrated feelings. Nor could she face the idea that she was both full of longing *and* full of bitterness. Nothing I said seemed to shift Anne's sense of despair at the realization that I was not the idealized maternal object she longed for. Anne's defensive vigilance and tendency to scan for danger reflected early experiences of having been taken by surprise. That insight, however, had little impact on this pattern.

It is now a decade later. The cycle, which repeated endlessly, began to shift almost imperceptibly a few years ago. I do not believe that this shift was the result of profound interpretations or moments of special insight or connection between us. Rather, it seems as if our mutual commitment to living through these cycles has very, very gradually effected a shift in Anne's experience of herself and me. That shift has allowed Anne both to use the holding space and to move beyond it.

Anne now uses the holding experience in a way that encompasses its paradoxical qualities (Ghent, 1992); she is no longer reliant on an inelastic illusion of my holding capacity. Anne has me and does not have me and seems to have let go, bit by bit, of the fantasy that she could find an idealized maternal relationship that repaired what she felt she lacked. Anne no longer enters the treatment room ready to subject the viability of our relationship to an acid test. She can suspend disbelief and tolerate the paradox of psychoanalytic work (Pizer, 1992, 1996), and this capacity supports her as we move in and out of moments of holding. While there are still times when Anne becomes highly reactive to shifts in my affective presence, by and large we are able to talk about these without precipitating a traumatic collapse. We laugh together now, and, as she contemplates my upcoming vacation, we marvel at how freely she can let me go.

My work with Anne tested the limits of my willingness to hold myself and to maintain a holding stance. I was confronted, almost daily, with my inability to be present in a way that Anne could take in. At moments, my need for self-holding seemed as great as Anne's; it was not easy to find that, despite my best efforts, I continually failed her. There was a danger that, with Anne, I might lose hope, in myself and in our work, and "forget" the powerful and positive moments we had shared.

I struggled to hold on to a memory of Anne's capacity to feel held by me in the face of her more pervasive feelings of disappointment and to sustain my awareness that my failures with Anne were not absolute, that she had other feelings about our work. By holding on to those moments, I began to do what Anne could not as yet do: carry an affective memory of the doubleness of our relationship. In this sense, I held the repetitive hopelessness that came out of Anne's constant spoiling of good experience while holding on to hope.

For a patient to experience and use a holding process, she must be able to sustain an illusion of analytic attunement in the face of the inevitable fluctuations and momentary nature of that attunement. That capacity requires an ability to tolerate and enjoy illusion, that is, to suspend disbelief and live within the paradoxical boundaries of the analytic relationship without questioning its essential affective vitality. However, people like Anne are highly reactive to issues of deception in a way that makes such exclusion dangerous. Anne's profound difficulty integrating the idea of her own "badness" resulted in a need to undo that badness through her connection with a loving, holding analyst. Her unconscious conviction that she was, indeed, bad pulled us into repetitive enactments that confirmed her worst fears about her unloveability.

In Anne's treatment, then, the illusion of attunement could not be sustained. Instead, repeated cycles of disruption and repair gradually supported the build-up for Anne (and me) of an affective memory of moments of holding. That affective memory created a structure into which my failures could slowly be integrated without altogether destroying the memory of our connection.

References

Aron, L. (1991), The patient's experience of the analyst's subjectivity. *Psychoanal. Dial.*, 1:29–51.

——— (1992), Interpretation as expression of the analyst's subjectivity. *Psychoanal. Dial.*, 2:475–508.

Balint, M. (1968), *The Basic Fault*. London: Tavistock.

Bassin, D., Honey, M. & Kaplan, M. M., eds. (1994), *Representations of Motherhood*. New Haven, CT: Yale University Press.

Benjamin, J. (1988), *The Bonds of Love: Psychoanalysis, Feminism and the Problem of Domination*. New York: Pantheon.

——— (1994), The omnipotent mother: A psychoanalytic study of fantasy and reality. In: *Representations of Motherhood*, ed. D. Bassin, M. Honey & M. M. Kaplan. New Haven, CT: Yale University Press, pp. 129–146.

Bion, W. (1959), *Experiences in Groups*. London: Tavistock.

——— (1962), *Learning From Experience*. London: Heinemann.

————— (1963), *Elements of Psychoanalysis*. London: Heinemann.

Bollas, C. (1978), The transformational object. *Internat. J. Psycho-Anal.*, 60:97–107.

Bromberg, P. M. (1993), Shadow and substance: A relational perspective on clinical process. *Psychoanal. Psychol.*, 10:147–168.

Burke, W. F. (1992), Countertransference disclosure and the asymmetry/mutuality dilemma. *Psychoanal. Dial.*, 2:241–271.

Chodorow, N. (1978), *The Reproduction of Mothering*. Berkeley: University of California Press.

Dimen, M. (1991), Deconstructing difference: Gender, splitting and transitional space. *Psychoanal. Dial.*, 1:335–352.

Ghent, E. (1992), Paradox and process. *Psychoanal. Dial.*, 2:135–159.

Harris, A. (1991), Gender as contradiction. *Psychoanal. Dial.*, 1:197–224.

Hoffman, I. Z. (1991), Discussion: Toward a social-constructivist view of the psychoanalytic situation. *Psychoanal. Dial.*, 1:74–105.

————— (1992), Some practical implications of a social-constructivist view of the psychoanalytic situation. *Psychoanal. Dial.*, 2:287–304.

Khan, M. (1963), The concept of cumulative trauma. In: *The Privacy of the Self*. New York: International Universities Press, 1974.

Klein, M. (1955), *Envy and Gratitude and Other Works*. New York: Delacorte.

Kohut, H. (1971), *The Analysis of the Self*. New York: International Universities Press.

Kraemer, S. (1996), "Betwixt the dark and the daylight" of maternal subjectivity: Meditations on the threshold. *Psychoanal. Dial.*, 6:765–791.

Little, M. (1959), *Transference Neurosis and Transference Psychosis: Toward a Basic Unity*. New York: Aronson.

Loewald, H. (1960), On the therapeutic action of psychoanalysis. In: *Papers on Psychoanalysis*. New Haven, CT: Yale University Press, 1980, pp. 221–256.

Mitchell, S. (1988), *Relational Concepts in Psychoanalysis*. Cambridge: Harvard University Press.

————— (1991a), Wishes, needs and interpersonal negotiations. *Psychoanal. Inq.*, 2:147–170.

————— (1991b), Contemporary perspectives on self: Toward an integration. *Psychoanal. Dial.*, 1:121–148.

Ogden, T. H. (1994), *Subjects of Analysis*. Northvale, New Jersey: Aronson.

Pine, F. (1984), The interpretive moment variations on classical themes. *Bull. Menninger Clin.*, 48:54–71.

Pizer, S. A. (1992), The negotiation of paradox in the analytic process. *Psychoanal. Dial.*, 2:215–240.

————— (1996), *Building Bridges: The Negotiation of Paradox in Psychoanalysis*. Hillsdale, NJ: The Analytic Press.

Sandbank, T. (1993), Psychoanalysis and maternal work—Some parallels. *Internat. J. Psychoanal.*, 74:715–727.

Sandler, J. (1960), The background of safety. *Internat. J. Psychoanal.*, 41:352–356.

Shabad, P. (1993), Resentment, indignation, entitlement: The transformation of unconscious wish to need. *Psychoanal. Dial.*, 3:481–494.

Slochower, J. (1991), Variations in the analytic holding environment. *Internat. J. Psycho-Anal.*, 72:709–718.

———— (1992), A hateful borderline patient and the holding environment. *Contemp. Psychoanal.*, 28:72–88.

———— (1993), Mourning and the holding function of shiva. *Contemp. Psychoanal.*, 2:352–367.

———— (1994), The evolution of object usage and the holding environment. *Contemp. Psychoanal.*, 30:135–151.

———— (1996a), Holding and the evolving maternal metaphor. *Psychoanal. Rev.*, 83:195–218.

———— (1996b), The holding environment and the fate of the analyst's subjectivity. *Psychoanal. Dial.*, 6:323–353.

———— (1998), Illusion and uncertainty in psychoanalytic writing. *Internat. J. Psycho-Anal.*, 79:333–347.

———— (1999a), Interior experience in analytic process. *Psychoanal. Dial.*, 9:789–809.

———— (2004), But what do you want? The location of emotional experience. *Contemp. Psychoanal.*, 40:577–602.

Stern, D. (1992), Commentary on constructivism in clinical psychoanalysis. *Psychoanal. Dial.*, 3:331–364.

Tansey, M. J. (1992), Psychoanalytic expertise. *Psychoanal. Dial.*, 2:305–316.

Winnicott, D. W. (1947), Hate in the countertransference. In: *Through Paediatrics to Psycho-analysis*. New York: Basic Books, 1975.

———— (1951), Transitional objects and transitional phenomena. In: *Through Paediatrics to Psycho-analysis*. New York: Basic Books.

———— (1954), Withdrawal and regression. In: *Collected Papers: Through Paediatrics to Psycho-analysis*. New York: Basic Books.

———— (1960a), The theory of the parent–infant relationship. In: *The Maturational Processes and the Facilitating Environment*. New York: International Universities Press, 1965.

———— (1960b), Ego distortions in terms of true and false self. In: *The Maturational Processes and the Facilitating Environment*. New York: International Universities Press, 1965.

Afterword

This essay addressed, and attempted to resolve, the apparent clash between contemporary relational thought and the concept of holding. I argue strongly against the assumption that mutuality is always clinically possible, and for the inclusion of holding within relational theory. By addressing the analyst's ubiquitous subjectivity and reframing the holding experience as a coconstructed one, I locate holding within the relational frame.

As relational thinking has come of age, the roles of enactment, self-disclosure, and spontaneity remain important, but more room now exists for the exploration of the internal. Holding is recognized as an additional clinical thread; the dichotomy of holding vs. intersubjective engagement has been replaced with a recognition of the complex interpenetration of these two clinical threads. Holding frequently represents a backdrop to interpretations or more explicit expressions of the analyst's subjectivity.

Where I originally argued that holding involves the analyst's capacity to contain her subjectivity, I now emphasize the analyst's *inability* fully to contain her subjectivity. Patients inevitably pick up things about us, even when we actively struggle to sustain a holding stance. An important dimension of the holding analyst's subjectivity is *embodied*, more than bracketed, by her capacity for restraint; the holding analyst remains quite present in the room, but in a particular way characterized by heightened affect resonance. Our patients' experience of us is *less absent than narrowed*; we are more likely to be experienced as even and resilient than as variable, vulnerable, or reactive. Thus, where I stated earlier that patients bracket their awareness of the analyst's dysjunctive subjectivity during holding, now I would say that patients bracket their awareness of those aspects of the analyst's presence that are incompatible with the holding illusion, most especially, the analyst's *variability, reactivity,* and *inability to hold,* and not her subjectivity per se. This is precisely what Anne could not do.

I continue to hold myself in the treatment context and, at times, to hold my patient, but with far more awareness of the permeability and shifting nature of these experiences. I would now say that holding involves a cocreated illusion of analytic attunement that is simultaneously stable and porous, that is, not easily shattered. The case of Anne illustrates the precarious nature of illusions tightly held, for here the vulnerability to breakdown pervaded and threatened to destroy the therapeutic frame.

My early writing on holding was very much tilted toward the patient's experience of the *other,* and I paid less attention to the relationship between holding and the patient's inner life. More recently, I have focused on the processes by which interior experience is accessed, articulated, and sustained inside and outside the holding frame (Slochower, 1999a, 2004).[1]

---

[1] These papers explore a range of therapeutic issues related to the psychoanalyst's professional development and experience, addressing the function and meaning of illusion (Slochower, 1998, 1999b, 2002, 2003a, c).

The clinical vignette I described illustrates how the illusion of analytic attunement can itself become toxic when its boundaries are rigid. Anne could not experience paradox or doubleness, could not encompass the ways that I *did* and *did not* care for her, *did* and *did not* remain attuned and present. The illusion of attunement central to the holding experience rested heavily on the undoing of a core, grim unconscious belief (that no one could care for her). The power of that conviction led Anne to repetitively reexperience a collapse of the holding illusion. It was not until Anne was able to hold the illusion of analytic attunement *lightly* (rather than tightly) that the holding experience opened up a more permeable, porous, protected space that was less fragile and thus less easily disrupted. The holding process that was at once both necessary and toxic became a crucial therapeutic dimension of our work, but only one such dimension. Anne's capacity to use the holding experience, to enjoy illusion without negating its edges, has allowed us to move into a far more open psychoanalytic arena. And so, after many years, Anne finds us both to be more human than otherwise, and we are increasingly free—to move, to breathe, and to *be* within the psychoanalytic context.

Old and New Objects in Fairbairnian and American Relational Theory

(1998)

Steven H. Cooper
David Levit

▼   ▼   ▼   ▼   ▼

Editors' Introduction

Among the most pressing issues for contemporary theorists of psychoanalytic technique is the question of the analyst's role in the psychoanalytic situation: What kind of object is the analyst to be? Does the analyst encourage projections and displacements that facilitate his being perceived as the "old," "bad," or "traumatizing" object? Does the analyst do anything to encourage the patient to perceive him or her as a different, "new," "good," or "better" object? What does it mean to be neutral in relation to these options? Does the analyst adopt any "role" in the patient's internal drama?

In this significant essay, Cooper and Levit explore the conceptualization of old and new objects in Fairbairnian (British object relations theory) and American relational theory. Although American relational theory itself draws on Fairbairn's contributions, there are, nevertheless, differences in approach and sensibility with regard to these critical concepts. Where Fairbairn emphasized the patient's tendency to hold on to old objects, the relationalists accentuate the complexities of interpersonal interaction.

This article also appeared as a central chapter in Steve Cooper's (2000) *Objects of Hope: Exploring Possibility and Limit in Psychoanalysis* (The Analytic Press). In that work, Cooper provides a thorough comparative analysis of contemporary psychoanalytic models and develops an integrated relational position with respect to issues of hope and hopefulness. Cooper's task is challenging, given that the most hopeful aspects of human growth frequently entail acceptance of the destructive elements of our inner lives; objects of hope, after all, may also be objects of disappointment, danger, competition, and envy. The analysis of hope, then, implicates what Cooper sees as the central dialectic tension in psychoanalysis: that between psychic possibility and psychic limit. He argues that analysts have historically had difficulty integrating the concept of limit into a treatment modality dedicated to the creation and augmentation of psychic possibility. And yet it is only by accepting limit as a necessary counterpoise to possibility and clinically embracing the tension between them, that analysts can further their understanding of the therapeutic process in the interest of better treatment outcomes.

What is it that the analyst may hope for the patient, and what is the patient encouraged to hope for himself or herself? What kind of object is the analyst to be for the patient? What is it in our theory that may prevent analysts from seeing the ways in which they are new objects for their patients? Similarly, what is it that keeps a patient from seeing how the analyst is new and different? What is the role of self-disclosure in facilitating the analyst's role as new? Is the "old object" inevitably the "bad object?" Is the "new object" always the "good object?" Are these categories themselves useful, or do they oversimplify the inner world? These are the significant questions that Cooper and Levit tackle in this chapter.

Old and New Objects in Fairbairnian and American Relational Theory[*]

As true as in 1983 with the seminal contributions of Greenberg and Mitchell, some of the most fascinating issues confronting American psychoanalysts today involve points of divergence and convergence between

* Originally published in *Psychoanalytic Dialogues*, 8:603–624. © 1998 The Analytic Press, Inc.

American relational theory and British object relations theory. In this article we take up a few points of theory related to specific comparative conceptualizations of the new and old objects and the implications for working in the analytic situation.

American relational theory has beneficially emphasized the importance for the newness of the analyst to emerge experientially as a contrast to a historically held object through a variety of interventions, including interpretations of transference and defense, as well as expressive uses of the countertransference. Currently, there is tremendous variability within relational theory (e.g., Mitchell, 1994; Stern, 1994; Tansey and Burke, 1989) as to whether the patient looks for newness in the old or whether the search for newness emerges from repetitive patterns with the old. These differences involve several other important dimensions of analytic process related to theories of development and the value of regression in analytic work. We believe, however, that it can be said, as it was by Hirsch (1994), that relational theory has generally emphasized that the patient is looking both to repeat old experience and to be exposed to new experience.

Much of a patient's experience of the analyst as old and new has little to do with specific technical procedures of the analyst and more to do with subtle nuances of the interaction and the patient's particular state at the time, including the organizing principles activated at the moment. Yet, at times, aspects of the analyst's disclosure, expressive participation, clarification, and interpretation direct the patient toward the difference between the contemporary object of the analyst in contrast to the historically held bad object. At times, the way we emphasize or construct ourselves is more along the lines that the patient has experienced past objects; at other times, it has more to do with the contrast we construct between our purpose, activity, or behavior and the past objects or historically held transference. At other times we construct ourselves or the patient in terms of who the patient or the dyad might become—a kind of anticipation of the patient's psychic future (Loewald, 1960; Cooper, 1997b). Part of the ways the analyst poses these constructions refers to modality of intervention (traditional interpretation, disclosure, or inquiry), and part of it relates to a style of intervening, including seriousness, humor, play, schtick, and the like. In a sense, negotiation (e.g., Russell, 1985; Mitchell, 1988, 1991; Pizer, 1992) refers to augmenting the patient's internal dialogue regarding these old and new experiences as well as in interaction with the analyst.

The notion of the new object was used initially by Strachey (1934) to describe how the patient, having become aware of the lack of aggressiveness in the real external object (in contrast to the patient's archaic internalized fantasy objects) is able to introject a new, more benign object. Subsequently, the aggressiveness of the patient's superego will be diminished. Strachey emphasized that the analyst's newness consists of the detoxification of troublesome affects before being communicated back to the patient. Loewald (1960) similarly referred to the ways in which the analyst, through his systematic analysis of the transference "distortions," was gradually experienced and observed as a helpful and therapeutic agent for change for the patient. For Loewald, the analyst is conceptualized as a new object to the extent that he or she offers the opportunity for a rediscovery of the early pathways and patterns of object relations leading to "a new way of relating to objects and of being oneself" (p. 22). Newness also includes aspects of the way the analyst holds a vision of the patient's future (Loewald, 1960) and comes to represent psychic possibility.

Although a new object experience is a major focus for all contemporary relational theorists, there are diverse perspectives on how newness develops. For example, a positive new object experience may be faciliated by the analyst's capacity to monitor and assess the relative degrees of safety and danger in the patient's transferential experience (Greenberg, 1986) and elements of repetition that threaten stagnation or impasse. Newness may also include the possibility that the analyst will make his subjectivity more known to the patient so that a contrast may be better established or developed between experiences of the analyst that at least correlate with historical experiences and the ways in which the analyst may provide or represent new and different relational experiences. In a sense, the patient cannot allow himself to trust that the new object is different from the old object.

Another form of newness emphasized in the American relational tradition occurs when the analyst acknowledges to the patient ways in which the patient has behaved very much like the old object. Here, the analyst offers what may be a new opportunity for more open mutual exchange and dialogue about such an occurrence (i.e., in which the analyst engages in repetition of a problematic old object experience).

Sometimes this newness is established less directly by drawing the patient's attention to his or her own revealed and concealed ideas and perceptions about the analyst's subjectivity (Aron, 1991, 1992). At other times, newness comes in the form of the analyst's expressing or disclosing aspects of psychic possibility that may catalyze new realms of experience of self and other. To some extent, any interpretation "virtually discloses" (Cooper, 1996) some aspect of the analyst's view of psychic possibility.

In contrast to American relational theories (which portray these various routes to potential newness), British object relations theory, particularly Fairbairn's (1952) work, has emphasized the attachment to old figures in order to control toxic affects and environmental failure. The old object—abandoning, persecutory, or exciting in nature—is internalized so that it can be controlled. To the extent that it is internalized and clung to as familiar, it is good because it brings safety and has adaptive value. The new object in the form of the analyst is bad or threatening to the extent that it represents the unfamiliar. Analyst disclosure in this context expresses psychic possibility related to the patient's renouncing old object experience or transforming it from persecutory or hurtful into something that can be grieved or mourned. The patient's resistance or reluctance can take the form of seeing the analyst as new from the get-go and being threatened by it or of maintaining a bedrock experience of the analyst as old object despite surface rumblings of newness.

The question explored in recent developments in American relational theories partly involves how and why this new object is able to become less threatening so that the old object ties can somehow be relinquished or substantially mitigated. The patient's potential relational pathways have become constricted or collapsed into a one-lane road. The analyst is trying to "tell" the patient that there can be a multiplicity of roads and connections. The patient sees or experiences that the relationship can be affectively colored in one way only. The analyst sees more than one color, although the colors seem sometimes faint or fleeting—fugitive coloring that quickly moves back into one color, the color of historically held transference.

Several authors have begun to delineate these differences between British object relations and American relational perspectives. In a recent article, Mitchell (1995) usefully examined various modes of interaction between patient and analyst within British and American relational theory. He discussed, in particular, the analyst's role of processing and containing affect, emphasized more in contemporary Kleinian theory, and aspects of the analyst's personal expressiveness and participation within interpersonal and American relational theory. Interestingly, Steiner (1993), from a contemporary Kleinian perspective, has also recently discussed the value for the analyst in maintaining certain aspects of tension between expressiveness and restraint within all interpretive processes. Each of these models actually differs in some ways from "developmental tilt" (Mitchell, 1988, 1991, 1993) models, Kohut's and Winnicott's which emphasize more the need of the analyst to meet certain aspects of the patient's experience of impingment and deprivation.

As is so often true, looking at analytic stance in a broad sense (i.e., expressiveness/containment/provision) necessitates looking more fully at a variety of central relational issues, such as the construal of new and old and safe and dangerous objects, all of which has many implications for understanding interaction. We discuss some of these definitions of old and new, safe and dangerous, mutual and asymmetrical, from a constructivist perspective, trying to explore some of the analyst's assumptions as to their meaning. The construal of new and old, like "need and wish" (Mitchell, 1991) has to do with both patient's and analyst's experiences. We believe that both Fairbairn and the recent developments in American relational models can assist in these complex construals and constructions of affect and idea for the analytic dyad.

In a sense, in all of our theoretical conceptualization, we often have a tendency to characterize what is new and old, mutual and asymmetrical, safe and dangerous, more in terms of the analyst's intentions than through the amalgam of analyst's and patient's conscious and unconscious experiences. For example, in the concluding section of his article on therapeutic action, Strachey (1934) schematically attempted to characterize a variety of interventions by focusing on the analyst's intentions, without access to the notion that any of these interventions are determined by unconscious enactments as well as construed in any one of several ways by the patient.

In more contemporary literature, many authors get into a similar pattern, linking the analyst's intentions as a way to characterize an intervention or construal on the part of the patient. For example, there has been a great deal of useful emphasis within the disclosure literature on disclosure as constructing the analyst as a new object differentiated from the historical transference object. Burke's (1992) fascinating article explores how in his view disclosure is more related to aspects of mutuality, whereas relative degrees of anonymity are more associated with asymmetry. We, along with Aron (1996), however, find this equation of disclosure with mutuality most dubious because, as with Strachey, there is a more exclusive focus on the analyst's intentions. Accordingly, an analyst may disclose with a conscious intention to mutuality that is not matched either to the analyst's unconscious motivations (Gill, 1983) or to the patient's experience of this intervention. In fact, we find that there are aspects of privacy, boundedness, and solitude within the analytic situation, which are among the most mutual aspects of the analytic situation, just as disclosure can resonate in experiences of asymmetry for particular patients. Not all circumstances in which disclosure proves useful can be explained as having been so because of the analyst's mutuality with the patient.

Underlying much of our discussion is the belief that there are useful tensions between, on the one hand, Fairbairn's emphasis on our attachment to bad and old objects and refractory clinging to these bad objects in the face of receiving something new and, on the other hand, a construal of a push or willingness toward integrating externality and newness of objects (e.g., Winnicott, 1969; Benjamin, 1988). There are several ways to understand these divergent formulations of basic developmental processes and their implications for psychoanalytic treatment. One is that each of these formulations is to some degree accurate and has greater or lesser degrees of applicability to particular types of patients. Another is that each formulation describes aspects of a more universal process that need to be integrated by the analyst. We are more sympathetic to the latter view.

Constructivism and the Continuum of New–Old Objects

It may seem commonplace to assert that patient's and analyst's experiences of the analyst's newness or oldness are constructed by each analytic dyad. Yet, analysts from widely divergent theoretical orientations have a tendency toward somewhat concrete construals of newness and oldness and safety and danger. We begin with some of the analyst's obstacles to seeing newness in contrast to repetition, and vice versa, and then turn our attention to some of the patient's obstacles to seeing newness.

Analysts' Obstacles to Seeing Newness

It seems to us that analysts who begin with a Fairbairnian theoretical bias toward hearing clinical process from the perspective that the old object is clung to for familiarity and safety might minimize instances in which new object experience is sought or expressed. Perhaps the patient engages in "object probing" (Ghent, 1992) in ways that are overlooked by the analyst because the patient's affects or attributions toward the analyst seem familiar when assessed against the patient's parental objects. For example, a patient who expresses negative feelings toward the analyst often seems to be seeing or experiencing something in relation to the analyst that resembles what he has felt toward a parent. However, what can be conspicuously or subtly overlooked in such formulations is the previously unavailable opportunity for expressing feelings with such an object. At other times, the analyst is likely to focus on certain ways in which the patient seems identified with the parent in forms such as identification with the aggressor or the victim. Although this may provide a useful way of understanding these old and familiar processes, there are also ways in which sadomasochistic identifications occur simultaneously with the new opportunity for communication patterns with others.

Winnicott (1965) and Casement (1985) have each emphasized how the patient creates a "real" or new opportunity to use an analyst to represent old object experience. Winnicott stated:

> Corrective provision is never enough. What is it that may be enough for some of our patients to get well? In the end the patient uses the analyst's failures, often quite small ones, perhaps maneuvered by the patient . . . and we have to put up with being in a limited context misunderstood. The operative factor is that the patient now hates the analyst for the failure that originally came as an environmental factor, outside the infant's area of omnipotent control but that is now staged in the transference. So in the end we succeed by failing—failing the patient's way. This is a long distance from the simple theory of cure by "corrective experience" [p. 258].

It is only over time that the analyst can come to see whether a particular kind of enactment of the transference is used in the ways that Winnicott is describing here. During this process, however, it is easy to see these forms of repetition as only part of the old object experience. Stern (1994) has described this kind of experience with the analyst as the "needed" object experience (even when it appeared initially as a repeated experience), but the problem is that Stern's descriptions can become teleological, as if the patient somehow knows how to work something through that was stuck. An alternative explanation is that as old object experiences are worked through, new object experiences are more accessible over the course of analytic work (e.g., Tansey and Burke, 1989; Mitchell, 1994). What we emphasize here is how much the analyst's theoretical biases influence how she constructs these experiences and determines what might be new in the patient's expressions. Here is an example.

Sarah was a 25-year-old woman who had been chronically depressed when she began analysis several years earlier. She was now in a phase in which she had been able to work through a great deal of her anger and sadness related to feeling rejected by her father. She had experienced him as always "too objective" rather than more openly effusive about her appearance and intellect. We were examining her current predilection for involvement with married or otherwise unavailable men and avoidance of men who might be more readily available for a relationship. We agreed that, despite her frustration with unavailable men, she remained attached to an opportunity to persuade her father to change his mind and throw all caution to the wind in order to be with her.

In the earlier phase of analysis, she had experienced me (SHC) as more globally unavailable and rejecting toward her. Over time, we had developed a warm, friendly way of being together, one in which she was still visited by feelings of my rejecting her, though in a more focused way. Sarah would adamantly tell me about my unsatisfactory ways of wording interpretations or observations and would propose comments that would be more affirming to her. At one level that was quite accessible to her, she recognized her "already ready" responsiveness to me as her unavailable and critical father. We also began to understand her instructions and corrections of my interventions as a new opportunity for her that she had not experienced during her growing up—namely, to give expression to her feelings of anger and complaint about her wish to have her father be less objective and more enthusiastic or passionate about her developing body and mind. We also understood her instructions as expressing a kind of nihilistic and despairing display of her sense that, if she did not tell me what to do, I would never comply with her wishes and needs to be affirmed. There were elements of punishment and sadism in the ways in which she would hypervigilantly discover one example after the next of my tendency to be critical or more reserved in affirmation than she wished. She had been able to experience her wishes for retaliation against me, including wishes to hurt me and make me feel as rejected as she felt by men. Often, as we spoke of these feelings, she would smile or laugh uncontrollably as she recognized the intensity of her anger.

Sarah agreed with my sense that she selectively perceived and experienced my remarks in terms of what was less affirming or supportive, and at times she minimized how I had acknowledged her achievements and strengths. She agreed with my observation that, at times, her selective perception represented a repetition of her relationship with her father, to which she painfully held. At times, I conveyed to her my agreement that she had a good point to make about my insensitivity to her need to feel affirmed, even as we took up something about her selective perception.

In this phase of analysis there were several threads of experience and enactment that help in thinking about the complexities of the new and old object experience. One complexity relates to enactment and the likelihood that the analyst will repeat painful aspects of the patient's earlier experience. Thus, the old object is reexperienced and repeated in the present. The patient's expectations and tendencies to repeat are forged onto the new experience with the analyst, and the analyst in various ways is likely to respond to or cocreate these repetitions. Enactments often involve the ways in which we unconsciously participate in a repetition of an earlier failure that was close to the patient's experience of an earlier trauma (Casement, 1985). The patient is skeptical to believe that the analyst can become a new object partly because the patient sees the ways in which the analyst is the same as the old object through repetition and enactment.

However, there are ways in which our tendencies to see repetition may overlook how new capacities for relatedness are emerging. Sarah's ability to feel safe enough with me to criticize, correct, evaluate, and complain constituted part of a new object experience. This observation is very much in keeping with the notion that negative transference often involves the deepest kind of trust and safety (e.g., Greenberg, 1986). Conversely, there are many instances in which positive and especially erotic transferences involve intense sadistic and negative affective experiences. It is easy to see how our theoretical constructions of Sarah as holding onto the old, bad father (safe) so as not to be threatened by the new might deter the analyst from viewing Sarah as exploring a new opportunity and pathway with the anlyst, as she gave repeated expression to very familiar feelings of rage and sadism toward me. The attempt to analyze how she is holding onto the old can potentially minimize how she indeed is taking in something new.

It is not uncommon and sometimes inevitable for us to repeat aspects of the old object whether we focus ostensibly on what seems to us old or new in what the patient is expressing or feeling. For example, if the analyst more rigidly sustains a stance toward emphasizing the newness in the patient's expression of negative feelings toward the analyst as something not previously allowed within the parent–child dynamic, then the analyst may be repeating aspects of the old. On the other hand, the relentless interpretation of Sarah's attachment to the old might have similarly constituted a repetition of Sarah's sense of being unrecognized by her father.

The case of Sarah raises an interesting question about whether or to what extent the sadism directed toward the analyst derives from the sense of threat from the new object or the sadism is the expression of feelings toward the old expressed by the new subject. We believe that there is something useful about the notion of an object representation's containing aspects of self and object that helps to understand some of these processes. We have already posed the more familiar question raised by Fairbairn's work—namely, whether the sadism is a response to the threat posed by a new object on the horizon that disrupts a tenacious gravitating toward the old. However, both British and American relational models have emphasized the ways in which the patient may enact aspects of the old object, requiring the analyst to adapt aspects of the patient's self in relation to the object. In these circumstances, the question is always whether the analyst will be or can be a new object and/or a new subject. Will the analyst feel beleaguered, helpless, sad, furious, or retaliatory in response to the patient's communications? If the analyst experiences these feelings and expresses them, can he do so in a way that differs from the ways the patient had done so? This can be accomplished through the analyst's containment and reintroduction of these feelings (speaking from an effectively processed internal emotional state) or through his judicious self-disclosure.

Although it is difficult to make general guidelines about how to determine whether patterns of old or new object experience are more dominant at any time, it is probably a good idea to keep each possibility in mind. The analyst needs to balance the need to stay with the experience of the analyst-as-old-object-in-effigy with the attunement to possible ways in which the analyst may emerge from the old object experience. We believe that, in Freudian analysis, there was too much of a resistance or reluctance on the analyst's part to interfere with the development of the old object experience. This position minimized the value of (a) the analyst's drawing attention to some of the ways in which the patient might be using the analyst in a new and different way from the old object, for fear of mitigating or diluting the power of historically held transference; (b) the analyst's using disclosure to differentiate the analyst at times from the old object experience; and (c) the analyst's using aspects of his subjectivity as a construction that might allow further interpretation (Cooper, 1997a, 1998).

Furthermore, the classical position paradoxically minimized the refractoriness and resilience of transference phenomena; that is, the transference is not necessarily diluted by addressing old and new object phenomena at the same time.

The points of reluctance or resistance for analysts within the relational model involve a potential to too quickly determine that the analyst needs to do something in order to act as a new object. Speaking about patients and analysts, Greenberg (1986) drew attention to the potential of both patients and analysts to defensively embrace aspects of the new object. It is quite understandable to seek relief from the unrelenting repetition of problematic relationships. The problems here, well documented by Gill (1983, 1994), relate to the possibility of either diluting or diverting aspects of transference or similarly being influenced by several unconscious factors. There is value in the patient's being able to find and create the object (Winnicott, 1969) in the form of the new-object-analyst. If the analyst harps on the theme of newness, the patient's experience may shift to staleness or compliance. Keeping in mind these complexities may help the analyst to determine whether interpretations or disclosures by the analyst regarding newness seem useful or whether interpretations that relate primarily to the patient's experience of the analyst as an old object may be more resonant or generative.

Patient's Inner Obstacles to Seeing Newness

There is a variety of components to the patient's clinging to the safety of the old object and his or her reluctance to accept the new object, in addition to those posited by Fairbairn's theory. These aspects relate more to aspects of immediate, contemporary experience and the person of the analyst emphasized in interpersonal and relational-conflict theory and much less to early experience and mechanisms of internalization, which were a point of focus for Fairbairn.

Most analysts would agree that patients are likely to see the analyst as similar to the old object because of the power of transference and the likelihood that enactments will affirm the patient's worst fear about the resemblance between the analyst and the parental object. Two other factors seem salient as well. The first is that everything we know about the tendency to repeat should lead us to the expectation that patients will unconsciously choose analysts who may in some ways psychologically resemble the parental object. In this way, the patient may be attuned to all sorts of things that they have seen before. A second factor may relate to what we call the "He or she can't be as good as they look" phenomenon. Regarding the first point, there are many ways in which it is easy to repeat neurotic aspects of object choice in every relationship—romantic, professional, and in terms of choosing an analyst. One of the things that is particularly perplexing for all of us in making choices is that we often believe we are choosing only on the basis of consciously experienced and observed phenomena. A man chooses a lover who is more easygoing and quiet than his intense and intrusive mother and then discovers that she is just as intrusive—she just seems to take longer to get to it. This is a good example, because it brings up the complexity of analytic work. In analysis, analyst and patient ask themselves whether this pattern is reflective of repetition in object choice and/or repetition in the ways the patient's experience of his intrusive and demanding mother is more likely to rear its head in any romantic relationship, particularly over time. The lines are rarely clear, particularly because the repetition in object choice may not necessarily be a choice of the same kind of object but rather may be an object who is willing to accept the processes of role induction and role responsiveness that the patient is needing or likely to enact. In addition, the patient may "be able" to find a familiar position for the self in the relationship, even when there are significant differences between the current other and internal objects. All of the issues discussed here are often confusing because they are likely to reflect overlapping and concurrent processes.

All of these processes are obviously applicable to transference in the analytic situation. The patient's experience of the analyst is colored with aspects of the historically based transference. The analyst sometimes acts in ways that confirm the patient's expectations that the analyst is like the parent. Then, to make matters even more confusing, the patient may often actually choose an analyst who resembles some of the most problematic aspects of the parent. These circumstances present great obstacles and opportunity for any analysis. Summarizing many of these observations, Greenberg (1986) wrote, "Unless he [the patient] has some sense of the analyst as a new object, he will not be able to experience him as an old one. The inability to achieve this balance is responsible for many analytic failures. If the analyst cannot be experienced as a new object, analysis never gets under way; if he cannot be experienced as an old one, it never ends" (p. 98). The resemblances help create the potential to experience the analytic situation with great depth and authenticity. Here, the inverse of Greenberg's statement is also relevant; that is, unless the analyst is enough of an old object, treatment cannot begin. For some patients, however, the similarity between the analyst and parental figures makes it difficult to experience the new opportunity the analytic situation offers for symbolic and interpretive play. In this case, Greenberg's original statement applies; that is, unless the analyst is enough of a new object, treatment cannot begin.

We believe that another factor in the patient's reluctance to experience newness in the analyst derives from the patient's skepticism about whether the analyst can really be as good as he seems. Hoffman (1994) has suggested that the analyst's "self" is in most instances relatively unknown to the patient. He states that one of the aspects of ritualized asymmetry in the analytic situation is "fostered partly by the fact that the patient knows so much less about him or her than the analyst knows about the patient" (p. 199). Hoffman further argues that the analyst is in a relatively protected position, one likely to promote some of the most tolerant and generous aspects of his or her personality. This protection exists despite the analyst's authentic participation and sense that he or she has particular feelings or experiences with the patient. Hoffman emphasizes how this relatively protected position tends to foster idealizations. Renik (1995), in contrast, sees these idealizations of the analyst as potentially problematic if they are insufficiently analyzed. Hoffman (1994, 1996) sees these idealizations as potentially a part of the analyst's authority and influence and potentially facilitative of the patient's use of the analyst.

The radical nature of the social context in analysis is one in which personal participation is an inevitability, but it is inherently contextually defined by the work task, both unique and overlapping with other social contexts. Thus, the interactive matrix (Greenberg, 1995) borrows from and is partly separate from the larger social context. This view is compatible with Hoffman's (1994) elaboration of the asymmetrical arrangement that partially protects the analyst's anonymity and how he or she will be known by the patient.

However, the tensions between what is unique about the analyst's participation and the overlap with the larger social context is of key importance to understanding another element of the patient's reluctance to experience the analyst as a new object. We believe that the patient is always partly aware that the analyst's modal responsiveness can not really be as good as he or she is able to be with the patient. We agree (Cooper, in press) with Hoffman that the analyst is in a sense protected by the patient and that many aspects of the analyst's self, despite the analyst's authentic engagement, remain in the background or are simply not well known by the patient. Yet, patients are often aware of this (they know what they do not know), or at least they know that there is much that they do not know. Although illusion is a necessary part of every analysis, many patients are aware of the tensions between the real and intimate and illusory nature of analytic engagement. Many analyses pursue as a central task the patient's inability to form such illusions in the analytic and nonanalytic relationships, just as for some patients the work is organized around how easy it is for the patient to form such illusions.

We are suggesting that, in many analyses, the patient, even as he suspends his disbelief, is aware of the possibility that he is getting some of the best of the analyst. Part of the patient's trepidation in moving to a new object can be expressed in seizing on this observation and applying it to a skepticism or reluctance to seize the possibility that anyone can be new, different, or this good. For example, part of the work involves trying to explore why anyone has to be that good in order to engender trust, love, wishes for intimacy, and the like. The patient's inability to trust the new or even to see the new is never entirely separable from his or her attachment to the old object or the old representations. Yet, we are emphasizing that there are built-in dimensions in the analytic setup that are a part of the patient's attachment to the old. It is important to note too that, given the tremendous vicissitudes of everyone's emotional states and of interpersonal relating, the patient is bound to have had experiences of the parent's being different from some position that became crystallized as a central old object position. Thus, patients have experienced parents as loosening particular old object experiences. Often, this variation is followed by the parent's resuming a central or primary (modal) affective stance. With repeated experiences of being seduced by the appearance of a "new object" in the parent, only to be disappointed, the patient would be that much less likely to trust any new signs of "newness" in the analyst. The patient sustains the tension around the question, "When is the other shoe going to drop?" The analyst's awareness of this dimension can be helpful in analyzing the patient's attachment to the old.

Thus, the Fairbairnian model in its pure form may at times minimize contemporary factors that further contribute to the basic Fairbairnian appreciation about the individual's need for attachment to the old object. In other words, there are ways in which the contemporary American emphasis on relational processes in the immediacy of analytic engagement has elucidated factors that reinforce an understanding of the patient's wishes to hold on to the old object. The patient is aware at some level that the newness or goodness of the analyst is related to the analyst's function—the analyst's role within the asymmetrical arrangement of analysis—and the analyst is so not to be believed entirely. Although Hoffman emphasizes the ways in which we are idealizable and not real (ways that foster idealization), there is also a question about whether there are ways in which the patient never fully believes this to be real. This is one of the forms of play in analysis that involve transference and countertransference. The patient is reluctant to take in a new experience that is viewed as artificial, not real. Obviously, this discussion is at the level of discourse that involves generalities. We know that some patients are prone to idealization, others to cynicism about whether the analyst can be a good object. Most of us operate on multiple levels of reality in the analytic situation (Modell, 1991), suspending our disbelief in some ways and less so in others.

American relational models reflect a great deal of awareness of contemporary factors in the analytic situation. The analyst would pay attention to how much the patient observes, perceives, and experiences the analyst, which might influence the patient's trepidation or reluctance to trust the analyst. The danger in this model is that the patient's "need" to repeat, or predilection to impose the old object situation, could potentially be minimized if the analyst becomes overly focused on the patient's immediate perceptions of the analyst as behaving in particular ways and especially if the analyst valorizes newness for therapeutic action. Obviously, there are many instances when the analyst is responding in ways that confirm the patient's expectations. There are other instances when the analyst may even be inducing certain roles and behaviors in the patient. However, there are also many instances when, in line with more classical views of transference, the patient repeats the old object experience with the analyst.

Disclosure and the Continuum of New–Old Object

Another issue related to the notion of constructivism and the continuum of old-new objects is the analyst's assumptions about the stimulus value of his interventions (if there ever is such a thing as stimulus value in analysis apart from the patient's and the analyst's psychic view of reality). For example, disclosure may offer the patient a perspective that aspects of disclosure are to be more axiomatically equated with mutual aspects of the analytic situation (Aron, 1996; Cooper, in press). In most cases, disclosure by the analyst is fairly selective and remains at quite a distance from how intimately the patient might want to know the analyst. We believe that disclosure usually involves a tension between aspects of mutuality and asymmetry in the analytic situation. Similarly, we believe that aspects of anonymity by the analyst may often include aspects of mutuality—those parts of both patient and analyst that are separate, that have secrets from each other, boundedness and privacy. Bion's (1977) statement about the analytic situation gets at these aspects of separateness, even if it is embedded in particular assumptions about the degree to which personalities involve separate intrapsychic structures rather than intersubjectively intertwined organizations: "We're both in this alone" (p. 65). It is overly schematic to say that disclosure involves mutual aspects of the analytic situation, just as it was for Strachey (1934) to draw clean lines of distinction between interpretation and suggestion.

Similarly, disclosure can be used to emphasize the analyst as either a safe or more dangerous object. The use of disclosure often involves a presentation of the analyst as a new object that is meant to be safe in ways that form a contrast to the dangerous or destructive feelings associated with the old object. This use of disclosure can be especially helpful if the patient is prone to experience the historically held transference in a way that is so extremely scary or depressing that the analytic process becomes limited or stagnated. The analyst essentially uses a form of clarification or differentiation of himself from the parental object with the hope of supporting the patient's capacity for self-observation, titrating or modulating affect. However, it is useful to be equally focused on the value of using disclosure as a way of presenting danger. The analyst often interprets or queries directly or virtually discloses a construction of himself in order to pose what is most threatening for the patient to consider. For example, the analyst says, "As angry as you are that the only reason I see you is so that I can charge you money for our visits, perhaps it is threatening to think about any other reasons that I might talk to you."

It is not easy to assess the effects or implications of the analyst's holding these biases in understanding interaction. One reason we emphasize that disclosure or constructions of the analyst as a new object cannot be prospectively categorized is that the patient usually experientially integrates, uses, or rejects our constructions in accordance with his or her readiness to visit new and old object experiences. Cooper (1997a) tried to examine aspects of how disclosure involving constructions of the analyst as a potentially new object often recapitulate for the patient aspects of the historically held transference. One possible implication is that, if the analyst approaches these disclosures as intertwined with aspects of mutuality and asymmetry, there may be more readiness to work with the complex texturing that the patient experiences in response to this or any other intervention.

Holding the Psychic Future: Future Object and Self

Every psychoanalytic theory of growth, either in describing development or the analytic process, involves aspects of benevolent disruption. Even "developmental tilt" (Mitchell, 1988) theories emphasizing the analyst's need to stay as close to the patient's psychic reality as possible (e.g., Winnicott, Kohut) stress the inevitability of failing the patient and the resultant tensions, which can be productive in terms of growth. Other theories, including classical, interpersonal, and relational-conflict theories, have built-in notions about how tensions between the participants produce change—it is just a question of how you go about the process, what the unit of analysis is (e.g., a mind or an interaction), and what the goals of analysis are about.

In a sense, every theory has a mode of benevolent disruption that partially constitutes the new object—either through survival of the patient's reactions to these failures or through psychic possibility, which emerges through interactional tension or shifts in intrapsychic organization. In Kohut, the new object is one that will not empathically fail around the responsiveness of healthy narcissistic needs. Winnicott's new object is able to meet the moment of hope expressed in the patient's authentic or true self. In the classical view, the new object is one that can offer a crucible for the patient's old experience, an opportunity for repetition to become visible, heartfelt, and tamed through neutralization of drives. In most relational models, analysis involves the opportunity for a combination of the new and repeated relationships. Relational models offer ways of thinking about the balance of new and old as well as technical approaches that help to construct the analyst and the interaction. In turn, this process aims to provide different perspectives on repetitive patterns in relating—a new relational opportunity.

We view the new object, partially in Loewaldian terms, as holding a version of psychic possibility for the patient. In most ways, this is also akin to Greenberg's (1986) emphasis on the analyst's needing to strike a balance between safe and dangerous, old and new. Loewald, however, did not address the complexity and variety of ways that the analyst need go about holding psychic possibility except through more classical interpretation. We have tried to emphasize that it is not universally useful to equate the newness of the object with safety. Although Fairbairn's theory allows for a deep appreciation of this observation, his theory is less attuned to interpersonal and immediate aspects of analytic interaction, which can help the analyst attend to how the new object is unsafe. Sometimes psychic possibility is provided or maintained by containment and restraint on the analyst's part, allowing the transference in the form of the old object to unfold. At other times, providing or underscoring psychic possibility involves the analyst's attempts to construct a view of how the analyst can be distinguished from the old object. At other times, this may involve drawing attention to how the patient is reluctant to let the analyst be viewed as an old object.

For example, Sarah's treatment was characterized by a tension between the analyst's consciously experienced hopes for the patient—an opportunity for her growth and capacity to form a relationship that would be more satisfying to her—and a kind of enactment of the old object, co-constituted by the two of us. My (SHC's) enactments were often manifested by saying things in ways that seemed overly evaluative to her. At times, this was quite "true" (i.e., her identifying an evaluative attitude in me in a given moment, which I later could see as well), as was her hypervigilance to these aspects of how I and others approached her. In fact, we were able over time to understand her intense reluctance to believe either that I was not critical of her or, that, if and to the extent that I was, it need not overshadow many other feelings and attitudes toward her, including ways in which I cared for and about her a great deal. What was of note was her readiness to experience me as a familiar object and my tendency, at times, to act in ways that would elicit this feeling in her. The analyst's inevitable participation in aspects of repetition can sometimes fuel the patient's tendency to cling to attachments, even though the analyst might at other moments be doing something quite new.

The analyst's interpretive anticipation of where the patient might go also often enacts something that is an amalgam of the old and new objects coconstituted by the patient and the analyst. Thus, holding onto the notion of the patient's psychic future often combines apsects of the old and new objects. This mirrors the ways in which the patient's experience of the old object may sometimes involve something new—in Ghent's (1992) terms, object probing. We are emphasizing the ways in which the new object functions to hold a view of psychic possibility for the patient. For some patients, psychic possibility has less to do with consciously experienced hope and more to do with the capacity to face and integrate painful experience that underlies consciously experienced hope. For others, psychic possibility has much more to do with the threat of trying to be more consciously hopeful in the face of loss or disillusionment.

The relational model not only emphasizes ways in which the newness of the analyst can be helpful but also has potential to deepen our understanding of why patients remain attached to the old. To some extent, examples of disclosure and constructions by the analyst in our literature emphasize the analyst as a new object who is safe relative to the historically held bad, dangerous object. Yet, sometimes disclosure involves useful constructions of ourselves as distinguished from the old, which are more threatening and more unsafe, as emphasized by Fairbairn. For example, it can be terrifying for a patient who has never trusted to increasingly confront an object who seems worth trusting, thereby imperiling all his extant systems and patterns of defense and withdrawal.

There is a fundamental paradox in Fairbairn. Despite his radical assertion that there is a drive called object relating, Fairbairn, like Freud, views the individual as not wanting to recognize a new person for fear of threatening an attachment to an old object. Obviously, for Freud, the old object is clung to because it reduces instinctual tension—there never really is a new object, only the refinding of an old object. For Fairbairn, the individual wants to hold onto the object he has known and internalized in order to create or maintain safety. Furthermore, the object with whom he visits and revisits in therapy is in many ways a bundle of the projected, previously internalized object images. Contemporary relational theory describes the hoped-for negotiations that can go on between the patient-subject with the analyst-as-new-object, amid the collaborative experience and clarification of the analyst-as-old-object in the transference. In some ways, this challenges Fairbairn's basic assumptions. Although we have attempted to incorporate the rich legacies of British and American perspectives, we believe that American relational theory provides a necessary supplement to a Fairbairnian view, particularly in its elaboration on a variety of factors that make the renunciation or exorcism of the old object so difficult.

The notion that the patient can really trust someone new in the face of bedrock patterns of relating is indeed an outrageously ambitious goal.

The patient works and hopefully learns to play with experiential and transferential tensions in believing that the analyst can be different from the person the patient has known; at the same time, the analyst, by necessity, is also similar in some ways to the patient's objects—similar either because the analyst repeats and re-creates what has happened or because the patient's experiential overlay inevitably comes into play. The analyst is always partly a construction based on who the patient has known and who he wishes to know as well as who the patient is and who he wishes and strives to become. Through these tensions and multiple levels of reality, the analyst has the opportunity to influence. Psychoanalysis tries to help people engage in deep experience, exploring their tendencies to trust and mistrust others, to playfully construct the real and illusory, the old, new, and future self and object.

References

Aron, L. (1991), The patient's experience of the analyst's subjectivity. *Psychoanal. Dial.*, 1:29–51.

———— (1992), Interpretation as expression of the analyst's subjectivity. *Psychoanal. Dial.*, 2:475–507.

———— (1996), *A Meeting of Minds: Mutuality in Psychoanalysis*. Hillsdale, NJ: The Analytic Press.

Benjamin, J. (1988), *The Bonds of Love*. New York: Pantheon.

Bion, W. (1977), *Seven Servants*. New York: Aronson, Inc.

Burke, W. (1992), Countertransference disclosure and the asymmetry/mutuality dilemma. *Psychoanal. Dial.*, 2:241–271.

Casement, P. (1985), *On Learning from the Patient*. London: Tavistock.

Cooper, S. (1996), The thin blue line of the intrapsychic–interpersonal dialectic. Discussion of papers by Gerson and Spezzano. *Psychoanal. Dial.*, 6:647–670.

———— (1997a), The analyst's construction of psychic possibility. Presented at meeting of Division on Psychoanalysis (39), American Psychological Association, Denver, CO.

———— (1997b), Interpretation and the psychic future. *Internat. J. Psycho-Anal.*, 78:667–681.

———— (1998), Countertransference disclosure and the conceptualizztion of analytic technique. *Psychonal. Quart.*, 67:128–154.

———— (in press), Analyst-subjectivity and analyst-disclosure. *Psychoanal. Quart.*

Fairbairn, R. (1952), *Psychoanalytic Studies of the Personality*. London: Routledge, 1981.

Ghent, E. (1992), Paradox and process. *Psychoanal. Dial.*, 2:135–160.

Gill, M. (1983), The interpersonal paradigm and the degree of the therapist's involvement. *Contemp. Psychoanal.*, 1:200–237.

———— (1994), *Psychoanalysis in Transition*. Hillsdale, NJ: The Analytic Press.

Greenberg, J. (1986), Theoretical models and the analyst's neutrality. *Contemp. Psychoanal.*, 6:87–106.
———— (1995), Psychoanalytic technique and the interactive matrix. *Psychoanal. Quart.*, 64:1–22.
Hirsch, I. (1994), Countertransference love and theoretical model. *Psychoanal. Dial.*, 4:171–192.
Hoffman, I. (1994), Dialectical thinking and therapeutic action in the psychoanalytic process. *Psychoanal. Quart.*, 63:187–218.
———— (1996), The intimate and ironic authority of the psychoanalytic presence. *Psychoanal. Quart.*, 65:102–136.
Loewald, H. (1960), On the therapeutic action of psychoanalysis. *Internat. J. Psycho-Anal.*, 41:16–33.
Mitchell, S. (1988), *Relational Concepts in Psychoanalysis*. Cambridge, MA: Harvard University Press.
———— (1991), Wishes, needs and interpersonal negotiations. *Psychoanal. Inq.*, 11:147–170.
———— (1993), *Hope and Dread in Psychoanalysis*. New York: Basic Books.
———— (1994), Something old, something new. Response to S. Stern's "Needed relationships and repeated relationships." *Psychoanal. Dial.*, 4:363–370.
———— (1995), Interaction in the Kleinian and interpersonal traditions. *Contemp. Psychoanal.*, 31:65–91.
Modell, A. (1991), The therapeutic relationship as a paradoxical experience. *Psychoanal. Dial.*, 1:13–28.
Pizer, S. (1992), The negotiation of paradox in the analytic process. *Psychoanal. Dial.*, 2:215–240.
Renik, O. (1995), The ideal of the anonymous analyst and the problem of self-disclosure. *Psychoanal. Quart.*, 64:466–495.
Russell, P. (1985), The structure and function of paradox in the treatment process. Unpublished manuscript.
Steiner, J. (1993), *Psychic Retreats*. London: Routledge.
Stern, S. (1994), Needed relationships and repeated relationships: An integrated relational perspective. *Psychoanal. Dial.*, 4:317–346.
Strachey, J. (1934), The nature of the therapeutic action of psychoanalysis. [Reprints]. *Internat. J. Psycho-Anal.*, 50:275–292, 1969.
Tansey, M. & Burke, W. (1989), *Understanding Countertransference: From Projective Identification to Empathy*. Hillsdale, NJ: The Analytic Press.
Winnicott, D. (1965), Communicating and not communicating leading to a study of certain opposites. In: *The Maturational Processes and the Facilitating Environment*. New York: International Universities Press, 1965.
———— (1969), The use of the object and relating through identifications. In: *Playing and Reality*. New York: Basic Books.

Afterword

This paper originated with a series of discussions between the authors about Jay Greenberg's writings on neutrality. We began with Greenberg's (1986) equating the new objects with good objects, and old objects with bad objects. We went on to think more about the differences between British object relations theory and American relational theory with regard to the concepts of good and bad objects. At the time, we both noted how Americans tended to equate newness with safety; in contrast, Fairbairn (1952) appreciated patients' comfort with old, albeit bad, objects, and their anxiety and fear of new objects. We then explored how analysts' theoretical expectations regarding these matters tend to influence how they listen and integrate what takes place within the interaction.

Very recently, American relational theory has seen an upsurge of interest in the analyst as a new, bad object (e.g., Mendelson, 2002; Davies, 2003; Cooper, 2004). This is not the Fairbairnian bad object, which is bad for its newness, but, rather, the American relational bad object, which is bad for its badness. Mendelson (2002) emphasizes the analyst's "bad-enough" participation as a prerequisite for establishing useful tensions between oldness and newness and danger and safety. This idea is similar to Greenberg's (1986) noting the pitfalls of an analyst's striving to make things too safe. Davies (2003) has illustrated that, although we have known for some time that analysts contain aspects of their patients' disavowed self-states, we are only just beginning to recognize that patients at times bear the burden of containing elements of their analysts as well. Cooper (2004) has focused on the analyst as a new bad object insofar as patients must reckon with and abide their analysts' limitations as an intrinsic part of treatment.

In retrospect, thinking about our paper, we see three different versions of Fairbairn that we and others have considered. The version on which we focused is the one probably closest to Fairbairn's original writing, namely, that each of us internalizes early traumatic experiences in order to control them. This internalization is meant to detoxify the painful affects associated with these traumatic experiences. Here, the danger of a potential new object experience with the analyst is that it threatens to open up old longings and holds the possibility of the repetition of the same traumas that occurred before the developing child was able to internalize them to control them. In Fairbairnian terms, the antilibidinal ego preemptively and protectively slams the door on receptivity to something new.

A second version of Fairbairn can be found in Mitchell's (1988) focus on the importance of loyalty in Fairbairn's theory. Here, connecting to a new object (or, equivalently, connecting to an object in a new way) is dangerous for the terrible feelings of disloyalty and guilt that such a connection evokes because this new connection endangers a sense of enduring internal attachment to the old object. Still a third version of Fairbairn, related to loyalty, is our motivation to cling to the old in order to stay with what is familiar and known.

This is territory that Mitchell explored. Mitchell (2002) elucidated how familiarity, as a construction, can be used in interactions to minimize or preempt the terrors of newness, as we confine our experience of love relationships within old object parameters. One of us (Cooper, 2004) has put it that "infatuation means never having to be an old object." Fairbairn was attuned to how a potentially new object experience brings feelings of disorientation, including the need to examine how old object experience contains elements of new and possible frontiers. The newness leaves us feeling lost and unmoored, isolated in an alien world. The devil you know is better than the devil you don't know, which is better than no devil at all.

In addition to these perspectives on the new object experience in the analytic situation, we also want to highlight here another theme from the original paper. While we took up instances when patients begin to experience the analyst as good for the first time, we also addressed those situations, later in the analysis, when the new object emerges but not as a "brand new" object. In some extremely poignant moments, patients have discovered or rediscovered, in relation to their analysts some long-forgotten good experiences that they had with their parents. We are reminded of Mark Twain's words about the transition in his perceptions of his father during his adolescence: "When I was a boy of 14, my father was so ignorant I could hardly stand to have the old man around. But when I got to be 21, I was astonished at how much the old man had learned in seven years." So, while a major contribution of relational theory is its elucidation of the aspects of newness and goodness that occur through enactments and reciprocal communications of self-states between patient and analyst, many instances of finding newness and goodness have to do with refinding something good from the old object (an old and good point made by Freud).

Finally, we emphasize that the vocabulary of old and new, good and bad, safe and dangerous is at best a primitive lexicon for describing complex affective experience. We are probably holding on to aspects of Freud's original dual drive theory by using this dichotomous terminology. We hope that analysts will strive to cultivate new ways of describing old and new that do justice to a richer, more nuanced way of characterizing affective/transferential experience in the analytic situation.

References

Cooper, S. (2004), State of the hope: The new bad object and the therapeutic action of psychoanalysis. *Psychoanal. Dial.*, 14: 527–551.

Davies, J. (2003), Whose bad objects are these anyway? Repetition and our elusive love affair with evil. Presented at conference of International Association for Relational Psychoanalysis and Psychotherapy, Toronto, January.

Fairbairn, R. (1952), *Psychoanalytic Studies of the Personality*. London: Routledge, 1981.

Greenberg, J. (1986), Theoretical models and the analyst's neutrality. *Contemp. Psychoanal.*, 6:87–106.

Mendelson, E. (2002), The analyst's bad enough participation. *Psychoanal. Dial.*, 12:331–358.

Mitchell, S. (1988), *Relational Concepts in Psychoanalysis*. Cambridge, MA: Harvard University Press.

—— (2002), *Can Love Last? The Fate of Romance over Time*. New York: Norton.

Why the Analyst Needs to Change: Toward a Theory of Conflict, Negotiation, and Mutual Influence in the Therapeutic Process

(1998)

Malcolm Owen Slavin
Daniel Kriegman

▼　▾　▾　▼　▾

Editors' Introduction

In this fascinating article, Slavin and Kriegman build on their coauthored book, *The Adaptive Design of the Human Psyche* (1992), in which they introduced evolutionary issues and concepts as they relate to the question of what is primary about the human mind and the relational world in which it functions. Slavin and Kriegman drew on contemporary evolutionary biological theory and its overall dynamic theory of human motivation in order to revise modern psychoanalysis.

In that book, Slavin and Kriegman described how our intricate inner psychodynamic system may have evolved to guide the ongoing negotiation and renegotiation of the self in the ambiguous, inherently conflicted relational world. In that world our minds are powerfully constructed within the family and the larger culture by others whose interests inevitably diverge from our own. Within this model of the evolution of mind, dealing with conflict, mutuality, and deception is part of the normal family matrix.

In the chapter "Why the Analyst Needs to Change," the authors extend their ideas to demonstrate why it is essential to the patient that the analyst be open to change within him- or herself as part of the analytic process. In contemporary evolutionary theory, the overall dynamic system of human motivation is adaptively designed to operate in a self-interested fashion. For these authors, self-interest is a natural organizer of human motivation and the patient's skepticism is a natural evolutionary adaptive capacity. It functions in the service of evaluating the degree of overlap and divergence of interests of the patient and the analyst. This perspective places internal conflict and interpersonal conflict center stage. Resistance is viewed as an essential adaptive function that protects one from influence by someone whose interests conflict with one's own. Patients are therefore highly motivated to observe therapists' ways of dealing with their own inevitable internal conflicts as well as with conflicts of interest between themselves and their patients.

It is inevitable that the subjective worlds and personal interests of patient and analyst will conflict. These inevitable conflicts of interest between patient and analyst are regularly hidden within all versions of psychoanalytic technique. Slavin and Kriegman persuasively argue that it would not make sense for patients to surrender to analysts' influence unless and until the patients were convinced that, in spite of these inevitable conflicts, the analyst's interests were sufficiently aligned with his or her own. From this point of view, ongoing mutual influence in analysis is generated by the need to test these conflicts of interest. Since "the power to influence" is generally granted only to those with whom we experience real, long-term, stable reciprocity, it is the patients' experience of the analysts changing that convinces each patient that there is a genuine working negotiation occurring.

In the course of developing their argument, Slavin and Kriegman take up and revise many fundamentals of psychoanalysis, including empathy, authenticity, conflict, resistance, and the therapeutic action of psychoanalysis. The crux of the matter is that, from a relational point of view, therapeutic action requires mutuality—we can expect our patients to reorganize their identities only if we are open to revising our own.

Why the Analyst Needs to Change: Toward a Theory of Conflict, Negotiation, and Mutual Influence in the Therapeutic Process*

▼   ▼   ▼   ▼   ▼

As we thread our way through the patient's brambles, we trip over the big feet of our self interest, then stumble to those same feet to resume the quest for the other (McLaughlin, 1995).

This essay addresses a basic dimension of the therapeutic process, something that lies at the very core of it and is a central feature of all human relating: the experience and role of conflict—inner conflict (within both patient and analyst), and interactive (interpersonal) conflict. We cannot talk about conflict without addressing, simultaneously, what we believe is a realm of experience that is inextricably linked with it, namely, the ubiquity of deception and self-deception.

We are going to try to discuss conflict, deception, and self-deception in a fairly generic way, by which we mean a way that cuts across the specific languages of particular psychoanalytic traditions. Our views will be most familiar and compatible with readers who have moved away from the classical assumption that all conflict and defense derives from drive/defense structures—away from viewing transference and resistance as necessarily or primarily equated with individual intrapsychic distortions of reality. Yet from this relational and intersubjective springboard we propose some assumptions about the nature of conflict that differ from the customary focus of theorists working in the relational, inter-subjective, and constructivist paradigms. Specifically, we develop a way of talking about conflict in the therapeutic relationship as deriving from the inherently *diverging interests* (identities and needs) of analyst and patient. We shall describe the deceptions and self-deceptions surrounding the conflicts of interest and the complex negotiation process that is often required to deal with it.

Conflict as an Essential Constituent of Relating

Consider Winnicott's (1950) incredible assertion, "The mother hates her infant from the word go" (p. 201). Winnicott was not talking about bad

---

* Originally published in *Psychoanalytic Dialogues*, 8:247–284. © 1998 The Analytic Press, Inc.

or less than adequate mothers. He was talking about all "good-enough," devoted mothers. We don't think Winnicott was even talking simply about "hate" (the affect, or affective state) per se; certainly nor primarily about the manifestation of a destructive instinct" pressing for expression. We believe he was alluding to the affective dimension of something broader and more fundamental in the nature of human relating: the absolutely inescapable, major conflicts of interest that exist in the background between *even* the two individuals who share in the closest, most mutualistic relationship on earth—the relationship in which, without question, a natural empathy and love normally constitute the predominant affective bond.[1]

Consider what Winnicott says:

> The baby is not [the mother's] own (mental) conception. . . .
> The baby is a danger to her body in pregnancy and at birth. . . .
> To a greater or lesser extent [she] feels that her own mother demands a baby, so that her own baby is produced to placate her mother. . . .
> He tries to hurt her, periodically bites her, all in love. . . .
> He is ruthless, treats her as scum, an unpaid servant, a slave.
> He shows disillusionment about her.
> [After] having got what he wants he throws her away like an orange peel. . . .
> He is suspicious, refuses her good food, and makes her doubt herself, but eats well with his aunt. . . .
> She must not be anxious when holding him. . . .
> If she fails him at the start, she knows he will pay her out forever [p. 201].

The paper in which Winnicott wrote these lines, "Hate in the Countertransference," is, of course, *not* about mothers and infants (although

---

[1] The reader can basically interpret "conflict of interest" and "self-interest" in terms of the familiar, social meanings of these terms. Psychoanalytic readers may assume that self-interest as a motivational principle implies goals that are more conscious, calculated, and rational than those we observe in analytic work. *We make no such assumption.* The framework in which we understand self-interest as an overarching organizer of human motivation ultimately derives from contemporary evolutionary theory, in which the *overall dynamic system of human motivation*—not necessarily particular needs, wishes, or affects—is adaptively designed to operate, as much as possible, in a self-interested fashion (Slavin and Kriegman, 1992). The reader may also wish to see Trivers (1974) for a fascinating discussion of the biology of conflicts of interest (parent–offspring conflict) in human development and the wider world of nature and Slavin (1985) for a discussion of the function of repression in the context of parent–offspring conflict.

they are never far from Winnicott's mind). Immediately following the foregoing list of observations about mother and infant, Winnicott states, "The analyst must find himself in a position comparable to that of the mother of a newborn baby" (p. 202). Winnicott then introduces his notion of an "objective countertransference"—by which he means those aspects of the therapist's feelings about the patient that derive not from pathology in the therapist, nor from pathology in the patient, nor even from the specific character and style of the therapist as it interacts with the character and style of the patient.

Rather, the so-called objective countertransference seems to refer simply to a level of feelings, often fear and hate, that coexist with love. The fear and hate that Winnicott finds central to human relating seem to arise from what we see as the "psychic undertow' that operates between any two distinct beings who are attempting to interact in an intimate way. In an overarching, often unconscious way, each attempts to use the other, to pull the other into his or her subjective world, and to *resist* the pull, the undertow, in the *opposite* direction. Simultaneously, though, each needs to "use" the other to construct his or her own identity and thus wants—must want—to take in aspects of the other's subjectivity. Each tries to redefine the other in his or her own terms (and both to accept and to resist redefinition in the terms of the other). We call these universal relational tensions an undertow because they operate inexorably beneath whatever crashing of waves and ebbing and flowing of behaviors catch our attention on the surface.

Beginning with Winnicott's mother, "who hates her infant from the word go," we are also, as Havens (1997) puts it, confronted with the fact that "we stare forth from individually shaped and genetically different nervous systems onto a world seen from this time and place by no one else" (p. 526).

This innate individuality is nor simply a function of having different histories (although it is, of course, immensely elaborated and developed by different sets of experiences). From the word go, as it were, our individuality derives, in part, from the fact that each of us must have access to inner signals that will prompt and guide us to construct and reconstruct our individual world in accord with our self-interest (including most prominently inner signals that guide the actual process of constructing a viable subjective sense of what constitutes our own self-interest in relation to the interests of others).

As Winnicott (1963) observed, "There is a core of the personality that never communicates with the world of perceived objects and that the individual knows . . . must never be communicated with or be influenced by external reality" (p. 187).

This "core" can be seen as not only referring to an inevitable effort to protect the vulnerable aspects of the self, but also as signifying *an adaptive capacity to create and sustain the self in face of the average, expectable conflict, bias and deception that comes along with communication and influence in a relational world that, despite considerable mutuality, always includes significant competing interests.* There is a continuing tension, a web of conflicting and coinciding aims in the normal relational world that are sustained and amplified by our human capacity, as Havens (1993) notes, to use speech (not only to convey and communicate but also, regularly) for the purpose of concealing our thoughts, shaping them according to one or another prejudice. "Every human encounter is therefore a collision of viewpoints in which language both connects and conceals differences in outlook (Havens, 1997, p. 526).

Winnicott (1963) went on to say, "Although healthy persons communicate and enjoy communicating, the other fact is equally true that *each individual is an isolate, permanently non-communicating, permanently unknown, in fact unfound"* (p. 187).

Again, we read Winnicott (and Havens) as attempting to capture a very basic human tendency to construct our communications unconsciously in complex ways that, despite genuinely shared aims, are nevertheless inevitably biased toward our own interests; we naturally anticipate that the communications we receive from others will be similarly biased.

Winnicott's "core" is thus not a mute, defensively shut-off fortress but an adaptive aspect of how the self is configured, an aspect that serves as an innate, inner reminder that prompts us with something like the following message: monitor every communication, every relationship, that exerts a potential influence; despite significant overlap, my self-interest is unique and only partly shared by others; and even if they love me, they will often tend to act more in their own interests than in mine.

The core (as we see it) is not a "thing," or set of contents that exists in a fixed, immutable way within us; it is a metaphor that captures the essence of a process by which we organize all interactive experience, selectively coding outgoing and decoding incoming communication. This process limits the vast shaping potential, the influence, that interactive (social) experience can have on the highly plastic human psyche. The core reflects our inner design for managing the paradoxical nature of the human adaptation to the relational world: namely, in order to create and maintain a sense of self—including a sense of our own self-interest—we must continually learn from and incorporate aspects of the relational world. We must be influenced and feel this influence to become ourselves. Yet the intrinsically ambiguous relational world will, in even the best of circumstances, be biased toward its own interests, will tend naturally to represent its constructions as" reality" and its aims and ties as more closely and altruistically aligned with our own aims and interests than can ever, in fact, be the case.

Winnicott's observations about the "hate" that is present "from the word go" and the "core that must never be communicated with or be influenced by external reality" relate to fundamental aspects of our psychological being, *vital constituents of relating*. As we see it, Winnicott was not referring to an attunement to the realities of conflict that is reducible to "endogenous drives that need discharge" in the Freudian or Kleinian sense (although his Kleinian training certainly sensitized him to the existence of inherent conflict "from the word go"). Nor was he referring to hateful and defensive responses to environmental failures as self-psychological or intersubjective perspectives stress (Kohut, 1972; Stolorow, Brandchaft, and Atwood, 1987). Nor was he simply referring to reactions to the inevitable vicissitudes and disappointments in relating as other relational perspectives would emphasize (Mitchell, 1988). We believe he was talking about a universal *dialectic* between all individuals and the relational world, a dialectic that a) is rooted in the existence of implicit conflicts of interest, b) is represented innately in basic affects like hate and the existence of a private core of the self, and c) is vitally linked to the complex innate strategies we employ to "use" the relational world in order to create and maintain our individuality.

Clinically, this dialectical conflict within and between individuals involved in intimate forms of relating will also operate "from the word go" (see Benjamin, 1988). In myriad forms and innumerable deceptive ways, our subjective worlds and our interests will conflict with those of our patients. The crucial dimension of conflict we are referring to is intertwined with yet does *not* derive from and is not fully graspable or understandable in terms of a) the patient's *pathology*, projected or displaced onto a blank screen neutral, or even an affectively resonating therapist (as traditional analytic theorists and contemporary classical theorists might hold); b) the therapist's countertransference response to the patient's pathology, the experience evoked by a projective identification into the roles of others who were in conflictual relationships with the patient in the past (as many object relations and interpersonalist theorists might hold); or c) the failures of therapists to adequately empathize or sustain an attunement with the patient's subjective reality (as the self psychologists would have it).

What we are saying is that—like any two individuals (strangers, close relatives, intimate friends, lovers, parent and child)—therapist and patient operate through subjective worlds, needs, agendas, ultimately interests, that, to some extent, always diverge. At times their interests will inevitably clash. Woven into the most loving and cooperative motives (over and above the influence of professional roles) every individual organizes—really must organize—his or her subjective world to communicate and promote his or her own interests. From birth onward our subjectivities are naturally and inherently biased toward our own vital agendas. This bias is basically adaptive; it underlies the meaning of human individuality in a world of conflicting interests; and it may operate consciously or unconsciously.

The Adaptive Resistance to Influence in the Analytic Relationship

We develop here a perspective in which the centrality of the conflict between the patient's and analyst's needs and identities leads to continuing efforts to break down each other's identity: to reveal and examine each other's biases (identities, loyalties, agendas) and the inevitable conflicts between them. Patient and analyst continuously experience each other doing this. They experience and evaluate the integrity of each other's effort to engage in this process. The process is highly mutual and reciprocal (Ferenczi, 1932) although not symmetrical (see Aron, 1992; Hoffman, 1994; Beebe and Lachmann, 1988). Indeed the substantially different roles of patient and analyst invariably heighten certain aspects of the inevitable conflicts between them and what they ultimately need to negotiate (Slavin, 1996a; Kriegman, 1998).

The analytic literature grapples with facets of this negotiation process using the technical frameworks of transference, countertransference, empathy, holding, affective resonance, role responsiveness, projective identification, enactment, resistance, and so on. But all these clinical conceptualizations lead to discussions of conflict in the therapeutic relationship in ways that, we believe, often obscure crucial aspects of how and why conflict is central to human relationships, how it operates inexorably within every thoroughly "good-enough" therapeutic encounter and is integrally tied to the therapeutic action.

Most of our clinical conceptualizations of conflict (over the whole spectrum from classical to object relational, interpersonal and self-psychological/intersubjective perspectives) exaggerate the difference between the therapeutic relationship and other intimate human interactions (Bromberg, 1991). Our concepts tend to restrict us to viewing conflict in the therapeutic relationship as arising from the patient's pathology, from the analyst's pathology (countertransference), from fail-

ures in technique, or simply from differing individual, subjective organizing principles (Stolorow and Atwood, 1992), interpersonal patterns
(Aron, 1992), or the complexity of human relating (Mitchell, 1988).

We believe that all analytic traditions overemphasize the extent to
which differences in the subjectivities of patient and analyst result from
either instinctual clashes, relational failures, or the accidents of an imper-
fect world. Rather, intersubjective disjunctions are often ultimately rooted
in genuine conflicts of interest. In a variety of ways, it is conflicting interests that generate the continuing (self-interested) efforts at *mutual* influence that can be found within most therapeutic communications, and
these conflicting interests are, inevitably, deceptively hidden within all
versions of analytic technique. Consider the following kinds of clinical
situations that, in one form or other, most of us have encountered.

Nancy and the Analyst's Newborn Child

Nancy was a very troubled young woman who had been characterized
by many other therapists as "very primitive." She became agitated and
depressed in response to hearing that her current therapist was about to
have a child. Her therapist responded warmly to her, yet tried to articulate what he felt was idiosyncratic in her perspective on the situation.
He conveyed something like the following thought: "We've seen how
much you tend to feel that there is a limit to the amount of love and
concern available in the world; so what I give to my child will reduce
what is available for you."

The implication was that the most significant dimension of Nancy's
current experience was a set of internalized assumptions carried over from
a childhood during which she suffered enormous deprivation and frequently felt intensely envious, jealous, and rivalrous with her siblings. The
emphasis on her past—although communicated in a compassionate way
without any direct implication of "distortion"—implied that her views did
not fit the reality of the current situation. Nancy seemed to contemplate
the therapist's words. But, following this session, she became more dis-
traught and angry (in his view she regressed further) and became suicidal!

A careful continuing look at this case revealed that the therapist was
deeply invested in his assumption that Nancy's fear, rage, and regression
came predominantly from her pathology, that is, that the threat to her
emerged essentially from her characteristic way of organizing experience
and was fundamentally at variance with his own basic sense of the
world. He knew, too, that, to some degree, his experience of Nancy also
arose from his analytic identity. He sensed that his analytic training and
theory were biased toward his interests, geared to developing and

protecting his therapeutic identity, his healthy need as a professional to feel that he had adequate, valuable resources to give.

For example, in supervision on this case, he was reassured that, of course, he would have enough to give and that the crucial therapeutic question was why Nancy could not experience his caring. He was encouraged to look at how she had even managed to project her doubts and anxiety into him—managing to enlist him emotionally in the reen-actment of her relationship with her rejecting patents—making him feel as though he were abandoning her. It was also pointed out that this was, simultaneously, a reversed side of the enactment: Nancy was now in the role of her abandoning parents (with whom she was identified) engaged in a rejection of the vulnerable child (projected into the therapist).

The analyst recognized that Nancy's characteristic readiness to expe-rience changes as threatening was clearly at play in the disruption that had occurred in the treatment. Yet the very power of Nancy's "regres-sion"—her intense transference—had set in motion an interactive process that led (with the help of further consultation) to a deeper reappraisal by the analyst of his own beliefs, specifically, of the way in which his views of Nancy shielded him from recognizing the elements of self-decep-tion and self-protection in his own initial response to her. During this process, he also had the opportunity to experience the birth of his child—his own joyful preoccupation with it and the very real drain it created on his resources.

In subsequent meetings the analyst found himself needing to acknow-ledge the vital, inherent truth that Nancy's "transferential anxiety" had ultimately brought him to hear: that, of course, his life energies were and would be significantly absorbed by a child of his own flesh and that his relationship with his child did represent a different—in many ways, far more powerful—investment than his bond with her. He acknowledged and discussed the reality of these conflicts, including his own struggle to recognize and articulate them. Nancy seemed to experience something in these discussions as genuine. She began, as she put it, to feel "real" again; she no longer felt that her therapist had "disappeared." She became less afraid and—in her inimitable way—quipped that "maybe her analyst would actually learn something about nurturing that might be of use to her." As she recompensated, they went on to explore many of the additional, painful, and highly defended personal meanings that his becoming a father held for her.

Tanya: Paying to Be Cared About

Consider another familiar therapeutic conflict. Tanya was experiencing recurrent, extreme distress at "having to pay to be cared about" by her analyst. Very careful attempts to use the analyst's empathic understanding to clarify the personal meanings of Tanya's distress in terms of either her ongoing experience in the analysis—or prior painful disappointments in her life—were met with doubt, sometimes by withdrawal, sometimes with an understanding that ultimately seemed compliant. The analyst thought he had already reached a workable resolution regarding the complex meanings of money through his own personal treatment, supervision, and extensive clinical experience. He also seemed to be closely attuned to the painful way in which paying for therapy replicated Tanya's individual history of being taken from and used by others, of never having experienced a generous and genuine giving.

Yet, Tanya's persistent "transferential anxiety" over the meanings of the fee eventually evoked a broader range of thoughts and self-confrontations in her analyst. Tanya's persistent distress eventually compelled him to confront his sense that the disappointment, shame, and rage associated with paying for treatment could be analyzed in a way that would essentially transcend the painful sense of their differing investment in the therapeutic relationship, that understanding the individual subjective meanings of paying could somehow allow them to override the way in which these real differences in participation signaled the existence of their painfully conflicting interests. The analyst ultimately conveyed to her that he could see that money was an indication of one of the ways in which their interests did, in fact, diverge. In charging her, he acknowledged, he could see that he was clearly pursuing his own interests—which, in this respect, were quite different from and actually in conflict with hers.

The analyst's earlier attempts to explore the issue of money with Tanya were cast in what he believed were the meanings that historically had shaped her subjective world. That her analyst did not initially grasp the inherently conflicting interests that pervaded their relationship lent weight to the implication that her reactions to the rules of exchange in the analytic situation were rooted in her idiosyncratic unconscious organizing principles. As carryovers from her past, this old set of meanings undoubtedly needed to be explored empathically in the present therapeutic relationship.

Yet Tanya needed more than to have the analyst empathically acknowledge and help her articulate her painful distress about "paying to be cared for" and her suspiciousness about the genuine character of the caring thus received. She seemed to need him to recognize that her feelings were, in part, responses to certain real implications of paying him for maintaining their current relationship. That is, she needed to have a firmer sense that her analyst was going to be able to acknowledge the existence and potential implications of the existential dilemmas created by inherent conflicts of interest. She seemed to benefit not only from a sense that her analyst could become aware of how these existential dilemmas were woven into their relationship, but from a sense that he could grasp how her sensitivity to this conflict represented an essential adaptive capacity on her part.

We believe that Tanya essentially used this aspect of her transference (her capacity to mobilize and express her anxiety and suspiciousness) to probe the therapist's capacity to become more aware of the inevitable "background of conflict" that formed the context for their mutual work together. She seemed to need to see if he could face the ways in which his interests were clearly different from hers and, in fact, were naturally biased toward himself. She initiated (and he engaged in) what we would call a transferential dialogue about it, a dialogue in which she compelled some real change in his views (see Slavin and Kriegman, 1992; Slavin, 1994).

The cases of Nancy and Tanya illustrate two of the most common clinical arenas in which the analyst's interests clearly diverge from those of the patient: the existence of the analyst's real kinship ties and the exchange of money for the analyst's attention. As a function of the real, conflicting interests that pervade these arenas, interactions within them are fraught with significant deception and self-deception. The relational conflict and deception seen in the cases of Nancy and Tanya go well beyond the idiosyncratic aspects of these particular analysts' and patients' subjectivities. Beyond the recognition that we inevitably "trip over the big feet of our self interest" (McLaughlin, 1995, p. 435) and ultimately encounter the "hate" in our countertransference (Winnicott, 1950), we need to understand (in much broader, more basic terms) *why* these dimensions of the treatment relationship universally arise.

These cases illustrate the operation of a deep, natural, human sensitivity to the ways in which our needs and identities conflict with those of others. This universal awareness forms a context in which a range of other personal, historical, and intersubjective meanings take shape. While the existence of these conflicting interests is a painful reality that must slowly be grasped and lived with over the course of treatment, the process of arriving at a relatively less deceptive and self-deceptive discourse about such conflicting interests is fundamental to the viability of the analytic relationship. Beyond the obvious and direct acknowledgment of the conflicts experienced during mini- "crunches" (Russell, 1973) like those with Nancy and Tanya—in virtually all long-term, intensive therapeutic work, there is a subtle process by which analyst and patient struggle with seeing and acknowledging the real conflicts in their needs and identities. This process is central to the therapeutic action.

How the Analytic Situation Heightens the Experience of Conflict and Deception

Analytically oriented treatment is designed to be a process by which an unrelated person (someone without the depth of commitment of a family member or a close friend) is given extraordinarily privileged access (and power potentially to influence) very deep layers of the mind. Given the view of the relational world we have been presenting, an inherent, "adaptive skepticism" is likely to exist between any two individuals— including a patient and an analyst—concerning a new situation where an unrelated person invites the establishment of an intense transference and potential renegotiation of identity. As we see it, a patient's skepticism is a crucial adaptive capacity. It balances the equally vital capacity for a "willing suspension of disbelief." It serves as a means of evaluating the particular texture of the overlap and divergence of the interests (the identities) of patient and therapist. That is, patients must assess the likelihood that the potential activation of archaic longings and other repressed or disavowed aspects of themselves will be occurring in the context of a truly safe and promising relationship. Patients are likely to call into question only what they experience as their essential, ongoing sense of self (and self-interest)—likely to allow themselves to "use" (be influenced by) their analyst only when they experience the analyst as genuinely allied with their interests (see Weiss and Sampson, 1986).

Yet, as Nancy's and Tanya's analysts repeatedly discovered, there exist a range of ways in which the interests of patient and analyst regularly clash. The inherent tendency of both to construct their experiences and communicate in a biased fashion means that a patient's sense that the analyst is fundamentally allied with the patient's interests can be achieved only in an elusive, intermittent way. We think a crucial aspect of the therapeutic action lies in an ongoing, two-way negotiation process by which patients come to experience—then inevitably doubt, lose, search for, and repeatedly re-create with the analyst—the vital sense that the analyst is willing and able to become sufficiently allied with their interests.

Quite apart from individual, pathological mistrust carried into the analytic relationship by the patient, the fact is that, in all naturally occurring human relationships, the "power to influence" that we grant to persons outside our closest family relationships normally depends on our tangibly experiencing real, long-term, stable reciprocity in our interactions with them. We may significantly change in the context of marriage, intimate, enduring friendships, and, occasionally, some mentor, collegial, and business relationships. Yet, in each of these relationships, the other partner makes major tangible investments or takes close to equally large risks. In virtually every sphere of our lives, we humans basically operate through such experienced, carefully monitored and evaluated reciprocity (Trivers, 1971).

Yet the analyst is an unrelated individual who asks the patient to pay (sometimes dearly) for what is always experienced (at times by even the most grateful patients) as a relatively small investment in terms of visible costs to the analyst. With an analyst there is little tangible, reciprocal sharing or exchange and—for long periods of time—usually ambiguous and subtle results.

In this light, consider the implicit message we deliver to our patients:

> Though I, as analyst, give you little that is tangible in return—and, in fact, insist that you pay me—I expect you to trust me, open yourself up to my influence, and give free reign to powerful fantasies and wishes. I imply that the interpersonal negotiating power, as it were, that the activation of these forces within you confers upon me will ultimately lead us to reorganize you in ways that are more aligned with your real interests than you can at this point even imagine (and that, right now, either of us can actually know).[2]

The Therapeutic Transference as a "Mimicry" of the Parent–Child Relationship

Consider also some of the larger meanings of the analysts interest in evoking an intense transference attachment and potential regression. We expect a therapeutic transference to develop: we create a setting and a way of relating designed to revive aspects of early experiences in the context of which the patient constructed basic conclusions about who he or she is and what can be expected from interactions with others. The analytic relationship is essentially designed to mimic, as it were, the unique emotional power and influence that early familial ties naturally hold for the child in the human life cycle. Through this mimicry, the transference creates a highly emotional human situation in which it may be possible to revise some of one's fundamental conclusions about oneself and the world.

Because we live and breathe the life-cyclical realities of our species every instant of our lives, we should not take for granted (absurd as it may seem to question it) the fact that children "allow" their parents and the familial environment to develop the degree of influence, the power as internalized presences (introjects) that they normally exercise in con-

---

[2] Also see Kindler's (1995) references to the therapist's "entitlement to intimacy" and Friedman's (1991) notion of the intrinsic "seductiveness" of the analytic situation.

structing the child's self organization, that is, in molding the child's basic definition of self and self-interest. Yet, despite the mother's "hate for her infant from the word go"—the very real conflicting interests and psychic undertow that operate between parent and child—the fact is that in a natural environment parents can be expected intrinsically to share their child's interests very deeply and to invest in them (more than anyone else) over a long period of time (Trivers, 1974). This seems to mean that the child's "core personality" (in Winnicott's [1963] sense) is, in fact, predisposed to allow more communication and influence (to modulate its innate skepticism to a greater degree) in early interactions with related individuals than at any other time in the life cycle. The therapeutic transference relationship essentially mimics these formative, developmental relationships in which there is a far different form of investment than in the analytic situation. It is thus inconceivable that our patients would not have an underlying sense that the experience of heightened transference expectations and longings exposes them to a dangerous deception and invites them to engage in a perilous self-deception.

However we conceive of the meaning and function of the transference, patients are apt to feel within it the potential for a tangible, reciprocal investment in their self-interest that is seductively similar to what natural, formative relationships could entail. And, yet—despite much in the analytic relationship that is as heartfelt and genuine as in any relationship—this therapeutic version is not the same as what occurs in most other reciprocal relationships that give rise to such powerful emotions. The pain of paying for concern, the constant reminder at the end of each hour of the limits of the therapist's involvement, all signal a much broader and more basic reality of the analytic situation: the therapeutic relationship does not carry with it the inherent investment in the patient's interests that kin and other natural, reciprocal relationships regularly entail. Patient and therapist must negotiate ways by which the patient may come to experience that, despite its painful "unrealness," the treatment relationship is, in fact, real enough to justify the patient's fully engaging himself or herself with its potential power and influence (Slavin, 1996b).

Just what is the analyst's investment in the patient? How far reaching is it in comparison with the natural context of familial hate and love in which the child's "core personality" may be designed to allow relatively greater communication and influence? Analysts tend not to define their core self-interests in a fashion that includes the self (and self-interest) of a specific patient to a great degree. Indeed, many of the *rules* of therapy are structured precisely to ensure that, the analyst's self-definition does *not* include the patient's self-interest to an overly great degree.

Consider the relative experience of a therapist and patient if, for some unavoidable reason, the relationship is prematurely lost. Given the risks the patient is asked to assume and given the analyst's relative safety and comfort, it is hard to imagine any human situation more likely to elicit a vigilant readiness to detect signs of potential conflict and deception. Beyond this imbalance in risk and safety, the analyst often tends to equate his or her subjectivity with reality; what is tilted toward the analyst's interests is often subtly conveyed as really in the patient's benefit.

The Patient's "Innate Skepticism"

Like Tanya and Nancy, all patients tend ultimately to compel us to face the fact that there is something fundamental in the relational structure of the analytic relationship, which, in a real sense, should make the patient suspicious. In the thick of the struggle with the unique transference–countertransference complexities of out relationship with a particular patient, we tend to ignore the fact that the therapeutic negotiation process probably carries the natural human capacity for self-revision (in the context of a powerful relationship) to an unusual—perhaps, in some ways, unnatural—extreme. This is why something tantamount to an "innate skepticism" is activated in most patients concerning this almost unparalleled new situation in which an unrelated person deliberately offers him- or herself as a vehicle for profoundly influencing and altering a patient's identity. This adaptive skepticism is, for us, a kind of backdrop to all discussions of "resistance." It refers to a general, adaptive core in all forms of resistance. This core is distinct from (although perhaps intertwined with) the "dread to repeat" (Ornstein, 1974) particular, painful relational scenarios that have thwarted development in the past.

As we see it, a patient's innate skepticism is the adaptive phenomenon that Winnicott was trying to describe when he struggled to articulate what he experienced as a "core that must never be influenced." It signifies a fundamental, universal form of "resistance to influence"—one that by no means aims to bar all influence, but, rather, subjects all potential influence to the scrutiny of a basic relational test: what is the texture, the subjective feel, of the overlap and divergence of this other person's interests and my own? Is this relationship actually sufficiently geared to my interests to (re)awaken my deepest longings? Is there enough of a sense that the analyst is willing and able to gear this relationship to the enhancement of my genuine interests—and consistently maintain that biased focus in my favor—for me to open up those aspects of my inner experience and desire that I long ago concluded were not safe to expose to relational influence? In a way that both analyst und patient dimly sense, because the analyst is an Other, whatever the analyst can offer will come wrapped in who he or she is—his or her needs, identity, biases. And, therefore, the patient is going to have to lose parts of him- or herself, compromise his or her interests, be hurt in the inevitable adaptation to the analyst.

Transference as an Adaptive Probe

The human capacity to develop and interactively use transferences may actually be geared, in significant part, to expressing and probing the potential for recognizing and negotiating the ambiguous mixture of real conflict and mutuality in human relatedness. Tanya repeatedly used her sense of the unreality of the "paid-for caring" in the treatment relationship to find out whether her analyst could see and accept his own needs as distinct from—even, at times, inimical to—hers. The analyst's recognition of his need to use her for his own ends did not diminish her longing to be cared for without reciprocating financially—indeed to be given more unconditional love than probably even a very good parent would provide. Yet the greater clarity about their conflicting interests significantly diminished the deceptive and self-deceptive blurring of their interests—the "insult added to injury"—that made the "unrealness" of the analytic relationship, with its painfully real limits on the expression of love and investment, even more painful and dangerous than it needed to be.

Nancy also responded intensely to her sense of this potential deceptiveness in the transference. She was not part of the analyst's life in a way that permitted her to observe or directly influence his investment in her even to the extent that a child can affect the relative investment in a sibling. She thus needed to mobilize fantasy and emotion within her transference as a way of probing the analyst's capacity for candid reflection on their conflicting interests over the investment in his own child. Tanya reacted to one of the most thorny areas of conflicting interest and potential deception in the analytic situation: that, in the early part of the analytic work, there may be, for some patients, a strong sense of the situation as tilted toward the fulfillment of the analyst's needs—financial, certainly, and also in terms of professional identity. If treatment is successful, the balance in the exchange is restored in the (very) long run. But, meanwhile, the painful experience of adapting to a relationship that is, indeed, structured in the short run to benefit the other person is one major way in which the "asymmetry" of the treatment relationship becomes experienced as problematic. Real diverging interests and the accompanying potential for deception and self-deception are amplified by the analytic context.

In many respects therapists must sustain an exquisite alertness to self-deception and avoidance of deception. For not only is the analytic relationship basically prone to the same complex web of conflict and deception as are other human ties, but the analytic relationship must ultimately justify its potential influence without making the same kind of real investment in the patient's life that is often found in other, naturally occurring reciprocal bonds. The negotiation between analyst and patient must continuously transform the deceptive part of the relationship, the unreality, into its benign form, something that is experienced as play and creative illusion (Winnicott, 1969). Ultimately, it must be real-enough on its own terms and in its own way (Greenberg, 1986) to justify the patient's using it effectively to question and revise fundamental conclusions about, and ways of interacting with, the relational world.

As Tanya, Nancy, and the case we are about to present compelled their analysts to recognize, one of the major ways in which therapists fail their patients revolves around the therapist's use of self-deceptive strategies for protecting or enhancing his or her interests in a fashion that is cast in terms of the interests of the patient. In our view, the danger that many patients sense in such a "confusion of interests" is not simply the dread of a repeated traumatic experience of major boundary confusions in their past. Within many ordinary enough, everyday deceptions lies the potential for further loss and erosion of the vital capacity to define, know, and promote one's own interests. *We believe that this tendency to engender a confusion of interests is the central feature of many less than good-enough, traumatizing, pathogenic family environments.*[3] And it is not uncommonly replicated in many therapies woven into what therapists codify as "technique."

By focusing on relatively isolated moments during a long, complex treatment process, the brief vignettes of Nancy and Tanya may suggest that we believe there can exist a clarity and simplicity in such analytic negotiations. There are, of course, many dimensions to the process of mutual adaptation that signal to patient and analyst alike that a genuine negotiation is taking place. In the following case example, we hope to

---

[3] This "confusion of interests" can be very destructive to the child, and we would probably tend to call its effect "traumatic." However, it can operate in subtle ways over a long period of time and can lead to a very familiar event: our dealing with very troubled and confused patients who continually exclaim, "What's my problem? I had a good family/childhood. Nothing *really* bad happened to me."

convey a bit more of the enormous complexity in this process of negotiation and mutual adaptation.

Edward and His Analyst

Edward was the most intensely and tenaciously depressed person his analyst had ever known. Trials of virtually every known medication had been almost totally ineffective. After a few years of treatment, on occasion the analyst felt that there were small, momentary brightenings in Edward's mood, brief periods of improved concentration, and, from time to time, moments of interest, intense passion, and insight. To his analyst, Edward seemed in these moments to be noticeably more alive.

The positive moments, the flickerings of hope and passion, were linked to the analyst's highly consistent efforts to remain closely attuned to Edward's subjective world, to remind herself that, more than anything else, he needed to establish (and continually restore) the sense that someone could grasp his experience of deadness and impossibility in which he constantly lived. They had come to construct a picture of his having grown up as an unwanted child—a child of a removed, depressed mother and a distant, critical father—who felt that he existed only insofar as he corresponded to and validated everyone else's expectations for him. He was tortured by an unresolvable dilemma: although he craved intimacy, attempts at closely relating with other people invariably left him feeling lost, trapped in what he called "the black hole." There he was bereft of meaning, lived only for the other person, and virtually lost all sense of himself as a real, living being.

Although in some ways the treatment relationship had become a kind of sustaining bond through which he seemed to feel more understood than he had ever felt in any other relationship, Edward's intense, deadening hopelessness always returned. He felt that he could never have the sense of aliveness that other people felt. Nor could he tolerate the deceptiveness, the hypocrisy, the self-deceiving "mechanical social ritual" that he astutely observed in the lives of others. Yet the more he removed himself from "meaningless social contacts," the lonelier he became.

Over time, Edward's analyst became regularly aware of living with a powerful, anticipatory dread within herself, a dread of what felt to her like the repeated undercutting and undermining of all good feelings. Early on in one session, Edward seemed to be fighting off the horrible tug of another slide into hopelessness. For an instant, the analyst was aware of silently siding with what she sensed as Edward's effort not to lapse, once again, into a state of angry despair. She attempted to remain closely attuned to the story he was telling about a perennially frustrating problem at work. As the hour proceeded, however, it became clear, that Edward's despair was gaining the upper hand. Nothing was helping. Whatever they might come to understand, he still had no life.

"Can't you see," he said, "I am dying more each day. This is futile."

In the midst of this hopelessness, it seemed as of something inside her begun to talk. She heard herself saying, "At times like this, I sometimes feel that all I can do is to be here with you in your despair." And then, as she realized it, she added, "Yes, there is something more, maybe more important. I, I have to try to deal with the part of me that really doesn't want to feel it."

In the next session, Edward said that something "sort of strange" had happened: "That image of you had a different sense to it. Different from the ways I think about this . . . you as a person who's enduring the despair . . . it puts you inside the image rather than outside it. Do you know what I mean?"

"I think so."

"As opposed to me being desperate, and you trying to know what to do about it. And me convinced that you can't do anything about it—enduring the desperation together. I think it's probably the only real comfort you can give me."

In many moments like that, it became clear to the analyst that her arduous and careful effort to remain attuned to Edward's subjective world clashed painfully with her own sense of life and hope. At a very profound level, her sense of hope for Edward was rooted in her own need to maintain a basically positive view of herself and of life, as well as her need to feel hopeful about the analysis itself. To the extent that Edward seemed to sense this conflict between them—and particularly that he sensed any tendency in her to deceive herself about whom the hope was really for—his despair and rage intensified.

Note that "whom the hope was for" was often quite ambiguous, even paradoxical. Edward's analyst felt a need to be hopeful about the analysis in a way that she felt compelled to acknowledge was *for her*, after all, analysis was part of her identity. Yet she also felt an ethical demand that she not fall prey to some projective identification (or pull toward an enactment) and allow Edward's despair and hopelessness to fill her: wouldn't she be failing her patient if she lost hope? The powerful, emotionally charged, paradoxical ambiguity threatened her identity in a destabilizing manner that added significantly to her simpler defense against despair and hopelessness about aspects of human existence. Thus, the conflict between Edward's need to have her "decenter" and experience the legitimacy of his subjectivity (his despair) and her need to find ways to stand outside the hopelessness was quite complex.

When she allowed his experience to move her to confront these aspects of the real conflicts between their identities (and her own need to keep the conflict out of her awareness) she could "hear herself" saying something to him that had a very different feel to her than her usual, careful, consistent empathic inquiry had. In a way that pathologized neither him nor herself, she communicated her own struggle to join him. Her response was spontaneous and authentic because it reflected her direct struggle with the conflict between them; and she conveyed something crucial about her ongoing capacity and willingness to be moved, changed, by him, despite countervailing pressures within herself.

She essentially demonstrated her willingness to experience her own internal struggle over hope and despair, an inner conflict that was induced, in part, by the conflict between them. She needed to reopen her own efforts to come to terms with some of the grief and despair she had felt in her own life. Having a genuine relationship with Edward required her to reimmerse herself in painful realities for which she had successfully and adaptively found a working resolution. It seemed as though she conveyed something crucial about her ongoing capacity and willingness to be moved away from something that had been provisionally settled in her own identity.

Deepening Conflicts with the Analyst's Identity

Despite these moments in which they negotiated a greater psychological "realness" in their relationship, Edward felt that the closer they became, the more he was condemned to live with a bitter, frustrated longing to be a real part of his analyst's life, her real life, like the "real" people in her life, her family and friends. Most painful was that while they could recognize and talk about his need to be held, she could never really hold him.

His earliest memory was of being in his mother's arms but sensing that she was vague and distracted. Mother didn't put him down, yet it felt as though she didn't really want to hold him. The analyst's closeness now only makes him more painfully convinced that, as in every relationship he has ever had, he is being tortured by getting something but not getting what he really needs. He clings to her while she pursues her real life; he stands on the sidelines.

If she actually (physically) held him, he believes it would destroy her life. So the only way he can feel held by her is if she admits and accepts his hopelessness, their hopelessness together—that is, the hopelessness of analysis and of life itself. They must accept that they have to stop engaging in a futile process. What can analytic understanding accomplish? He has no life. Can't she see, he is dying more each day? He wants to die. He realizes (when she points it out) that this Catch 22 is the essential dilemma he experiences at every turn, the "black hole" of relationships: he desperately needs to feel that she is genuinely with him, yet he can feel her to be genuinely with him only if she accepts his reality, his belief that analysis is futile. And if she does, their relationship must end.

She knows that in some way it *is* a Catch 22: a paradox that ultimately derives from the fact that their needs are in conflict. And his need for her to feel his despair profoundly conflicts with his desperate need for her to sustain her—and his—hope. She must recognize his inner conflict. But she has come to realize that, first and foremost, she must wrestle with the real conflict between them, not gloss over the ways in which analysis is, in a real sense, a seduction, a tease, bringing him to experience his needs intensely yet not providing the real loving holding that he ultimately needs.

Over the years, the analyst became increasingly aware that their relationship entailed enormous risks, risks for which, when it came down to it, she was not prepared by her training or her own long and productive analysis. Sometimes the risks and dangers were felt as largely external: when Edward seemed more desperate and suicidal, she feared being accused of driving him crazy by doing analytic treatment with a man who could not tolerate it. Frightening images of Margaret Bean-Bayog (and the personal and professional catastrophe that had befallen her in her "regression" treatment of Paul Lozano) drifted through her mind.[4] She knew that some of her valued colleagues and teachers might well fault her for pursuing an intensive analytic treatment with a man so disturbed. The conflict felt like disloyalty (her abandonment of them and their teaching) as well as like a direct danger to her interests (her professional reputation and livelihood). Not only might she fail to help him, she might hurt him. She might also deeply hurt herself in the process.

With countless reiterations of this theme, the analyst came to a wrenching, emotionally complex appreciation of what Edward was compelling her to see. On numerous occasions, she began to try to communicate her grasp of this to him. Indeed, in many ways, she would not (analysis, as she practiced it, could not) give him what he needed: to be held, to be a "real" part of her life. Nor could she fully accept the legitimacy of his despair and fully decenter into a complete empathic union with his hopelessness; as long as she was functioning as his analyst, she

---

[4] The widely publicized Boston case of a psychiatrist whose career was destroyed over her work with a severely disturbed man who eventually killed himself.

could never fully accept that psychoanalysis with him was futile. Yes, these were, in significant ways, limitations of her method, not simply his inability to adapt to the limitations, or her failure to attune herself thoroughly and consistently enough to him. The realities of her own life and her way of working created the limits in their relationship. These limitations might be more than he could take. His life might not improve; and the heightened longings stimulated by the analysis might be so unbearable that he would kill himself.

Then, on several occasions, she conveyed to him that she knew he would feel acceptance and relief if she acknowledged the hopelessness and futility of their work: "It would even bring me real relief from the feeling that I am engaging you in something that benefits me while it perhaps endangers you and brings you (and me) more pain and little gain. But, at many moments, I feel a life within you, something that responds to me and stirs a feeling of life in me; and when I feel this, the hopelessness and futility is not the only thing in the picture. I can't ignore that life, despite my own uncertainty about the ultimate outcome."

These clearly painful realizations on her part were conveyed to him as she understood them. They seemed to make him feel that she was less deceptive with herself, and that was of some importance to him. Soon after this, the analyst saw an uncharacteristic flicker of a smile on his face at the beginning of an hour, a smile that he quickly aborted. When she asked about it, he said, "I come in the door and look in your eyes and see you smile and it's like I'm inside it, inside the smile. If I don't 'stay in your smile' I'll have nothing to say. If I stay in it and smile back, I'll begin to lose myself in you. But if I don't see you smile I'm completely alone and lost."

Through all these episodes, the analyst came to appreciate further that, beyond the frustrations produced by her maintaining professional and personal limits, it was, in many ways, her life itself—her feelings, hope, needs—that was dangerous to him. He desperately needed to feel her life, but, simultaneously, it threatened to rob him of himself, to kill him. Ultimately, it seemed to be her continuing, inevitable self-deceptions (that is, her unwitting tendency to confuse their interests) that drove him into a quietly raging despair. And it was her open revelation to him, each time, of her dawning realizations about her need to remain hopeful (*for herself* as well as for him) that restored the sense of realness and authenticity to their relationship.

Near the seventh year of treatment, Edward commented that he thought she had begun to move her hands a lot more. Only when he said this did she become aware that she had, in fact, been dimly aware of feeling this shift herself.

"Is it true?" he asked.

"Yes. As you say it, I can see it."

"What does it mean?" Edward asked.

She said she feels as if she were groping toward him and groping around herself, searching in the dark. She had, she told him, begun to try to express things with him that she didn't really understand but was trying anyway.

Soon he began to question her frequently whenever he felt that she might be holding back. He said he wished she could "push him more."

"Do you even know what to do to push me anyway?"

"I feel as if I'm pushing you when I respond in some way that you'll feel is for me, not for you. You know, based on my belief in analysis, my agenda."

Surprisingly, he now seemed genuinely *unconcerned* about this major issue.

"Look," the analyst said. "It often feels as if there is one kind of pushing that feels as if it is for you but that I realize is for me. And another kind that feels as if I'm taking some kind of risk for myself."

"You? What do you mean, risk?"

Moving her hands helped a lot here. Edward averted his eyes, as though he could not stand to see her make a false step.

"Sometimes," she said, "I start to worry that we're doing things here that are really my agenda—that it is going too far for you. It can feel essentially cruel, that it will hurt you, make you 'regress,' less able to work and function. The risk for me often comes when I say to myself, 'Don't let this fear control you. You know you believe more and more that what you're trying to do is basically right. Be more active with him, go ahead, put it in words, try whatever it is out.' I think it's when I take this risk of hurting you that something feels like a good kind of pushing."

Edward's face opened gradually as she spoke. He nodded. Something was clearly getting through, but it often did. After a pause, he burst out, "So all these years I've been thinking you're sitting there thinking about me—and you're actually thinking about you!"

They both laughed very hard.

"This is such a strange relationship," he said. "We're here to understand me, but we have to understand you in order to understand me."

Slowly, over much time, through this kind of negotiated understanding, Edward began to develop a sense of realness in the relationship with his analyst that, for the first time, seemed to endure despite the annihilating pull of the "black hole." He reported that he felt somehow that something more solid had come into his experience and that he thought he had perhaps chosen to live.

The relationship between Edward and his analyst was fraught with deepening experiences of conflict and the continuing uncovering of a web of unwitting deceptions and self-deceptions. No doubt Edward's pathology —the tenuousness of his self-organization and his entrenched, unrelenting beliefs in the danger and hopelessness of relationships— contributed heavily to the extreme complexity of negotiating a greater closeness with him. Equally, aspects of his analyst's struggle derived from rigidities and blind spots within her self-organization. Yet we believe a very significant dimension of this conflict, deception, and self-deception was not attributable to his pathology or to idiosyncratic countertransference obstacles or to significant technical failures on the part of his analyst.

In the course of the negotiation process, Edward and his analyst challenged each other's identity on many different levels. His primitive transference (in both its pathological and adaptive elements) served to create and sustain a relentless series of challenges to his analyst's identity.[5] But these challenges were—had to be—quite real to her; they entailed a deep and consistent questioning, and revising, of the way she organized aspects of her personal world. Yet only in the course of her sustained negotiation with Edward did these features of her identity take on meaning as "countertransference obstacles" that needed to be overcome. In other words, aspects of her personal and analytic identity needed to be reopened in order to negotiate an authentic relationship with Edward, not because they were especially problematic in her own personal or professional life.

At the same time, the challenge and negotiation were not simply an "enactment," a replay of pathological relational scenarios induced or recruited (by projective identification) into the mind of the analyst. The negotiation was over real conflicts between Edward's identity and the analyst's personal and professional identity, conflicts that were clearly intensified by the tremendous natural seduction (Friedman, 1991) and potential for deception in the analytic situation. Yet this conflict served as an indispensable vehicle for creating a meaningful negotiation process.

---

[5] Pizer (1992, 1996) has developed an interesting perspective in which negotiation and "mutual adjustment" are central to the analytic process. His emphasis is on the process of negotiation of many of the paradoxical aspects of the patient–analyst experience. Although a full discussion of his concept is beyond the scope of this paper, we believe that the "negotiation of paradox" invariably takes place within the *context* of the negotiation of conflicts interest and may represent a clinical emphasis that is potentially complementary to our own.

Implications

In the first section of this article, we presented a view of internal and intersubjective conflict as fundamentally rooted in a *normal, adaptive bias that pervades our subjectivity*—a bias that will inevitably clash with the subjectivities of others. The existence of such "evolved, existential conflict" is an ancient, enduring aspect of human development and adult life. It accounts for the existence of a *concomitant, evolved tendency to disguise (from others and ourselves) aspects of our subjective bias while anticipating and evaluating the motivated biases in the subjectivities of others.* We are, in effect, designed to open ourselves (but only partially and selectively) to the influence—the enormous shaping power—of an engagement with the relational world.

We talked about conflict, deception, and self-deception from a vantage point that lies a bit *outside* of the customary language and frameworks of tranference–countertransference, enactment, affective resonance, projective identification, and so on, in which contemporary analysts customarily discuss the complex intersections of the subjective worlds of analyst and patient. From this broader perspective we raised very fundamental questions about the therapeutic relationship as a human endeavor. These questions are touched on in much contemporary relational and intersubjective writing, yet, the language of our usual clinical-theoretical narratives keeps us from getting at this broader relational reality.

Now the question is, how do we relate what we have been describing in somewhat new language to more familiar analytic concepts and ways of talking about some of these same clinical phenomena?

Our view of conflict and deception—self-deception takes us far from what we believe is the classical analytic emphasis on conflict emanating from (ultimately drive-based) motivated *distortions* of reality. Yet we move well beyond the tendency of relational, intersubjective models to attribute conflict exclusively to the unfortunate vicissitudes of an individual's particular, problematic (or less than adequate) relational experience. Our perspective allows us to bring into focus a very important arena of inevitable, *motivated* conflict and deception within all relationships, including the treatment relationship. We focus on an aspect of conflict that is a function of *both* the therapist's and the patient's biased subjectivity. And while always intertwined with meanings derived from past experience (transference) and countertransference, a crucial element in this very real, ongoing conflict and deception is lost when it is reduced to either a) a "role-responsive" (Sandler, 1997) enactment of the patient's old pathogenic reality (through the necessary enlistment of inevitable countertransference); or b) the complexity and difficulty of the therapist's dealing with his or her own selfobject needs (Bacal and Thomson, 1996; Stolorow and Atwood, 1992) in the effort to sustain a sufficiently other-oriented, empathic stance. Let us look at some of the implications of viewing the familiar, analytic notions of projective identification, enactment, empathy, and authenticity from the point of view of the universal mixture of conflict, deception, and self-deception that we call evolved existential conflict.

Projective Identification and Enactments

In speaking of relational dynamics in which conflict is induced within the other, people often use the term projective identification. For us, this term is problematic when it refers to a process by which certain versions of self-experience, or of inner conflict, are somehow seen as "put into" the therapist or even simply as eliciting an affective resonance in the therapist's personal life. Such "induced" experience and role responsiveness (Sandler, 1976; Ogden, 1985) may well occur but do not capture the interactive and internal negotiation process to which we are referring. The related notion of enactment can be talked about in the same way: as though the transference–countertransference mix that is enacted (and, it is to be hoped, eventually understood) were a kind of as-if scenario in which the participants emotionally relive the *patient's* fantasy world— not the therapist's real (and fantasy) world—as it is activated by their relationship (Bollas, 1987; Jacobs, 1991).

We are referring to a more interactive process that is closer to those processes described in discussions about the patient's evocation of—and attunement to—the real inner life of the therapist (Searles, 1975; Hoffman, 1983, 1991; Aron, 1991; Blechner, 1992; Lichtenberg, Lachmann, and Fosshage, 1992; Pizer, 1992, 1996; Davies, 1994; Rogers, 1995). We are proposing that such interactive processes can be understood as operating within a broader "evolutionary biological" understanding of the inevitability of conflict in all human relationships. The experience of negotiation in the treatment relationship is activated by an adaptive striving by patient and analyst to engage teal conflicts—real multiplicity and inner dividedness—within the therapist in the treatment relationship. The evocation of conflict within the analyst and the recognition of the clash between the analyst's identity and that of the patient serves to create the necessary conditions for a genuine renegotiation of internal representations (beliefs, introjects, expected interactional patterns) that were forged in the context of mutuality, conflict, and deception within earlier formative relationships. Patients are highly attuned to the therapist's ways of dealing with the inevitable conflicts of interest experienced *within* his or her identity and *between* his or her identity and that of the patient. We believe that we are all equipped with an evolved, intuitive sensitivity to the natural self-deceptions and deceptions in which we all engage and (especially in the clinical setting) must tease out in ourselves and each other. Let us consider how this natural, adaptive sensitivity relates to the use of empathy as an analytic stance.

The Intrinsic Ambiguities of Empathy

Edward's analyst made a skillful effort to grasp consistently his experience—to maintain a consistently empathic stance (Ornstein, 1979; Kohut, 1984) or a "sustained empathic inquiry," as the intersubjectivists put it (Stolorow et al., 1987). This stance was crucial to keeping the conflict within tolerable limits for both of them by minimizing Edward's experience of the divergence of their subjective worlds. But, contrary to the impression given in much of the self-psychological literature, on many occasions the empathic grasp of Edward's experience, though crucial, was of limited effectiveness. We think the reason for this is that a consistent attunement to Edward's subjective world did not, in itself, go far enough as a genuine signal of the analyst's capacity to ally with Edward's interests. And at moments it even exacerbated his sense that she was deceptively evading the conflict that he knew existed between them.

If we understand the meaning of empathy in the context of the background of expectable conflict and deception in the therapeutic relationship (that is, beyond the self-psychological/intersubjective frameworks in which it is often embedded), we can see why an empathic stance is a vital, effective communication of the analyst's position regarding the patient's real interests. Yet, at the same time, we can see how the very sources of empathy's effectiveness as an interpersonal communication generate problems that necessitate *other* ways of relating.

Empathy is a fundamental interpersonal signal that lets patients know that a genuine alliance with their interests is a real possibility. Sustained empathic communication signals that the therapist is more likely than most perhaps to be willing to decenter from his or her own personally adaptive bias (and to be emotionally capable of doing so) in order to join in viewing things from the subjective point of view of the patient. The therapist's consistent decentering, or abandoning of his or her own (personally more adaptive) subjective view, even though only temporary and never fully achieved, signals the potential for a genuine investment that might be emotionally equated with the type of investment experienced outside of the analytic setting only with a true friend or close relative.

Yet no therapist can achieve a consistently empathic immersion in another's experience. Essentially the design of our psyche—the nature of human relating—mitigates against it. Even a largely consistent empathic stance is very hard to achieve.

In a discussion of the highly disciplined, consistently empathic inquiry written about and practiced by the analyst Evelyne Schwaber, Lawrence Friedman (1992) noted that in Dr. Schwaber's persistent struggle to share her patient's point of view, she

> shows us something that we might not see as clearly in Kohut: it is not just empathy that is powerful, but the wish and effort to empathize. Dr. Schwaber puts the spotlight on what is in the shadow of Kohut's theory: the negative aspect of empathizing is as important as the positive; the empathizer's willingness to give up his own investment. . . . The analyst is frustrating her own natural thinking style in order to . . . come close to the patient. Recognizing the magnitude of the sacrifice, the patient can probably feel the analyst's urge toward closeness almost physically. Ordinarily, only an unusually dedicated love would produce such a self-sacrificing devotion. . . . Most analysts want to know their patients well. But they are not all equally willing to discomfort themselves in the process, and not all theories encourage such discomfort.

We think Friedman has accurately captured some of the enormous meaning communicated within the struggle (see Schwaber, 1983) to maintain an empathic stance. We also suggest that Kohut and the self psychologists have, as Friedman notes, left the meaning of this struggle in the shadows. There has been a tendency in self psychology to discuss the empathic stance in ways that imply that it is largely a technical maneuver.

Attributing failures of empathy to individual countertransference or faulty technique (and successes to proper techniques and a lack of countertransference interference) can be very misleading; it is only one version of the story, a limited version that leaves out the fact that we experience consistently empathic responsiveness as a (usually very welcome) deviation from what is normative in virtually all human relationships—not simply from those relationships that have significantly failed us. Every child is prepared (from the moment of conception onward) to expect that the relational world will be filled with hard-to-recognize conflict, conflict that is likely to be hidden behind rules and views that are represented as more tailored to the child's own interests than in fact they are.

A consistently empathic stance is, in this sense, simply unnatural. A highly consistent attempt to communicate to the patient exclusively from a vantage point within the patient's subjective world (although absolutely crucial) will tend to be only cautiously accepted by some patients and, for others, will become suspect as a strategy for hiding the therapist's self. Some therapists may, in fact, use the empathic stance to remain defensively hidden from their patients. Over and above any particular individual defensiveness that may be attributed to the therapist, the overly consistent use of the empathic mode will, for some patients, be sensed as the therapist's hiding some aspect of himself or herself, possibly in the pursuit of his or her own interests. Often, an immersion in the patient's subjective world must be complemented by what is, in effect, the visible expression of the therapist's reality (Ehrenberg, 1992; Fosshage, 1995).

As Modell (1991) notes, there is an enduring set of paradoxes here: the therapist cares and listens deeply, and yet, when the hour ends, the therapist summarily dismisses the patient. The patient must believe in the reality of the powerful feelings that arise in the relationship and yet tolerate that, at the very same time, to a degree, there are limits and boundaries on the expression of these feelings that would be inconceivable in a naturally occurring relationship. A patient once referred to this as an ongoing sense that one lives with a "taboo" in therapy, a certain taboo of the real. Many aspects of a real relationship are there but never fully touchable. Like all taboos, the forbidden fruit of the real heightens the power of the situation and also makes the situation quite precarious. For some patients, this particular heightened longing is unbearable. For most patients (and therapists) there are times when it is barely bearable. It is always a background tension.

"Throwing Away the Book," Self-Interest, and the Process of Achieving "Authenticity"

There are inevitably times when, as Hoffman (1994) says, the therapist must "throw away the book" in order to demonstrate a genuine willingness to place the patient before some of the rules of therapy. Patients can feel the therapist's move away from a loyalty to teachers, belief systems, the hiding places afforded by rules and rituals. There is a palpable satisfaction—perhaps a corrective emotional experience—in the sense of "spontaneous deviation . . . shared by patient and therapist . . . when they depart from an internalized convention of some kind." The "taboo of the real" is broken, and the validity of the therapeutic relationship is affirmed when the therapist's struggle to engage with a particular patient calls into question some of the rituals, rules, and beliefs important to the therapist (in this case encoded in a whole style and tone of relating). It becomes a more real relationship as the "one size fits all" structures, rules, and expectations set in place before the two parties even met are renegotiated in the specific relationship between two individuals.

Throwing away the book, however, can and has, in some circles, "become the book" (Hoffman, 1994)! A certain idealization of therapeutic spontaneity or self-disclosure tends to emerge in which this behavior itself becomes a new agenda, an agenda that, as we see it, *will inevitably become biased toward the needs and views of those who come to advocate it*. As any new therapeutic approach (any new stance and version of technique, regardless of its content) emerges, it will often represent, in part, a movement away from the therapist's traditional preconceptions and loyalties toward the patient's subjective reality. Then, as the new approach becomes codified, it will tend to become more and more invested with the therapist's own personal identity and agenda as well as the collective agenda of the members of a new faction or school.

With a bit more historical perspective than analysts are accustomed to adopting, we can see how virtually any codified analytic approach will almost certainly come to yield a new set of rituals. In other words, the reason that "throwing out the book becomes the book" lies precisely in the ongoing, natural tendency of therapists to *bias* the process toward their own ends. Hoffman seems to be addressing some of the problems introduced by this tendency toward bias when he recommends the maintenance of a "dialectic" between the therapist's acceptance of ritual authority and anonymity, on one hand, and "spontaneous deviation" (including self-revelations) from those rituals on the other. Out of this dialectical tension and acknowledgment of the paradoxical realness and unrealness of the analytic situation a more genuine "authenticity" in the therapist's participation is expected to emerge.

We believe that, if we appreciate Hoffman's paradoxical dialectic, we are likely to practice with a new sensibility rather than a new set of rules and technical guidelines. Such a sensibility represents a higher level principle concerning the necessary struggle with (deviation from) authority with which each therapeutic relationship compels us to engage. Thus, Hoffman's views probably encourage the sort of grappling with inner and interpersonal conflict that enhances the therapist's authenticity. Though such a higher principle is less likely to become codified and ritualized into a "new book," we suspect that, over time, even such a broad dialectical principle is not likely to transcend the deeply rooted tendency (in the therapist, his culture, his therapeutic "school") to translate and ritualize the meaning of the principle in ways that are biased toward his own subjective ends. Thus, ultimately, we would expect that this very dialectical principle would come to be concretized and practiced in a way that, itself, would need to be "deviated from" and negotiated.

The natural and universal tendency to bias technique (often self-deceptively) toward the analyst's interests is an important aspect of why consistent attempts to apply many specific analytic, technical prescriptions are of limited value (see Greenberg, 1995). Any stance or set of techniques that is formulated prior to the engagement of specific individuals in a particular psychoanalytic relationship—be it neutrality, sustained empathic inquiry, relational authenticity (or even a broad appreciation of the dialectic between ritual authority and spontaneity)—may tend to become deceptive, a deception that is usually rooted in self-deception. In this sense, "authenticity" in our responses as analysts is a quality that can only gradually be achieved, or created, through our struggle with our patients' influence on us: the struggle to reopen aspects of our own identity (including our therapeutic frame), with minimal deception and self-deception, in areas that are elicited by and relate to our patients' conflicts.

Sometimes the changes, the needed deviations, are "spontaneous," as Hoffman (1992) put it, only *after* the therapists' prolonged immersions in their own subjective world as it is influenced by their struggle to relate intimately with their patients. Consider Ogden's (1994) description of the coming to life of an analysis that had seemed correct but lifeless:

> In retrospect, my analytic work with Mrs B to this point had sometimes felt to me to involve an excessively dutiful identification with my own analyst (the 'old man'). I had not only used phrases that he had regularly used, but also at times spoke with an intonation that I associated with him. . . . My experience in the analytic work . . . had "compelled me" to experience the unconscious fantasy that the full realization of myself as an analyst could occur only at the cost of the death of another part of myself (the death of an internal object analyst/father) [p. 16].

At the outset of an analysis, the analyst may start out as a "new object," a person whom the patient can experience as having views, needs, and responsiveness different from the patient's familial objects (Greenberg, 1986). We also know, however, that usually the analyst simultaneously starts out as an "old object"; both patient and analyst will, from the outset, reenact old relational patterns. Only through a prolonged interpersonal and internal negotiation with the challenge and influence of the patient can the analyst, cumulatively, *become* for the patient a more fully usable "new object," new to the patient because the analyst is—through the negotiation process—new to him- or herself!

From this point of view, it is the experience of the process of negotiating the real conflicts between the analyst's and patient's "otherness"—their differing needs and identities—that constitutes "what is new." It is the patient's experience of the analyst's changing—of the analyst struggling to come to terms with something new—that provides the crucial knowledge that there is a genuine working negotiation occurring. Because the relationship between analyst and patient entails real conflicts between their identities, the negotiation process, ultimately involving real changes in the analyst, provides the crucial experience for the patient to reopen and rework old conclusions about his or her self and the potential for effective negotiations with the relational world.

Some Concluding Thoughts

As our patients try to raise questions about their own entrenched, debilitating ways of experiencing themselves, they use the transference to ferret out and activate within the current therapeutic relationship precisely those areas of relational conflict and (failed) interpersonal negotiation in which old conclusions about themselves were formed. The transference may begin by creating an "as-if" reality, if you will, a "potential space" for activating and exploring the past in the present. But, although this reliving of the patient's transference is crucial, it *cannot* be an end in itself. Such analytic "play" leads, in turn, to a call for the opening up of real, often unseen but inevitable, conflicts within the analyst and the conflicting needs of analyst and patient. In this sense, transference is a vehicle, a means to arrive at an arena in which the therapist's own identity, own real strivings and interests, become deeply engaged in the negotiation process. Transference (or projective identification) brings the analyst into a realm in which the past is not simply enacted (or affectively resonated with by the analyst) in the present. The past is, in fact, rediscovered by the patient in the present in a very profound way—in the analyst's identity and the realities of being with the analyst. As Edward put it, after years of intensely confusing negotiation, "This is such a strange relationship . . . We're here to understand me, but we have to understand you in order to understand me." Here is where the process of interpersonal, intersubjective negotiation becomes most difficult—and most genuine.

From the word go, the therapeutic relationship is filled with many moments—from mini-"crunches" (Russell, 1973) like those illustrated in the cases of Nancy and Tanya to vast, conflictual landscapes like that described between Edward and his analyst. This is the arena in which patients look for and enable us to see some of the divisions and tensions in our identity, the multiplicity and bias in us. Wittingly and unwittingly, we let them raise questions about who we are. Through such adaptive probing, patients may palpably sense how they can influence us ("deconstruct" us). They can sense how, when faced with this challenge, we put ourselves back together (in a somewhat different way) in the context of our particular relationship with them.

A genuine renegotiation, reintegration (an increased experience of "realness") is far more likely to occur when our patients see what happens when—tapping into the fault lines in our identity, our conflicts—they take us someplace that is obviously hard for us to go. But we go there and often change in the process, because having a relationship with them requires it. They are worth it. All the time, our patients provoke in us (and read) the quality of *our* inner dialectic, our ways of experiencing and resolving internal and interpersonal conflict. And they assess its implications for renegotiating or reintegrating *their* selves in the context of inducing us to adapt to them—and them to us.

References

Aron, L. (1991), The patient's experience of the analyst's subjectivity. *Psychoanal. Dial.*, 1:29–51.

———— (1992), Interpretation as an expression of the analyst's subjectivity. *Psychoanal. Dial.*, 2:475–507.

Bacal, H. & Thomson, P. G. (1996), The psychoanalyst's selfobject needs and the effects of their frustration on the treatment: A new view of countertransference. In: *Basic Ideas Reconsidered: Progress in Self Psychology, Vol. 12*, ed. A. Goldberg. Hillsdale, NJ: The Analytic Press, pp. 17–35.

Beebe, B. & Lachmann, F. (1988), Mother–infant mutual influence and precursors of psychic structure. In: *Frontiers in Self Psychology: Progress in Self Psychology, Vol. 3*, ed. A. Goldberg. Hillsdale, NJ: The Analytic Press, pp. 3–25.

Benjamin, J. (1988), *The Bonds of Love: Psychoanalysis, Feminism, and the Problem of Domination*. New York: Pantheon Books.

Blechner, M. (1992), Working in the countertransference. *Psychoanal. Dial.*, 2:161–179.

Bollas, C. (1987), *The Shadow of the Object: Psychoanalysis of the Unthought Known*. New York: Columbia University Press.

Bromberg, P. (1991), Introduction to symposium on reality and the analytic relationship. *Psychoanal. Dial.*, 1:8–12.

Davies, J. M. (1994), Love in the afternoon: A relational reconsideration of desire and dread in the countertransference. *Psychoanal. Dial.*, 4:153–170.

Ehrenberg, D. B. (1992), *The Intimate Edge*. New York: Norton.

Ferenczi, S. (1932), *The Clinical Diary of Sandor Ferenczi*, ed. J. Dupont (trans. M. Balint & N. Z. Jackson). Cambridge, MA: Harvard University Press, 1988.

Fosshage, J. (1995), Interaction in psychoanalysis: A broadening horizon. *Psychoanal. Dial.*, 5:459–478.

Friedman, L. (1991), Address to the American Psychoanalytic Association.

———— (1992), Discussion of Evelyne Schwaber's paper, "Psychoanalytic Theory and its Relation to Clinical Work." Presented at Scientific Meeting of the Psychoanalytic Society of New England, East, October 24.

Greenberg, J. (1986), Theoretical models and the analyst's neutrality. *Contemp. Psychoanal.*, 22:87–10.

———— (1995), Self-disclosure: Is it psychoanalytic? *Contemp. Psychoanal.*, 31:193–205.

Havens, L. (1993), *Coming to Life*. Cambridge, MA: Harvard University Press.

———— (1997), A linguistic contribution to psychoanalysis: The concept of performative constructions. *Psychoanal. Dial.*, 7:523–534.

Hoffman, I. Z. (1983), The patient as interpreter of the analyst's experience. *Contemp. Psychoanal.*, 19:389–442.

———— (1991), Toward a social constructivist view of the psychoanalytic situation. *Psychoanal. Dial.*, 1:74–105.

———— (1992), Some practical consequences of a social constructivist view of the psychoanalytic situation. *Psychoanal. Dial.*, 2:287–304.

———— (1994), Dialectical thinking and therapeutic action in the psychoanalytic process. *Psychoanal. Quart.*, 63:187–218.

Jacobs, T. (1991), *The Use of the Self*. New York: International Universities Press.

Kindler, A. (1995), Discussion of A. Ornstein's "The Rocky Road Toward a New Beginning." Presented at 18th Annual Conference on the Psychology of the Self, October 21, San Francisco.

Kohut, H. (1972), Thoughts on narcissism and narcissistic rage. *The Psychoanalytic Study of the Child*, 27:360–400. New Haven, CT: Yale University Press.

———— (1984), *How Does Analysis Cure?* ed. A. Goldberg & P. Stepansky. Chicago: University of Chicago Press.

Kriegman, D. (1998), Interpretation, the unconscious and analytic authority: Toward an evolutionary biological integration of the empirical scientific method with the field defining empathic stance. In: *Empirical Perspectives on the Psychoanalytic Unconscious*, ed. M. Bornstein & J. M. Masling. Washington, DC: American Psychological Association.

———— & Slavin, M. (1990), On the resistance to self psychology: Clues from evolutionary biology. In: *The Realities of Transference: Progress in Self Psychology, Vol. 6*, ed. A. Goldberg. Hillsdale, NJ: The Analytic Press, pp. 217–250.

Lichtenberg, J., Lachmann, F. & Fosshage, J. (1992), *Self and Motivational Systems*. Hillsdale, NJ: The Analytic Press.

McLaughlin, J. T. (1995), Touching limits in the analytic dyad. *Psychoanal. Quart.*, 64:433–465.

Mitchell, S. (1988), *Relational Concepts in Psychoanalysis: An Integration*. Cambridge, MA: Harvard University Press.

Modell, A. H. (1991), The therapeutic relationship as a paradoxical experience. *Psychoanal. Dial.*, 1:13–28.

Ogden, T. H. (1985), *The Matrix of the Mind*. New York: Aronson.

———— (1994), The analytic third: Working with intersubjective clinical facts. *Internat. J. Psycho-Anal.*, 75:3–19.

Ornstein, A. (1974), The dread to repeat and the new beginning: A contribution to the psychoanalysis of narcissistic personality disorders. *The Annual of Psychoanalysis*, Vol. 2:231–248. New York: International Universities Press.

Ornstein, P. (1979), Remarks on the central position of empathy in psychoanalysis. *Bull. Assn. Psychoanal. Med.*, 18:95–108.

Pizer, S. (1992), The negotiation of conflict in the analytic process. *Psychoanal. Dial.*, 2:215–240.

——— (1996). Negotiating potential space: Illusion, play, metaphor and the subjunctive. *Psychoanal. Dial.*, 6:689–712.

Rogers, A. (1995), A *Shining Affliction: A Story of Harm and Healing in Psychotherapy*. New York: Viking.

Russell, P. (1973), Crises of emotional growth (a.k.a. the theory of the crunch). Unpublished manuscript.

Sandler, J. (1976), Countertransference and role-responsiveness. *Internat. Rev. Psychoanal.*, 3:43–47.

Schwaber, E. (1983), Psychoanalytic listening and psychic reality. *Internat. Rev. Psychoanal.*, 10:379–392.

Searles, H. F. (1975), The patient as therapist to his analyst. In: *Tactics and Techniques in Psychoanalytic Theory, Vol. 2: Countertransference*, ed. P. Giovacchini. New York: Aronson, pp. 95–151.

Slavin, J. H. (1994), On making rules: Toward a reformulation of the dynamics of transference in psychoanalytic treatment. *Psychoanal. Dial.*, 4:253–274.

——— (1985), The origins of psychic conflict and the adaptive function of repression: An evolutionary biological view. *Psychoanal. Contemp. Thought*, 8:407–440.

——— (1996a), Is one self enough? Multiplicity in self organization and the capacity to negotiate relational conflict. *Contemp. Psychoanal.*, 32:615–625.

——— (1996b), Analytic re-parenting (and parenting) as negotiated achievements. Presented to Annual Spring Meeting of Division 39 of the American Psychological Association, New York City, April.

Slavin, M. O. & Kriegman, D. (1992), *The Adaptive Design of the Human Psyche: Psychoanalysis, Evolutionary Biology, and the Therapeutic Process*. New York: Guilford Press.

Stolorow, R. & Atwood, G. (1992), *Contexts of Being*. Hillsdale, NJ: The Analytic Press.

——— Brandchaft, B. & Atwood, G. (1987), *Psychoanalytic Treatment: An Intersubjective Approach*. Hillsdale, NJ: The Analytic Press.

Trivers, R. (1971), The evolution of reciprocal altruism. *Quart. Rev. Biol.*, 46:35–57.

——— (1974), Parent-offspring conflict. *Amer. Zoolog.*, 14:249–264.

Weiss, J. & Sampson, H. (1986), *The Psychoanalytic Process: Theory, Clinical Observation, and Empirical Research*. New York: Guilford Press.

Winnicott, D. W. (1950), Hate in the countertransference. In: *Collected Papers: Through Paediatrics to Psychoanalysis*. New York: Basic Books, 1975, pp. 194–203.

——— (1963), Communicating and not communicating leading to a study of certain opposites. In: *The Maturational Processes and the Facilitating Environment*. New York: International Universities Press, 1965.

——— (1969), The use of an object and relating through identifications. In: *Playing and Reality*. Middlesex, England: Penguin.

Afterword

Malcolm Owen Slavin

On many occasions when I have presented later versions of some of the ideas in this paper a few people (often newer analysts) remark that "hardly anybody talks like you and Kriegman do about the clashes between the needs of analysts and patients—about the patient's skepticism concerning the *unnaturalness* of the analytic frame and the meanings of its *lack* of reciprocity. You talk about these things as, well, facts of life, without pathologizing, without faulting either participant. It's a relief," they sometimes add, "to put this aspect of the work on the table theoretically and, especially, to be able to think about our own experiences with patients in these terms."

Yet other colleagues—responding to the same emphasis on the ever-present role of the analyst's self-interest as well as to the inherent realism we attribute to our patients' wariness about our influence—are more disturbed by what they believe are the implications of our stance. Sometimes they confide that they are having a hard time with what they call a harshness or darkness in our view of human motives. Or they worry that our emphasis on a certain *universality* in our patients' "adaptive skepticism" about being influenced by us will lead away from an appreciation of the idiosyncratic, transferential meanings of resistance, rooted largely in individual fantasy or trauma; or that our focus on the multiple, *deceptive potentials* inherent in the analytic frame will detract from an appreciation of analysis as a unique, magical potential space, a cherished theater for psychic change. A bit sheepishly, others confess a puzzlement over what to them seems like a contradiction between the paper's emphasis on the ubiquity of conflict—its repeated references to the "dark side," as Irwin Hoffman (2001) puts it, of the analytic frame—and the fact, say these colleagues, that they perceive me as a basically empathic, hopeful guy.

So, for six years, my own thinking about this paper has developed in spontaneous as well as formal, often quite candid, interaction with a very wide range of audiences in which I am the discussed or the discussant. It has developed through many intense, sustained relationships with supervisees and patients whose experience and response have tested the paper's assumptions about analysts and patients and challenged and extended the whole notion that "the analyst needs to change." Because this ongoing dialogue is the main source of whatever changes have taken place in "this analyst" regarding the paper, I present here my reflections as responses to the kinds of questions that have animated me over these years.

Where did the notion of the "analyst needing to change" originally come from? And why are there several footnoted allusions—but no direct arguments—connecting the analytic process to evolutionary biology and to the book you and Dan had just recently written about analytic models from that broad perspective?

Frankly, putting "needs to change" in the title was partially chosen for the obvious hyperbole in it. Over time the scope and importance of change in the analyst has become increasingly apparent. Beyond dramatizing the need to appreciate the reciprocal aspects of the analytic relationship, we teasingly implied that change comes about *only* if, in some fashion, the analyst changes. Something, we felt, had to help shake us analysts out of our relentless tendency to diagnose quickly the tensions in the relationship between analyst and patient into a set of eagerly waiting, familiar categories—transference, countertransference, empathic or selfobject breaks, resistance, enactment, projective identification, and so on. As illuminating as these technical categories may be at many stages of our work—and as necessary as some of them seem to our identities as analysts—we felt that constructing analytic experience in those familiar terms actually takes on far greater meaning when a strong, ongoing sense of dialectical tension is preserved between the human realness of the relationship and its various transferential or technical dimensions. We set out to bolster what we saw as the weaker pole of this "analytic versus broadly human" dialectic in the minds of most analysts *without*, we ardently prayed, relying on any new version of the ever-proliferating technical jargon that, itself, often undercut the vital tensions analysts experience in this realm.

How Dan and I came to construct a different picture of human motives and relating—a bit different sense of what's real—on this issue is, of course, linked to our book. We had spent many years looking at our clinical experience in part with eyes conditioned by thinking broadly about human nature in terms of contemporary evolutionary biological theory, an emerging viewpoint captured in a series of papers through the late 80s and culminating in our book (Slavin and Kriegman, 1992). It was this weaving inside and outside analysis—the impossible task of standing in both places at the same time—that made it look as though *all* analytic clinical models had very seriously underestimated how much the tensions between analyst and patient are rooted in the existential facts of their naturally differing, individual human perspectives. In the initial setting-up and ongoing maintenance of a good-enough working analytic relationship—ironically, perhaps especially in the strongest working relationships—analyst and patient continuously negotiate their own somewhat differing conscious and unconscious agendas and (however they subjectively define them) their own individual needs.

Yet in this paper the influence of evolutionary theory on our thinking was almost entirely acknowledged in footnotes on the advice of a friendly *Psychoanalytic Dialogues* editor who was interested in our analytic views. The editor cautioned that, at that time, the aversion of some postmodernist, relational analysts to anything that seemed universalizing and linked to biology—albeit simultaneously constructivist—could create roadblocks to publication.

Is the evolutionary theory linked to the fact that some colleagues feel there is something unduly harsh and dark about your emphasis on the pursuit of self-interest in human relating, on potentials for deception in the treatment relationship?

What stands out in contemporary evolutionary theory is that *two* contrasting motivational currents, self-interested and altruistic, evolved into a kind of innate dialectical tension in the human heart—a stark contrast to earlier, one-sided, social Darwinist views of human competitiveness and aggression that perhaps overly influenced Freud. In our book, we tried to make it clear that, from an evolutionary perspective, there is absolutely nothing deeper (more primary or innate) about self-interested motives than there is about the inherently prosocial, cooperative, human concern for related individuals. Both are equally ancient parts of us, if you will.

So it isn't that the "dark side" is writ so large. It's not. Rather, it is precisely the immense interdependence and mutuality in a good analytic relationship—as in most basically good-enough families—that, paradoxically, makes the interwoven threads of self-interest and bias stand out as incredibly significant, sometimes as problematic. But, on the other side, the painful and poignant tensions with self-interest give far greater meaning to the kinds of mutuality and love that can emerge. For me, the ironies here are actually what is quite hopeful. But some of our colleagues, of course, view this broader tragic side of an evolutionary worldview as if it were more one-sided than I believe it is.

But what about that whole other reaction, especially of younger colleagues, who feel more directly relieved in some way by what they hear in your perspective on their motives?

Yes, the main reaction to our normalizing or naturalizing narration of conflict in the analytic relationship has been that it is "freeing" in that it openly recognizes a substantial, self-interested side of doing analytic work that most analysts seem very well to know they experience. Analytic candidates, especially, find it useful to have a way to conceive of the legitimate, adaptive role of the analyst's self-interested motives as they try to negotiate that complicated, uncertainty-racked transition from what they have been calling psychotherapy to an analysis with their first controls. Deeply questioning their own legitimacy as analysts, many find it liberating not to have to hide or soften the sense that—however useful the analysis may eventually turn out to be for the patient—it is not difficult to recognize that, in the shorter run, many of the benefits to the *candidate* (the major professional and professional identity gains) are palpably real.

Ironically, the frank recognition of this realness about the tangible, shorter term benefits to the analyst often argues initially for acknowledging the ways in which good-enough, self-interested analysts *do not* need to change—they do not have to disavow their sense of the often disproportionately self-interested short-term benefits to them of the move to the couch. Except, of course, that reorienting themselves to the self-interested realities of the analytic enterprise in this way initially entails a kind of de-idealizing of themselves and of the altruistic nature of analytic practice. Though initially this experience may seem freeing, I am repeatedly struck by the way in which de-idealizing the analytic process while struggling to retain hope and confidence in it is one of the most telling processes of "change" that analysts in training undergo. I think the occurrence of change within many candidates in supervision has a real effect on their relationships with their patients. Perhaps that accounts for some of what some see as the surprising success of some control analyses despite the inexperience of the analyst.

So there seems to be something a bit more ironic about the notion that "the analyst needs to change" than you realized. Have you shifted and changed as an analyst—let's say in your view of what "the analyst needs to change" means? And of the therapeutic action?

Yes, the whole analytic enterprise—especially the process of negotiating change—looks more ironic, more paradoxical, sometimes more blatant, sometimes more subtle, more "right there" and couched in endless guises, than we could recognize when we wrote the paper. Several astute writers who have commented on our work (Benjamin, 1998, 2003; Ringstrom, 1998; Pizer, 1999) have led me to see how —interwoven with the negotiation of real conflicting interests—the subjective experiences through which we know and wrestle with those conflicts are often organized centrally around human developmental and intersubjective paradoxes. For me, though, appreciating the subjective paradoxes of development and object-relating ultimately remains most useful—feels most grounded and honest— when it is rooted in an awareness, and emotional acceptance, of the background tensions, indeed the real limits and dangers of conflict-ing interests in all intimate relating.

If you look at your own work and extend that work with "data" from the (sometimes strikingly) different work of supervisees, you continu-ally see that patients ask us to try to go somewhere—emotionally, imaginatively, ethically—somewhere beyond where, in virtually any other relationship, we are ready to go. The analytic frame serves us and protects us for sure, but in a way that also puts us in greater emo-tional jeopardy. We must sometimes bear more, or differently, than what we bear in any other intersubjective context. Whether this bur-den creates crunchlike impasses or simply subtle, long-term shifts in the building of a relationship, I keep finding myself struck by just how much, and in how many different ways, analysts are called on to revisit their own basic, internal, existential issues in order to relate deeply to a given patient despite the fact that analysts may well have resolved those issues sufficiently to function in the rest of their own lives. Moreover, in the process of doing this, it seems to me that often the analysis itself (or the working frame of a given analysis) also needs to change as part of the therapeutic action.

For my supervisees, me, and several creative analysts whose work I have studied and discussed these challenges can sometimes be incred-ibly agonizing and confusing—fraught with contradictions (see my dis-cussions [Slavin, 2002, 2003] of Atwood, Stolorow, and Orange [2001] and Davies [2003]). They are moments when the analyst's reality is pushed and challenged. In one form or other we end up being asked for something we *cannot* refuse yet, often, *must* refuse. Perhaps it is joining a patient's ultimate despair or madness in ways that simply defy any simple empathic recognition. If we *do not* find a visible way to join the patient, we abandon him or her. Yet it *seems* that, for long periods, if we *do* join them we must somehow violate something connected to our own beliefs, impose unacceptably on our lives, even seem to aban-don some key aspect of our therapeutic identity.

As I see it, these are the moments when many contemporary analysts increasingly call on constructs derived from Kleinian theory because they promise to narrate these moments in ways that seem to capture some of their mysterious, bigger-than-both-of-us projective qualities. In these accounts, the story seems inevitably to entail patients' evac-uating unbearable affect and conflict from themselves by putting it into us. Doing this compels us to feel their pain and coerces us into reenactments of *their* old relational scenarios.

In a small but very significant variation on this story, I have come to see these moments far less as patients' aiming to colonize us with their (pathological) stories and far more in the larger adaptive context in which the projections occur—that is, patients' vital human need to see who we are and what kind of potentially "new" experience they can have with us (Aron, 1996). Basically what we call projections usually look to me as though they are in part designed to serve as communicative probes, or vehicles, tactics, for compelling us analysts to experience *ourselves* more fully—and, if we are capable—to confront and struggle with real tensions within ourselves. These aspects of ourselves, as I view it, represent the *analyst's own versions* of the same human dilemmas (over what is real, over love and hate, self and other, self-esteem, meaning and despair) that prove overwhelming for our patients (and are, for all of us, ongoing, lifelong human adaptive challenges with which we never cease to grapple).

This kind of negotiation is essentially what goes on around key developmental issues between parents and children as parents inevitably struggle with (and defend against struggling with) the reopening of what are their own inner working solutions to the same issues faced by their children. The personal realness of this mutual challenge in analysis is what replicates the interactive context in which the patient's maladaptive solutions were shaped. The very realness of it for the analyst is, paradoxically, what allows the patient to develop deep, intense transferential meanings as the issue is relived, for real, with the analyst.

In other words, my sense is that I have become a usable, transferential version of a parent when, in some measure, I have allowed myself to become a bit lost at my version of that parenting place where a patient's earlier experience in the family failed. Together we may refind and revise something old in them, in part through my willingness to reopen and, I'll say it, *to suffer anew* something *old* in myself.

Though it is much clearer to me now than when the paper was written that there is a lot of basic healing of the analyst that goes on when we engage in this way, I still think that Searles (1975) too narrowly construed this process as therapeutic rather than more broadly, as two individuals engaged in an adult developmental process (P. Crastnopol, personal communication). Sometimes what seems key is the particular kind of love that is signaled by our willingness to suffer alongside the patient for stretches of time creating a more a level playing field— a field of two fellow sufferers—each dealing with their own version of the same human dilemmas.

So where in all this, as you said, does the analytic frame itself need to change?

What I am referring to is something that closely complements the analyst's very real, very personal willingness to struggle internally for and with the patient. In tension with the elements of intimate human relationships, all analytic approaches probably need to include some degree of ritualized authority (Hoffman, 1998)—a certain heightened dramatic structure that is intertwined with basic boundaries, rules, and roles but, in a sense, goes beyond rational technique into the realm of something that conjures a bit more mystery.

Set strictly apart from other relationships and deliberately wrapped (even by very open, interactive relational analysts) in a transference-inducing ambiguity, this aspect of the treatment relationship is particularly prone to being (and being experienced as) *deceptive*. Put bluntly, because the analyst's interests and belief system naturally infuse the design of the analytic frame, the patient needs to probe, explore, and establish how much and in what way the more mysterious qualities of the ritual and frame are, in this case, useful illusions versus well-meaning, but deceptive, hocus pocus.

In most of the successful analyses I have seen (and markedly not in the unsuccessful ones), there is a flexible process of negotiation over aspects of the analytic frame and process itself—aspects that, at first, were assumed by both analyst and patient to be in some way integral, sacred, essential to the analytic process. Just as our personal openness to reexperiencing our versions of the issues with which patients struggle enables them to trust that we truly grasp their interests, so our readiness to reopen, examine and alter our relationship with some sacred aspects of the analytic process (to which we have been wedded) often seems indispensable to generating a sense that the analytic process is aligned with who they are.

Sometimes it is literally impossible for very fine, otherwise flexible analysts to move far enough within the timeframe of the analysis. I recently heard of two analysts who were able to do so *after* the analysis and were lucky enough to have second chances when, later on, the patients returned (Cooper, 2003; Pizer, 2004). I hope it is clear that I am *not* advocating an automatic, unreflective "giving in" to our patients' views or accommodation to their pressures for changes in the frame. Remember, Dan and I strongly emphasize analysts' need to look out for their own interests, and their interests are often embedded in, and protected by, the analytic frame. Indeed, as Glen Gabbard (personal communication) has said, a clear understanding that there are inherently differing, sometimes conflicting, needs of patient and analyst may ultimately be our best protection against regressive pulls toward boundary blurring, even boundary violation.

I *am* advocating that—after struggling to grasp deeply the differences between our experiential world and that of our patients—we make many of our complex decisions about what to preserve or modify in the frame in terms of what we ultimately believe is essential for *us* at this moment as well as for *our* broader way of working—not in terms of various abstractions about analytic authority. The frank recognition and expression of our own interests, combined with our understanding that our needs will sometimes strongly conflict as well as coincide with those of our patients, preserves a vital kind of tension and realness in our work. We believe that this stance inclines us toward an overall analytic sensibility (and way of negotiating) that differs from most efforts to preserve the frame based primarily on particular, theoretically rooted understandings of what kind of limits, containment, selfobject needs, spontaneous disclosures, and so forth are presumed to be in the *patient's* interest.

Six years after publication, it seems clearer that the vital role of flexibility and change in the frame—like change in the analyst—must emanate from an acute awareness of how our own investment in the analytic frame is, itself, a very complex human commitment, tied to some of our own needs, to our professional identity and beliefs, as well as to our attachment, empathy, understanding—growing intimacy with—a particular patient. We must allow the multiple, sometimes contradictory, strands in our commitment to be challenged and *partially disassembled*. Each strand shifts in relative weight and meaning, yielding new experience for the analyst and patient, as well as a revised version of the frame. The analytic process comes to tap the power of an ancient, evolved human imperative—the yearning for genuine reciprocity. What is inevitably a generic, off-the-shelf analysis at the start is partially dismantled and, with luck, within a time period both parties can tolerate, changed into a novel, idiosyncratic engagement.

References

Aron, L. (1996), *A Meeting of Minds: Mutuality in Psychoanalysis.* Hillsdale, NJ: The Analytic Press.

Atwood, G., Stolorow, R. & Orange, D. (2001), Shattered worlds/psychotic states: A post-Cartesian view of the experience of personal annihilation. *Psychoanal. Psychol.*, 19(2).

Benjamin, J. (1998), Finding the way out: Commentary on papers by Slavin and Kriegman and Ringstrom. *Psychoanal. Dial.*, 8:589–598.

——— (2003), Discussion of "The analyst's otherness as a source of hope" by M. O. Slavin. Presented at spring meeting, Division 39, American Psychological Association, Minneapolis, MN, April.

Cooper, S. (2003), The new bad object and the therapeutic action of psychoanalysis. Keynote address, Division 39, American Psychological Association, Minneapolis, MN, April.

Davies, J. M. (2003), Whose bad objects are these anyway? Repetition and our elusive love affair with evil. Presented at conference of International Association for Relational Psychoanalysis and Psychotherapy, Toronto, January.

Hoffman, I. Z. (1998), *Ritual and Spontaneity in the Psychoanalytic Process.* Hillsdale, NJ: The Analytic Press.

Pizer, S. (1999), *Building Bridges: The Negotiation of Paradox in Psychoanalysis.* Hillsdale, NJ: The Analytic Press.

———— (2004), Impasse recollected in tranquility: Love, dissociation, and discipline in the analytic process. *Psychoanal. Dial.,* 14:289–312.

Ringstrom, P. (1998), Therapeutic impasses in contemporary psychoanalytic treatment. *Psychoanal, Dial.,* 8:297–315.

Searles, H. F. (1975), The patient as therapist to his analyst. In: *Tactics and Techniques in Psychoanalytic Theory. Volume II: Countertransference,* ed. P. Giovacchini. New York: Aronson, pp. 95–151.

———— & Kriegman, D. (1992), *The Adaptive Design of the Human Psyche: Psychoanalysis, Evolutionary Biology, and the Therapeutic Process.* New York: Guilford Press.

Slavin, M. (2002), Post-Cartesian thinking and the dialectic of doubt and belief in the treatment relationship: A discussion of "Shattered worlds/psychotic states: A post-Cartesian view of the experience of personal annihilation" by G. Atwood, D. Orange, and R. Stolorow. *Psychoanal. Psychol.,* 19(2).

———— (2003), How we struggle to become "new objects." Discussion of Jody Messler Davies's "Whose bad objects are these anyway? Repetition and our elusive love affair with evil." Presented at conference of International Association for Relational Psychoanalysis and Psychotherapy, Toronto, January.

Show Some Emotion: Completing the Cycle of Affective Communication

(1999)

Karen J. Maroda

▼   ▼   ▼   ▼   ▼

Editors' Introduction

With the shift from a one-person to a two-person psychology that has defined the relational turn in psychoanalysis has come a heightened attention to the personal involvement of patient and analyst and of the affective link between them. Karen Maroda has courageously called for emotional honesty and affective self-disclosure in the analytic encounter. While Maroda's work is profoundly personal and creative, however, more than others, she has also insisted that theorists of psychoanalytic technique articulate the principles that guide their clinical interventions so that these procedures can be taught and studied systematically. She began to outline her own systematization of psychoanalytic technique in her 1991 book, *The Power of Countertransference* (reprinted 2004 by The Analytic Press) and continued her exploration in *Seduction, Surrender, and Transformation* (1999, The Analytic Press), a sample from which follows.

What are the actual clinical implications of a relational approach for psychoanalytic technique and practice? In the chapter-sample that follows, Karen Maroda calls on psychotherapists to "show some emotion." Maroda proposes a thoroughly interactive model of psychoanalytic practice in which the patient learns through the medium of affective communication with the analyst. Maroda grounds her technical recommendations in a clinical theory of affect. Given that most patients have problems with affect management, completing cycles of affective communication between therapist and patient becomes vitally important in the therapeutic process.

Maroda's writing is consistently passionate, challenging, and provocative. Where psychoanalysis used to call for abstinence, neutrality, and anonymity, Maroda pushes for emotional honesty and personal availability. In the introduction to *Seduction, Surrender, and Transformation*, Maroda writes that "relational analysis requires both parties to examine how and why they are in conflict—what led up to this event, how each person experiences it, how each person's history sets the stage for the current conflict, and finally, how they must reveal their emotional responses to each other and resolve the conflicts as best they can" (p. 4).

While promoting radical mutuality and a thoroughly interactive clinical methodology, Maroda never avoids or neglects facing the role of power and authority within the analytic dyad. She remains carefully attentive to the asymmetries of power and to the need to develop psychoanalytic principles of technique that protect the integrity of the analytic process.

Show Some Emotion: Completing the Cycle of Affective Communication*

▼   ▼   ▼   ▼   ▼

Mutual surrender is a sine qua non for therapeutic action, that is, change. But what actually takes place in this moment of surrender that allows for change or transformation? In order to understand and facilitate a therapeutic surrender, we need to understand better the nature of affects and the role of emotion in individual growth and development,

---

* An earlier version of this chapter appears in Karen J. Maroda, *Seduction, Surrender, and Transformation: Emotional Engagement in the Analytic Process.* © 1999 The Analytic Press, Inc.

as well as in the therapeutic process. What follows is both a review of the relevant literature on emotions, and an application of this information to the therapeutic process. It appears that many, if not most, of our patients suffer from impairments in affective experience and regulation, and that there is evidence that we need to express our own emotions to facilitate our patients' affective development. Building on Stern's (1985) notions of *intereffectivity* and *affective attunement*, I propose that the analyst's affective responses are critical for completing the cycle of affective communication. This chapter concludes with an in-depth discussion of the clinical implications of the uses of emotion in analytic treatment.

Psychoanalysis and Affective Theory

First, what is the role of affect in classical analysis? Shapiro and Emde (1991) make the point that Freud and his followers "did not develop a coherent model accounting for affectivity in clinical theory and even less so in metapsychology" (p. iii). Blum (1991) adds that Freud focused rather narrowly on the notion of affective abreaction, or the notion of reliving a traumatic incident and catharting the disturbing emotions. (See Spezzano, 1993, for a comprehensive review of the literature on affect in psychoanalysis.) Little was known during Freud's lifetime about affective development, let alone the neurological foundation and locations for affective experience. I make this point not in the interest of criticizing classical theory or practice, but rather to emphasize the obvious: as research in human development and neuropsychology provide new information that has important implications for the therapeutic process, we have the opportunity to modify our ideas and interventions accordingly. And the topic of affect now affords us just such an opportunity.

The cumulative research over the past 30 years tells us much about affect development and the importance of affective communication. The essence of this chapter is that the *mutually affective moment* constitutes what is therapeutic between analytic therapist and patient. And that the therapist plays a critical role in helping patients compensate for early deficits in the ability to know, feel, name, express, and manage both the basic, innate affects (e.g., fear and anger) and the more differentiated and cognitively mediated affects (e.g., shame and love). Thus, just as the mother played this role in early childhood, the therapist facilitates the cycle of affective communication within the therapeutic relationship.

If we look at the child research for clues as to what our adult patients need, there is a plethora of information. Schore (1994) notes that as early as 60 years ago, the Russian psychologist Vygotsky, studying the basic mechanism under-lying the internalization of higher psychological functions, posited the general developmental principle that all psychological processes appear first at an interpersonal and only later at an intrapersonal level . . . all higher functions emerge as a result of social interaction [p. 358].

This is an amazing statement that, if true, validates not only the thera-peutic enterprise, but also the contemporary emphasis on the interper-sonal aspects of treatment. Vygotsky's theory supports the notion that intrapsychic change across a broad array occurs as a result of interper-sonal exchanges, lending credence to the concept of a more active, expressive therapist. But is Vygotsky's theory supported by modern research? To a great degree, it is. Stern (1985), in reporting his research results, says:

One conclusion is that the infant somehow makes a match between the feeling state as experience within and as seen "on" or "in" another, a match that we can call *interaffectivity*.

Interaffectivity may be the first, most pervasive, and most immedi-ately important form of sharing subjective experiences. Demos (1980, 1982a), Thoman and Acebo (1983), Tronick (1979), and others, as well as psychoanalysts, propose that early in life affects are both the primary *medium* and the primary *subject* of communication [pp. 132–133].

The primary importance of affect continues as the infant evolves, and at around nine months, according to Stern, mothers naturally change the nature of their affective responses, moving from mere imitation of the infants' affect to responding with their own affective expressions. Stern says that "what is being matched is not the other person's behavior per se, but rather some aspect of the behavior that reflects the person's feel-ing state" (p. 142). He refers to this affective matching between mother and infant as *"affective attunement."*

Although the literature on adults does not address the issue of affec-tive attunement per se, the longstanding recognition of the therapeutic benefits of high-level empathy can be understood as a similar mechanism for promoting affective development in the therapeutic relationship. The analytic theory most compatible with a notion of the need for a life-long affective attunement with others would be Kohut's (1984) ideas regard-ing the never-ending need for mature self objects who, by definition, pro-vide needed empathy and affective responding.

Stern (1985), Stolorow, Brandchaft, and Atwood (1987) and Stolorow and Atwood (1992) emphasize that infants and children are heavily depen-dent on affective responses from their caretakers. Without affective responses they lack internal organization and the ability to express and contain their own affective experiences. Stolorow and Atwood (1992) refer to Krystal, stating that

> Krystal (1988) has suggested that a critical dimension of affective development is the evolution of affects from their early form, in which they are experienced as bodily sensations, into subjective states that can gradually be verbally articulated. . . .
>
> [A]ffects may fail to evolve from bodily states to feelings because, in the absence of validating responsiveness, they are never able to become symbolically articulated. Hence the person remains literally alexithymic [pp. 186, 187].

Alexithymia, of course, is the inability to express, differentiate, and name emotions (with the exception of occasional angry outbursts) and usually results from childhood trauma. While most patients do not present with alexithymia, most patients are lacking in affect development in some significant way. Brown (1993) notes that developmental failures in affect may "manifest themselves in one or more areas: expression, experience, tolerance, verbalization, recognition, orientation, transformation, and consciousness of affective processes, respectively" (p. 43). So we are left with the knowledge that the "capacity for affective expression may be innate, but the capacity for affect experience unfolds in the course of development" (p. 6). As the child develops, he or she builds an increasing repertoire of emotions and learns that affects are a primary mode of communication, that they act as "signals for another person" (Krystal, 1988, p. 17). Children's abilities to accurately label and express their feelings are highly dependent on how often and to what degree their caretakers express their own feelings (Brody and Harrison, 1987). Krystal (1988) also tells us that a critical dimension of affective development is the "evolution of affects from their early form, in which they are experienced as bodily sensations, into subjective states that can gradually be verbally articulated" (p. 42). (He notes that alexithymic patients remain stuck at the level of experiencing affect only, or primarily, as physical sensations or symptoms.) The most significant aspect of affect that *does not change with development* is that "nothing becomes an emotion until it travels outside of the brain to the musculature and microcirculation of the face, there to be assessed and interpreted as an affective response" (Nathanson, 1996, p. 385). (Tomkins, 1962, of course, did the pioneering research on innate affect and its expression on the face.) So when we think we know what a patient is feeling by the look on his or her face, we are probably right. Just as the patient knows what we are feeling in the same way.

Much of the controversy regarding therapist self-disclosure has been based not just on the issue of "contamination" but also on the relative superficiality assumed in the verbal exchanges between therapist and patient. Where is the unconscious in all of this? Are we simply to assume that both analyst and patient actually know what each is feeling most of the time? The answer to that is no, of course not. An accurate reading of affect depends on both parties' trusting their visceral responses to, and sufficient ability to read, a variety of facial expressions. And these expressions will occur, even if one is unaware of them. My patient, Susan, who is alexithymic and almost always denies being angry, very often registers the facial expression documented by Tomkins (1962) as rage. And I find myself feeling uneasy and somewhat defended when she walks into her session wearing this facial expression, no matter what she says to me about what she is feeling. Her face and my gut reaction match each other and tell more truth than what she can always consciously know.

Another important aspect of the expression of emotion is that it is social (Parkinson, 1996) and, as such, often appears just as the patient enters the office. The expression has been saved for me, or occurs in response to me, for a specific purpose, whether or not the patient is aware of this purpose. Parkinson cites a study by Kraut and Johnston (1979), who observed bowlers and noted that they had one set of responses when they turned to face the other bowlers, the latter responses being much more animated and expressive. When they were facing the pins, there was no point in registering any facial expressions, because there was no one to receive them. Parkinson cites this as evidence that emotions are social and serve as a form of communication. He says,

> Many emotions have relational rather than personal meanings (e.g., deRivera, 1984) and the expression of these meanings in an emotional interaction serves specific interpersonal functions depending on the nature of the emotion . . . emotion is social through and through. Its fundamental basis in many cases is as a form of communication [p. 680].

Therefore, therapists and patients alike constantly register emotional reactions to each other, helping to inform each other of their true feelings, regardless of their conscious experience.

To summarize, infants and children learn to express their emotions freely, and ultimately, through their mothers' responses, learn how to name, differentiate, and manage them. Initially the mother typically only mirrors the child's rather basic expression, but as the child expands his or her repertoire the mother responds, not just with mirroring, but mixes in her own personal emotional response. As Thompson (1988) says, "Emotion is initially regulated by others, but over the course of early development it becomes increasingly self-regulated as a result of neuropsychological development" (p. 371). Since these experiences are universal, doesn't it seem likely that the therapist helping an adult with affective regulation problems would need to follow the same basic principles for facilitating affective regulation that are used in childhood? Both verbal and nonverbal interventions need to be appropriate for the adult patient, yet it is hard to imagine that the process for learning affect management would differ substantially regardless of the age of the patient. If we further consider that the route to intrapersonal development is relational, or interpersonal, then the affective attunement between analyst and patient becomes a critical variable in the therapeutic action.

Written on the Body

Although I concur with Stolorow, Atwood, and Krystal regarding the importance of reciprocal mutual influence for the regulation and integration of affective experience, I *disagree* with the implied conclusion that children evolve into adults who rely primarily on symbolic articulation of affect—words. Certainly, if all goes well, the acquisition of language facilitates the regulation of affect, in that it gives the individual the opportunity to label, discuss, understand, and mediate affective states. A basic analytic tenet says that we use our intellect to help organize and regulate our affective experiences. Verbal expressions also allow some form of affective communication in instances when strong displays of emotion might be considered socially inappropriate and would therefore be punished.

While acknowledging the inherent importance of developing the ability to label and discuss emotions rather than only experiencing them as bodily states, I disagree with the assumption that continued development negates the critical aspect of *physically experiencing emotions* to complete an affective communication. We all know that we experience feeling viscerally and that this is true throughout our lifetime. Our minds do not cue us that we are feeling something strongly; our bodies do. Our minds inquire as to the origin and meaning of that feeling, and help us to manage those feelings. But without the bodily sensation, there is no inquiry. (After all, even in adulthood the face remains the primary signaler of an affective event, rather than verbal expressions.)

Fast (1992) tried to recapture the importance of the body, as well as the mind, in her paper on mind-body and the relational perspective. She says that while Freud's notions of bodily involvement in emotional states were erroneous, he was correct in assuming a mind-body relationship. She notes that even though Freud understood well that infants cannot separate thought from bodily action, he chose to emphasize the later period when mental consideration preceded motoric action.

Fast credits Piaget for noting a mind-body period of development. But, like Freud, he proposed that normal development progresses to the point where the capacity for thought is free of the body. The implication is that emotion is registered intellectually, *in the mind*, rather than physically, *in the body*, if development occurs normally. Therefore, even though it is undoubtedly true that the capacity for verbalizing and cognitively mediating emotion evolves developmentally, the body never ceases to be a critical part of the emotion-signaling system, which Kelly (1996) describes as "critical for immediate, first-line survival" (p. 61).

Grotstein (1997), lamenting the separation of mind and body in analytic thinking, says they are

> always inseparable but that they *seem* to lend themselves to the Cartesian artifice of disconnection so that we can conceive of one or another for the sake of discrimination. Put another way, I believe that the *mindbody* constitutes a single, holistic entity, one that we can think about and believe that we can imaginatively experience as being separate but that is mockingly *nonseparate* all the while [p. 205].

Psychoanalysis, as it recognizes the importance of affect in human development, subsequently faces the task of re-integration of mind and body. What we know to be true is that patients who have been traumatized, and also the general population of personality disorders, demonstrate developmental failures in experiencing and managing affect. And these people represent a large percentage of those currently seeking treatment. Of course, it is no news to most clinicians that many of our patients suffer from the inability to experience and regulate their emotions. Much of the countertransference literature focuses on the affective onslaught one faces when treating many cases of narcissistic and border-line personality disorders. We have known for a long time that affect regulation is a problem that these patients bring to treatment and that presents a significant challenge to us as therapists. But I would have to add that I do not think we have been terribly successful in developing adequate theories and techniques for dealing with these patients. And the idea of using our bodily sensations as signals remains foreign.

To what extent do both our patients and ourselves use our bodies to register, and even communicate, deep emotions? I doubt that anyone could honestly say that he experiences a deep emotion without some observable accompanying physical sensation. And perhaps, in our desire to elevate the mind above the body, we have underestimated the role of the body in communication.

If we conceive of projective identification as primarily a body-to-body communication, then the simple containment of that affect by the analyst is insufficient on two grounds: one, letting the patient know that the communication has been received, and two, helping the patient to translate his emotional state into verbal representations—something that is essential to communication in the adult world. Understanding that the ability to verbalize affective states is a developmental achievement only partially acquired by many of our patients, we can naturally look more closely at body language, physical sensations, and projective identifications to help us understand and treat our patients. I think our resistance to "going first" when it comes to verbalized affective expressions often deprives our patients of the affective responding they need to further their own development.

We seem obsessed with the notion of "containment" of the patient's affect, which has limited value in terms of helping the patient with affect regulation. And I often wonder *who* or *what* we are really interested in *containing*. Discussions of therapist expression of affect at professional meetings often reflect a myriad of fears over what will happen if the analyst is overtly emotional. Terms like "out of control" and "potential for abuse" often drown out any serious discussion of how to use emotion constructively in the analytic setting.

Is Affect Inhibition Overvalued?

It seems that we have few problems diagnosing patients who suffer from the inability to contain and mediate their affective responses. These are the patients who often make our lives miserable as we attempt to cope with their emotional outbursts and impulsive behaviors. Unquestionably, treating people who are consistently out of control is challenging and stressful. But what about the patients who are *overcontrolled?* Do we worry less about them, and become complacent because they can provide an often much-needed respite from our patients who overwhelm us with their affective regulation problems?

In recent years Krystal (1988) and McDougall (1982) have raised our awareness of the patients who are alexithymic. Rather than presenting hysterically, these patients are very much in control and take pride in their cool, calm, collected manner, which society often rewards. Krystal says,

> What is deceptive to those unfamiliar with this disturbance is that these patients, who often function very successfully in their work, appear

"superadjusted" to reality and lead one to expect excellent intellectual function. However, getting past the superficial impression of superb functioning, one uncovers a sterility and monotony of ideas and severe impoverishment of the imagination [p. 247].

Susan, the aforementioned patient whom I have chosen to use throughout this volume, certainly qualifies as alexithymic, arriving for her first session immaculately dressed, polite, pleasant, and appearing to function at a high level. When I asked her if she had ever been in treatment before, she related a history of four previous therapists, although none for any length of time, all of whom deemed her to be quite sane. One simply dismissed her as not needing therapy. And another took her as a lover, in part because she perceived Susan as wealthier, more successful, and more in control than she. The therapist's wish to be taken care of by Susan emerged soon after they began their affair. What made me aware that there was more to Susan than met the eye was her history and her current lack of emotional distress or insight regarding her life situation. You may recall that she came for therapy because she was unable to look for work and did not understand why. She was also socially isolated, lonely, and had no insight into her past failed relationships, including the affair with her last therapist. She showed no emotion when I questioned her about her past and expressed what I considered to be an unnatural lack of anger or regret over her therapist's abuse of her. She said that she dumped the therapist and had felt in control of the whole affair, so there was no reason to be upset. These attitudes told me that Susan had some very serious emotional problems, no matter how cool she seemed. In the sessions that followed over the next few months, Susan showed the same lack of emotion when she described her rather traumatic childhood, which included daily verbal and physical abuse by her parents. She described her mother as being completely emotionless, a "blank screen" who would not tolerate any show of emotion by her children, deeming it a "sign of weakness." Susan never remembered her dreams and literally did not know what I was talking about when I asked her about her fantasies.

Patients like Susan often spend years in psychoanalysis, dully repeating the details of their lives, but rarely getting any better. However, unless they regress (in which case all hell breaks loose), these patients do not demand our attention. Krystal (1988) notes that they come on time, pay their fees, and are generally responsible and undemanding. Yet their problems are just as serious as the patients who constantly demand that we notice them. Averill (1994) points out that the person who cannot express emotion in an open and effective manner when appropriate is as much out of control as is the person who habitually "lets it all hang out." Control implies the ability to respond in the way one wants, whether that entails the inhibition or expression of a response [p. 267].

I would add that it is not only what the person wants that is important, but also what is emotionally honest and what is optimally desirable at the moment. But I agree with Averill that helping our inhibited, cooperative, and well-behaved patients to be more emotional should he as important as helping our over-emotional patients to contain themselves. The fact that society will reward the former but not the latter should not cloud our clinical assessment of the patient's capacity for healthy affect regulation.

Emotion and Cognition

First of all, all learning is facilitated through emotion. Contrary to what many people believe, cognitive processing is effected significantly by emotion. People are far more likely to remember something that elicited an emotional reaction (Bower, 1994). Panskepp (1994) cites research that demonstrates the critical role of emotion in all types of cognitive functions:

[T]he easiest way to light up higher mental processes—of thought, strategies, and conniving—is to activate basic emotional systems (Gray, 1990). When these basic systems have been aroused, then cognitive activity flows spontaneously [p. 313].

This information stands in stark contrast to the belief that emotions hinder or prevent clear thinking, reasoning, and problem solving. Certainly excessive emotion impairs reality testing and, good judgment, but the optimal condition is ongoing, manageable emotional stimulation, not the absence of strong feeling. Emotion plays an important role not only in the quality of cognition, but also in the type. Clore (1994) says that

findings suggest that emotion influences cognitive processing, perhaps in very fundamental ways. Positive affect appears to encourage unconstrained, heuristic processing, sometimes with creative results, while sad affect seems to foster a focus on more controlled, systematic processing [p. 110].

So the nature of our feelings also determines the nature of our thoughts, and vice versa. (The cognitive behaviorists have at least half of this right.) The essential role of emotion in effective information processing highlights not only the patient's need for ongoing, regulated affect, but also the therapist's. As I stated earlier in this volume, the analytic therapist who places too much emphasis on thoughts and interpretations, and avoids having strong feelings, cannot only fail to stimulate affective expression and management in her patients, but also will fail to *think optimally about the patient's condition and needs*. Just as mind and body cannot be separated, neither can feelings and thoughts.

Furthermore, the established relationship between emotion and cognition provides evidence that a good treatment needs to be an ongoing emotional event. If we accept that people change only when they can feel deeply and freely, when these feelings are responded to affectively by another person, and that both negative and positive affects provide opportunities for different types of cognitive processing, the responsibility for the analytic therapist to be emotionally involved, available, and expressive becomes greater.

What Is Emotional Memory?

Orange (1995) brought the concept of emotional memory to the forefront of analytic thinking. She says it "includes any form or part of experience that largely bypasses cognitive processes and carries significant residues from the intersubjective worlds of the past. Emotional memory has an unmediated quality that makes it feel compelling" (p. 113). She talks about how emotions can actually have a life of their own, which when I read it, seemed like a foreign idea to me. Didn't I just say that thoughts and feelings operate in concert? How then, can there be a strictly emotional memory? And what does emotional memory have to do with current functioning and the treatment situation?

For one thing, the concept of emotional memory is somewhat vague and unproven in the broad application that Orange provides. She built on the ideas of Emde, whom Clyman (1991) quotes regarding the idea of a recurrent pattern of affective experience. Clyman says that "Emde (1983) has suggested that there is a prerepresentational 'affective core of the self' which guarantees our sense of continuity across development in spite of the many ways we change" (p. 378). In other words, we have fairly stable ways of emotionally experiencing life that is not significantly altered by new experience. In this sense, a core affective pattern would he part of a necessary homeostasis, a notion supported by Schore (1994).

> Early object relational experiences thus directly influence the emergence
> of a frontolimbic system in the right hemisphere that can adaptively

autoregulate both positive and negative affect in response to changes in the socioemotional environment. . . . The core of the self lies in patterns of affect regulation that integrates a sense of self across state transitions, thereby allowing for a continuity of inner experience [p. 33].

So there is clinical and experimental evidence that stable affective patterns, as well as specific affective reactions, exist and are called forth by stimuli that somehow mimic the original event. And Freud, once again, turns out to have known quite a bit. He hypothesized that we tended to recreate the same emotional scenarios over and over again, although he did not know at the time that affect-laden experiences actually have their own independent storehouse in the brain, ready to be recalled at an instant. I would add to this that the re-experiencing of past, intense affect is always a visceral event that is part of what makes it so real in the present, even if it entails some cognitive distortion so that it can be ordered up. For example, in the case of Susan, when she lies down on the couch and talks to me about how abusive her parents were, she begins to have these feelings all over again. The fact that her parents would throw her down on the floor and stand over her, sometimes slapping her, only increases the intensity of her equating the analytic process (lying on the couch, with me slightly away and above her in my chair) with her most negative early childhood experiences. Susan honestly feels at those moments that I am abusing her just as her parents did. She is swept away by her emotional memories and the visceral reenactment she experiences. In her mind, I must hold and comfort her to prove that I am different from her parents and not taking sadistic delight in her agony.

LeDoux (1994) tells us that it is important to distinguish between emotional memory and memory of emotion:

The latter is a declarative, conscious memory of an emotional experience. It is stored as a fact about an emotional episode.

Emotional memory (mediated by the amygdala) and memory of emotion (mediated by the hippocampus) can be reactivated in parallel on later occasions. . . . In summary, emotional and declarative memory about emotion are mediated by different brain systems. These systems operate simultaneously and parallel during experiences. As a result, we can have conscious insight into our emotions and emotional memories . . . without emotions, one would have to learn the positive and negative stimulus value of situations through strictly cognitive means [p. 312].

So our emotional memory reminds us of the importance, or lack of importance, danger or safety, of everything in our environment. Emotional memory allows for homeostasis, but it is also a keystone of the phenomenon of "learning from one's experience." As LeDoux says, our emotional memory tells us immediately what to do, saving us the trouble of think-ing through every new situation. On the less adaptive side, it may also instruct us to avoid some person, place or thing that reminds us of some-thing unpleasant from the past that may, in reality, offer something pos-itive that our emotional memory blinds us to.

Once again, Freud has been vindicated, in the sense that he posited transference as an established pattern of relating and emotional respond-ing that is cued by something in the present, but oftentimes calls up both an affective state and thoughts that may have more to do with past expe-rience than present ones. And even though Freud intuitively understood the importance of reliving these affective states, he incorrectly concluded that the patient could *cathart* and achieve new insights and patterns of relating. Not being privy to the mechanisms for early affective expres-sion and regulation, he could not know that the analyst's emotional par-ticipation was critical to the patient's success in recognizing, expressing, and integrating affective states. He had half the equation, perhaps because the whole equation places such great personal demands on the analyst. (If eye contact was too stressful for Freud, how could he con-ceive of a day marked by one emotional exchange after another?) The type of emotional availability I am discussing requires so much energy and attention from the analyst, as well as self-awareness, that it severely limits the number of patients that anyone could see in a given day. Thus, practicing this way is not only potentially personally threatening, but also places significant limits on the analyst's personal income.

Affect, Alexithymia, and Trauma

The uses of emotion are particularly important when treating patients who have suffered early trauma. Krystal (1988, 1997) has alerted us to the needs of the patients he describes as alexithymic—those who cannot recognize, or label or express emotions other than occasional outbursts of rage. He says these patients typically have been traumatized in child-hood, causing them to develop into adulthood without the essential tools for expressing and containing emotions. Although the burgeoning liter-ature on incest and other "survivors" seems to place great value on recalling past abuses, it seems that the more essential hurdle facing an individual who suffered early trauma is the identification, expression, and management of affect in the present.

If we integrate what we know about individuals who have been trau-matized with Krystal's portrait of the alexithymic patient, we are left with the person who is hypervigilant, overattending to the slightest detail of the analyst's behavior or deportment, yet unaware of his or her own moods and feelings. These patients cannot answer when asked how they are feeling. As a result, they often defensively change the topic to some observation of the analyst, or they respond with what they know, usually a physical feeling or symptom. The patient may say he or she feels a weight on the chest, a stomach tied up in knots, or a current worry about having cancer, AIDS, or some other potentially fatal condition. Stuck at the level of physical processing of emotion, rather than integrating physical sensation with cognitive awareness and a language for feelings, the alexithymic patient stays away from the topic of his or her own emotions. Earlier I quoted Krystal's observation that alexithymic patients often present as "super-adjusted," preferring to remain cool and calm at all times, and often believing that any show of emotion is a sign of weakness that will be seized as an opportunity to destroy the patient.

Thus Krystal's alexithymic patient and McDougall's psychosomatic patient, as well as the myriad numbers of patients identified as having experienced early trauma, seem to have a great deal in common and be drawn from the same general pool. They somatize rather than cathart, are hypervigilant, and are lacking in basic trust. They often use projective identification as a way of communicating with their therapists, essentially letting the therapist know, "This is what I am feeling." They trust their intuition and their bodies more than their feelings, which are often just a blur of "feeling upset," and often need their analysts to self-disclose or make physical contact with them as a way of facilitating both trust and emotional communication. (See the final section of this chapter for more discussion of the clinical implications.)

Gender Differences

Finally, how are men and women different in their experience and expression of affect? Social stereotypes proclaim women as the emotional gender and men as the stoics, yet the literature on alexithymic patients refers primarily to women. If women who have been traumatized at an early age have little access to their emotions, then we have a rather large group of women who clearly defy the sexual stereotype. Yet Brody (1993) says that there is increasing evidence to support the idea that women express their emotions more intensely, both verbally and nonverbally (facial expressions), than men do. Another interesting finding reported by Brody is that "males are more intensely emotionally expressive through actions and behaviors than are females" (pp. 113–114). In other words, if a man feels strongly about something, he wants to act on that feeling in some way, while women are more content restricting themselves to verbal expressions of emotion. As I read this I couldn't help but wonder if this helps to explain why the analytic literature (overwhelmingly dominated by male authors) historically reflects fears of analysts being out of control and acting out if they attempt to self-disclose their countertransference feelings. Could it be that these fears of acting out reflect a gender difference in emotional expression, since women typically violate the boundaries less often than men do, and do not seem to be as concerned about self-disclosure as a slippery slope?

Of course, this does not mean that we should simply dismiss the male analyst's concern about acting out. It might be fair to say that women are more likely to be comfortable with expressing their emotional responses to patients, and less likely to commit boundary violations—yet this would certainly be less likely among female therapists who had their own history of trauma and/or alexithymia. It could be equally as fair to say that male analysts (knowing their own predilection for acting on their feelings) need to be more cautious and monitor their own inclinations more carefully to preserve the boundaries. Yet the many male therapists who know they are comfortable with verbal expressions of their feelings certainly would not need to concern themselves as much with the gender difference findings.

Clinical Implications

Whether or not the gender differences in expressing emotion account for the reluctance of analysts to be more emotionally expressive, there is no doubt that therapists' expression of emotion has been a very controversial topic in recent years. Even the intersubjective theorists such as Stolorow and Atwood (1992) remain convinced of the need for abstinence on the analyst's part, in spite of their recognition of the role of "reciprocal mutual influence" (p. 18) in any intersubjective field. While these authors criticize Mitchell and others for failing to acknowledge the influence of the analyst on the process, their case material reads much like any other, with their theoretical stand being used to enlighten the analyst's interpretations rather than create a field of mutual, yet asymmetrical, affective communication. Stolorow and Atwood seem to believe that empathy alone will provide the interventions needed for the emergence of repressed affective states. But my question remains, how do you relate empathically to an *unexpressed* emotion?

Basch (1991), with reference to a narcissistic patient he was treating, makes the point that more active interventions are needed to help the patient recognize and express split-off affect, although he is not explicit in his recommendations.

The analyst's affective abstinence that serves us so well with the psychoneurotic patient would only have played into the defense of a patient like Mr. W., a patient with a narcissistic character disorder. Since disavowal interferes with affective recognition and maturation in the area of the patient's pathology, it is pointless to play the waiting game and trust that, sooner or later, the patient will transfer what needs to be analyzed [p. 301].

In a similar vein, Krystal (1988) points to the limitations of conventional technique:

[C]onsideration of the energizing aspects of emotions provides both a rationale for and a recognition of the need to reintegrate and self-regulatory activities as part of the psychotherapeutic work. At the same time it alerts us to the fact that classical (perhaps more accurately, "conventional") psychoanalytic technique may he missing a vital aspect of the patient's and therapist's function. Rather than taking an idealistic view of the purity of technique, we might better direct that idealism to pursuing the goal of the patient's greater self-integration [p. 125].

Thus both Basch and Krystal have noted that many of the people we treat will simply not make very much progress in the area of affective recognition and expression without direct affective interventions by the therapist. Although I discuss the specifics of self-disclosure in the following chapter, there is no question that affective interventions certainly require therapists' disclosure of felt emotion. I previously (Maroda, 1991, 1995b) outlined guidelines for therapist disclosure that allow for both emotional responses elicited by the patient's question of "How are you feeling toward me right now?" and for revelation of affect experienced as the result of projective identification. The above authors' discussion of the patient's split-off affect lends itself to further discussion of how the therapist facilitates the patient's experience of his or her own disavowed feelings. McDougall (1978), in discussing the way some patients attempt to influence their analysts, says that

Rather than seeking to communicate moods, ideas, and free associations, the patient seems to aim at making the analyst *feel* something or stimulating him to *do* something: this "something" is incapable of being named and the patient himself is totally unaware of this aim [p. 179].

From my own experience, I would say that McDougall's "something" is usually the experience and expression of the patient's split-off affect. Unable to bear their own feelings, many patients seek to have their analysts feel and express these feelings for them, so they can find them acceptable and learn to do this for themselves. For the therapist to deny the patient this essential experience, which we can liken to the mother's early affective responding to the infant, is to deprive the patient of an essential step in his or her affective development. Interpretations given when affect is needed amounts to anti-communication, resulting in the patient getting worse.

That is why so many patients accuse their therapists of being unresponsive no matter how concerned those therapists might genuinely be, or how hard they try. Often anything short of an affective response does not count, or register, at all for the patient. He will behave as if no response was given by the therapist, or will accuse the therapist of deliberately withholding the sought-after response. Things become understandably complicated, as McDougall says, when the patient, asked what he wants, often says he does not know, due to his having repressed the affect he is seeking to find through his analyst.

Just as our early emotional development depended on receiving affective responses from others, so does our continued development. Most certainly for those who are seeking what amounts to a remedial emotional education when they come for treatment, the affective responses of the therapist are critical for completing the cycle of affective communication.

When I read case histories I am often dismayed to discover how often therapists describe getting control of themselves after being strongly stimulated by a patient, carefully making sure that they do not express emotion when responding. If the patient is stimulating anger, for example, the therapist will wait for the wave of anger to pass, and then as cooly and calmly as possible say, "I think you would like me to feel as angry as you do." Implicit in such a response is, "But don't think for a minute that I'm going to. You can spend your entire session trying to provoke me, but I will never give you the satisfaction of seeing me angry."

When I read things like this, I always think to myself, "Why not?" Why not show the patient exactly how angry you are? What is the point of withholding emotion and thwarting the patient in his quest for affective communication? As I have stated previously (1995) he will only have to up the ante next time, until he finally gets an emotional response or gives up in despair and subsequent depressed withdrawal.

Traditionally, analytic clinicians have believed that any personal responses would only detract form the patient's experience. This made some sense if you believed that analysis was primarily an intrapsychic event. But it makes much less sense if you believe that analytic treatment is not only both intrapsychic and interpersonal, but that (as stated earlier in this chapter) the order of developmental progression dictates that the interpersonal necessarily occurs first, with the intra-psychic following.

If the patient repeatedly stimulates a strong emotion or visceral response in the analyst, then it is probably time for an affective response. So long as the therapist is reasonably in control and behaves responsibly, the show of emotion should not be damaging to the patient. (In the next chapter I address questions regarding the analyst's pathology at work, potentially coloring his affective experience of the patient.)

In reviewing the literature on affect I found an interesting chapter on affect and intimacy (Kelly, 1996) that focused chiefly on couples' intimate relationships. In this context Kelly discusses the negative outcome that results when individuals do not respond honestly with feeling to each other. Yet when I read it I was struck by how much it equally applied to the therapeutic dyad.

> All close relationships require proximity that causes us to step on each other's toes. If, for whatever reason, one does not say "ouch" and communicate the distress experienced as a result of the other's actions, a complex dilemma is created. The need to disguise the distress causes the inmost self to be hidden from the other. The distress, if unrelieved, eventually triggers anger and resentment that must also be hidden. This causes further withdrawal and hiding of the inmost self. The other, perhaps not even aware of the offense, experiences feeling of rejection triggered by the withdrawal, without information adequate to allow reestablishment of the intimate bond. Now hurt, this other may also resort to withdrawal, thus setting in motion a recursive loop of rejection and hurt [pp. 87–88].

Looking at the research on affect necessitates the question: In thwarting our patients in their quest for an emotional response from us, have we unknowingly been withholding that which could be most therapeutic? We might be tempted to rationalize our lack of overt emotional expression, on the old grounds that we will detract from the patient's experience, but this fails to address the change process. I have claimed that the patient often will be unable to ever name his own affective experience if the therapist does not feel and name it first. Likewise, Schore (1994) says that

> The psychotherapist's establishment of a dyadic affective "growth promoting environment" influences the ontogeny of homeostatic self-regulatory systems (Greenspan, 1981). Towards this end, both positive and negative classes of affect need to be transacted and regulated in the therapist-patient relationship [p. 463].

In other words, affect research suggests that emotional exchanges between therapist and patient are critical to the patient's growth and development. He states further that

> affect regulatory dialogs mediated by a psychotherapist may induce literal structural change in the form of new patterns of growth of cortical-limbic circuitries, especially in the right hemisphere which contains representation of self-and-object images [p. 469].

It stands to reason that if emotional exchanges, or lack of, created the affective patterns that a person creates over and over again, that only new emotional exchanges could facilitate the altering of old affective patterns. Changes in thoughts affect cognitive patterns in the brain, and new emotional exchanges create new emotional memories and affective patterns in the brain.

If we remember that emotion is the most basic form of communication, and is essentially relational, then perhaps we can rid ourselves of the notion that the therapist's expression of felt emotion is somehow inappropriate or damaging. Krystal (1988) has suggested that therapists' difficulty in treating alexithymic patients may be due to the frequency with which they suffer from the problem themselves. Obviously only returning to treatment could address the problems of the alexithymic therapist.

From my experience there are more therapists who have painfully sat on their emotions, erroneously believing that they were doing the right thing. For these therapists, the prospect of using their emotional responses constructively for the patient's development is a potentially rewarding and mutually healthy experience. Understanding that the withholding of felt emotion can be just as harmful as any affective expression, given its covert nature, perhaps we can explore the therapeutic nature of affect, freeing both our patients and ourselves.

References

Averill, J. (1994), The patient's experience of the analyst's subjectivity. *Psychoanal. Quart.*, 1:29–51.

Basch, M. (1991), The significance of a theory of affect. *J. Amer. Psychoanal. Assn.*, 39(Suppl.):291–304.

Blum, H. (1991), Affect theory and the theory of technique. *J. Amer. Psychoanal. Assn.*, 39 (Suppl.).

Bower, G. (1994), Some relations between emotions and memory. In: *The Nature of Emotion: Fundamental Questions*, ed. P. Eckman & R. Davison. New York: Oxford University Press, pp. 303–305.

Brody, L. (1993), On understanding gender differences in the expression of emotion. In: *Human Feelings: Explorations in Affect Development and Meaning,* ed. S. Ablon, D. Brown, E. Khantzian & J. Mack. Hillsdale, NJ: The Analytic Press, pp. 87–121.

_____ & Harrison, R. (1987), Developmental changes in children's abilities to match and label emotionally laden situations. *Motiv. & Emotion*, 2:347–365.

Brown, D. (1993), Affective development, psychopathology, and adaptation. In: *Human Feelings: Explorations in Affect Development and Meaning*, ed. S. Ablon, D. Brown, E. Khantzian & J. Mack. Hillsdale, NJ: The Analytic press, pp. 5–66.

Clore, G. (1994), Why emotions are felt. In: *The Nature of Emotion: Fundamental Questions*, ed. P. Eckman & R. Davison. New York: Oxford University Press, pp. 103–111.

Clyman, R. (1991), The procedural organization of emotions. *J. Amer. Psychoanal. Assn.*, 39(Suppl.):349–382.

Fast, I., (1992), The embodied mind: Toward a relational perspective. *Psychoanal. Dial.* 2:389–409.

Grotstein, J. (1997), "Mens sana in corpore sano": The mind and body as an "odd couple" and as an oddly coupled unity. *Psychoanal. Inq.*, 17:204–222.

Kelly, V. (1996), Affect and the redefinition of intimacy. In: *Knowing Feeling: Affect, Script and Psychotherapy*, ed. D. Nathanson. New York: Norton, pp. 379–408.

Kohut, H. (1984), *How Does Analysis Cure?* ed. A. Goldberg with P. Stepansky. Chicago: University of Chicago Press.

Kraut, R. & Johnston, R. (1979, Social and emotional messages of smiling: An ethological approach. *J. Personality & Soc. Psychol.*, 37:1539–1153.

Krystal, H. (1988), *Integration and Self-Healing: Affect, Trauma, Alexithymia*. Hillsdale, NJ: The Analytic Press.

_____ (1997), Desomatization and the consequences of infantile psychic trauma. *Psychoanal. Inq.*, 17:126–150.

LeDoux, J. (1994), Memory versus emotional memory in the brain. In: *The Nature of Emotion: Fundamental Questions*, ed. P. Eckman & R. Davison. New York: Oxford University Press, pp. 311–312.

Maroda, K. (1991), *The Power of Countertransference: Innovations in Analytic Technique*. Hillsdale, NJ: The Analytic Press, 2004.

_____ (1995), Projective identification and countertransference interventions: Since feeling is first. *Psychoanal. Rev.*, 82:229–247.

_____ (2002), No place to hide: Affectivity, the unconscious, and development of relational techniques. *Contemp. Psychoanal.*, 38:101–120.

McDougall, J. (1978), *Plea for a Measure of Abnormality*. New York: International Universities Press.

Nathanson, D. (1996), Some closing thoughts on affect, scripts, and psychotherapy. In: *Knowing Feeling: Affect, Script and Psychotherapy*, ed. D. Nathanson. New York: Norton, pp. 379–408.

Orange, D. (1995), *Emotional Understanding*. New York: Guilford.

Panskepp, J. (1994), Subjectivity may have evolved in the brain as a simple value-coding process that promotes the learning of new behaviors. In: *The Nature of Emotion: Fundamental Questions*, ed. P. Eckman & R. Davison. New York: Oxford University Press, pp. 313–315.

Parkinson, B. (1996), Emotions are social. *Brit. J. Psych.*, 87:663–683.

Schore, A. (1994), *Affect Regulation and the Origin of the Self: The Neurobiology of Emotional Development*. Hillsdale, NJ: Lawrence Erlbaum Associates.

Shapiro, T. & Emde, R., eds. (1991), Affect: Psychoanalytic perspectives. *J. Amer. Psychoanal. Assn.*, 39 (Suppl.)

Stern, D. (1985), *The Interpersonal World of the Infant*. New York: Basic Books.

Stolorow, R. & Atwood, G. (1992), *Contexts of Being: The Intersubjective Foundations of Psychological Life*. Hillsdale, NJ: The Analytic Press.

_____ Brandchaft, B. & Atwood, G. (1987), *Psychoanalytic Treatment: An Intersubjective Approach*. Hillsdale, NJ: The Analytic Press.

Thompson, R. (1988), Emotion and self-regulation. In: *Nebraska Symposium on Motivation, Vol. 36,*, ed. R. Diensibier & R. Thompson. Lincoln: University of Nebraska Press, pp. 367–467.

Tomkins, S. (1962), *Affect, Imagery, Consciousness*. New York: Springer.

Afterword

Rereading this chapter, some five years after I first wrote it, I am still excited by the research on affect and its implications for treatment. Understanding that emotion is not the enemy of reason offers hope for both therapist and patient, freeing us to experience our deepest feelings without negative judgments. Understanding that the therapist's emotional response is both impossible to hide and critical to the emotional development of the patient also frees us. Discovering that we actually think more clearly when we are experiencing a freeflow of emotion confirms my own experience, both personally and professionally. When I am withdrawn or otherwise disconnected from my feelings, I can't think well about the patient or about how to intervene. I also can't write very well. I need to be "plugged in" emotionally to participate in the process, just as the patient does. As I stated in the chapter, it is only the state of being overstimulated emotionally that hampers cognition. At those times, I devote my energies to containing and soothing myself, just as I work to help my patients contain and soothe themselves when they are emotionally overwhelmed.

In a follow-up piece (Maroda, 2002), I pursued the issue of developing techniques based on our current knowledge of affect and make the case that the two-person approach cannot be a revolution in psychoanalytic thinking if it does not inherently demand a new body of two-person techniques. I believe that the research on affect I described in that article provides valuable information that can inform technique.

I understand and appreciate that it is difficult to experiment. We naturally want to feel we are doing right by our patients and that we are practicing responsibly. But we cannot have change without experimentation. As I have experimented over the years, I have discovered just how much change is an evolutionary process. In my follow-up article in 2002 I noted that, when I first started disclosing verbally to my patients, they responded very positively and wanted more. But over the years, as I have become more comfortable with *not* attempting to hide my own emotional experience and allow it to naturally register on my face, my patients have less need for me to verbalize what I am feeling. They often can see and feel what I am feeling and can silently receive the feedback they need. So, as I have become more comfortable with my feelings, my patients need less overt disclosure. I imagine this would prove to be universally true, but I would like to hear about other therapists' clinical experiences.

Controversy continues on issues of when and what to disclose, although I still maintain that my emphasis on disclosure of countertransference affect at the patient's behest or when stalemate occurs (Maroda, 1991) is most therapeutic. In recent years some therapists have sanctioned disclosure of sexual feelings, which I still think is rarely helpful. Interestingly, therapist hostility remains largely unexplored. There is some evidence that patients diagnosed with borderline personality disorder do better when their therapists express some anger (it may actually help them to contain their own). But, overall, therapist anger and disapproval have been the hallmarks of negative therapeutic action—often preceding a failed treatment. Yet anger in the therapeutic relationship is as inevitable as in any other relationship. The question remains: How much is therapeutic, to what extent should it be verbalized, and to which patients?

Clearly we have much work to do as we continue to revolutionize psychoanalytic theory and practice. Having acknowledged that the therapeutic dyad cannot transcend the conscious and unconscious emotional forces that shape all human relationships, we can look forward to continuing innovations that further humanize and expedite the therapeutic process.

References

Maroda, K. (1991), *The Power of Countertransference: Innovations in Analytic Technique*. Northvale, NJ: Aronson, 1995.
—— (2002), No place to hide: Affectivity, the unconscious, and development of relational techniques. *Contemp. Psychoanal.*, 38:101–120.

Psychoanalytic Supervision: The Intersubjective Development

(2000)

Emanuel Berman

▼   ▼   ▼   ▼   ▼

Editors' Introduction

Emanuel Berman's unusual "double" psychoanalytic training places him in a unique position to write about psychoanalytic education. Berman first received his psychoanalytic training at the New York University Postdoctoral Program in Psychotherapy and Psychoanalysis. This program began in 1961 and from its inception was dedicated to academic freedom, student activism and participation, a plurality of psychoanalytic perspectives, and to a comparative psychoanalytic approach to education. Later, moving to Israel, Berman undertook yet a second psychoanalytic training at the Israel Psychoanalytic Institute in Jerusalem. This program, begun by Max Eitingon in 1933, provided the more traditional psychoanalytic education founded on the tripartite approach of supervision, course work, and personal analysis. Berman went on to become an active faculty member of both programs and has written extensively about the history of psychoanalytic theory, training, and practice.

In a series of important papers, culminating in his latest book, *Impossible Training* (2004, The Analytic Press), Berman uses his own experiences in these contrasting centers of training to examine contemporary psychoanalytic education. Berman expresses concern about the inhibiting and persecutory potential of any strong "utopian state of mind" that may create an emotional climate dominated by perfectionist ego ideals and superego pressures. Naturally, as analysts, we strive to be as competent and effective as possible, developing various theoretical notions of what is curative in psychoanalysis. But this striving must be dialectically counterbalanced by our lively attention to what actually happens, much of which is beyond our choice or control. When the balance is tilted, a determination to be a certain way decreases our inner freedom and spontaneity and as a result reduces our capacity to understand. According to Berman, overconfident models of the desirable analytic role may paradoxically reduce the usefulness of psychoanalysis as an open-ended setting in which unexpected insights and new experiences can evolve.

In this article, Berman examines the implications of relational psychoanalysis for our understanding and practice of clinical supervision. Berman's intersubjective perspective on the analytic process makes the notion of purely didactic supervision untenable and shifts the supervisory process from its historic one-person approach on understanding the patient to a systems approach examining the various relations among the various dyadic systems: patient–analyst, analyst–supervisor, supervisor–institute. Supervision is portrayed as the crossroads of a matrix of object relations of three persons, of a complex network of transference–countertransference patterns. Supervision, much like analysis itself, is, for Berman, an intensely personal process in which the emotional responsiveness and individual subjectivity of the participants is central. The avoidance or denial of the supervisor's subjective role in it may make supervision stilted or even oppressive and stand in the way of resolving supervisory crises and stalemates. In the course of exploring a relational approach to supervision, Berman takes up the analyst's and the supervisor's reciprocal fears of exposing their weaknesses, the impact of the institute as a setting and the transferences it arouses, and the inherent conflicts of loyalty for each participant in the analytic/supervisory triad. Berman's article thus represents the extension of the relational approach beyond the clinical psychoanalytic situation and into the realms of psychoanalytic training and education.

Psychoanalytic Supervision:
The Intersubjective Development*

Our thinking about the analytic process has been strongly influenced in recent years by the notion of intersubjectivity in the analytic dyad. This notion has enormous implications for psychoanalytic supervision as well. If taken seriously, it points the way to potential radical changes both in the content and in the style of supervision.

What do 1 mean by *intersubjectivity?* My own thinking in this matter is an outgrowth of a long tradition (Berman, 1997c), including authors such as Ferenczi (Berman, 1996, 1999), Balint, Winnicott, Racker and Gill and from our contemporaries—Benjamin, Bollas, Casement, Mitchell, Ogden, Renik, Stolorow and others. Naturally, the specific formulations are my own.

Psychoanalysis is both a "one-person psychology" (studying intrapsychic processes) and a "two-person psychology" (studying interactions). The concept of intersubjectivity attempts to integrate both aspects. The psychic realities of both analyst and analysand, it implies, are involved in their encounter and are transformed by that encounter. Transference is both an outgrowth of the patient's life history and a reaction to the personality and actions of the analyst, who can never fully become a "blank screen" or an "empty container" (Aron, 1996). There is a continuous mutual influence between analyst and analysand, though this mutuality evolves in the context of a clear asymmetry that must be acknowledged (Aron, 1996; Berman, 1999).

Transference, in its broader definition, unavoidably combines displaced and projected elements with realistic perceptions and the analyst is never sufficiently "objective" to separate these out definitively. We can raise questions and offer ideas about the sources of different elements, but to attempt a definitive judgement as to what is true and what is distorted in the way we are viewed implies absolute knowledge of ourselves, i.e. a denial that there are unconscious aspects in our own psyche (Gill, 1982).

Likewise, countertransference unavoidably combines issues stemming out of the basic psychic reality of the analyst and aspects that are responsive to the specific analysand. Some authors have attempted to separate

* Originally published in *International Journal of Psychoanalysis*, 81:273–290.

these out into different categories (e.g. Springmann, 1986), but I suspect this attempt is futile. In my own experience, in self-analysis and in the supervision and analysis of candidates, every reaction that first appears as pure projective counteridentification (Grinberg, 1979) or mere role-responsiveness (Sandler, 1976), turns out upon further scrutiny to have aspects that are related to the analyst's unique personality (in other words, there are reasons why a projective identification can "catch on"). Conversely, the analyst may be certain he or she is reacting from a purely personal vulnerability, but fuller exploration reveals that a particular analysand powerfully activates that vulnerability, while others do not.

Transference and countertransference constantly activate and mould each other and are actually parts of one total cyclical process, which has no starting point. Studying each separately makes as much sense as studying a game of chess by analyzing the moves of the white figures alone. In this respect the "counter" in the word countertransference may be misleading, as *transference is also counter-countertransference* (Racker, 1968). The total transference/countertransference cycle generates a joint new reality, a transitional space with its own unique emotional climate, in which analytic work takes place.

Countertransference Cannot be Relegated to the Candidate's Analysis

Such an intersubjective view of the analytic relationship has, first of all, clear implications for the content of psychoanalytic supervision. It makes the option of *purely didactic supervision*, which avoids countertransference or relegates all of it to the candidate's own analysis, *untenable*. Discussing the dynamics of the analysand alone, or demonstrating "correct" technique, is of limited value. If we assume that important elements in the transference are reactive to the analyst's actual personality and behaviour, it follows that we cannot fully understand the analysand's experience if relevant aspects of the analyst's own personality and emotional reactions are not discussed in supervision.

I do not believe that the supervisor has the capacity to pass a final verdict as to the accuracy of the analysand's attributions, but the supervisor can become an invaluable partner in thinking about the possible validity of such attributions. It is potentially very helpful—though not easy—when a supervisor says, "You know, I also heard that interpretation as aggressive." Or the opposite direction may be relevant, as in the following example.

A supervisee raises his difficulty with the analysand's idealization of him. When listening to the material, the supervisor wonders about the choice of the term "idealization." The supervisor actually experiences the analysand as expressing realistic gratitude to this competent and empathic analyst. Raising the issue leads on to the analyst's low self-esteem, which made him blind to the progress this gratitude may signify for the analysand, a person who is harshly critical of his parents and almost everybody else and quite lonely.

If we assume that countertransference is both a clue to understanding the psychic reality of the analysand and is an influence on its further development in the course of analysis, it follows that *countertransference cannot be avoided in psychoanalytic supervision*, including its more personal sources, which cannot be separated out in advance. We need to know, to give a simple example, that the analysand reminds the analyst of her brother, if we are to help her in attempting to clarify for herself how this association affects her countertransference, uncover the ways in which this countertransference unavoidably colours the analyst's actions and verbalisations and therefore unknowingly influences her analysand as well, changing in turn his transference to her and the whole atmosphere in the consulting room.

In this framework, the idea of a standard technique becomes obsolete. Haynal speaks of "the illusion that there can be a technique that one needs only to learn and apply 'correctly'" (1993, p. 62). The alternative challenge is to follow the analytic interaction carefully, with close attention to minute details, pausing to consider the intersubjective implications of each verbal or nonverbal exchange. In this context interpretations, silences or slips of the analyst's tongue are examined in terms of their affective antecedents and consequences, rather than on the basis of their conscious intention; in this respect they are explored in a similar way to the associations, requests or jokes of the analysand.

The analytic impact of interventions can be evaluated only in retrospect. What was formulated as an empathic interpretation may be experienced as an insult; what first appears as the analyst's blunder may eventually lead to an important insight and so on. Beyond basic ideas about the setting and its boundaries, which are important in that they make this scrutiny possible, what needs to be learned is not a list of steadfast rules, but an introspective and empathic sensitivity to the actual sources and actual impact of our actions and non-actions. This is a most personal learning process that requires considerable personal exposure and is strongly influenced by the supervisory climate.

If we accept that analysis may, at some unique moments, benefit from the direct expression of countertransference (Bollas, 1987; Tansey and Burke, 1989; Aron, 1996), the exploration of such an option becomes another supervisory challenge. Many candidates are afraid to make any such interventions and their avoidance may be costly at times, especially when they attempt to side-track an involuntary expression of counter-transference already noticed by the analysand, in which case they are perceived as defensive and anxious. The potential encouragement of a supervisor, after thoughtful joint consideration of all risks and benefits, to express things—in some instances—more directly, may be an impor-tant step towards breaking a stalemate in analysis. Naturally, counter-transference disclosure cannot be considered if countertransference in general is not patiently explored first.

Let me give an example: a supervisee reports that his analysand con-stantly blames him for identifying with his wife rather than with him; all his attempts to interpret this as a fearful projection are ineffective. Fuller discussion in supervision makes it clear the analysand has a point: in the countertransference, the analyst experiences his analysand as a bully and the analysand's wife as a victim. This reaction turns out to have some sources in the analyst's life, but also to be moulded by the analysand's projective identification. This analysand consciously depre-ciates his wife, but unconsciously invites empathy towards her much more than towards himself. It becomes clear that the analyst's past inter-pretations, which implied denial of the analysand's complaints, made the analysand confused and even more suspicious. On the other hand, a judi-cious acknowledgement of the analysand's perceptions could become a springboard to the new understanding of his marriage, not as the exter-nal battlefield he consciously portrays, but as the stage of an inner drama, in which many of his own dissociated experiences as a battered child are projectively expressed through his wife.

Supervision as a Crossroads of a Matrix of Object Relations

An intersubjective focus cannot be limited, however, to the analyst and analysand alone. It also pulls us into *the intersubjective reality created between supervisor and supervisee*. Psychoanalytic supervision therefore becomes a task in which the psychoanalytic orientation is expressed not only in content, but in the nature of the process as well. Psychoanalytic scrutiny can be effectively directed towards our own work as supervi-sors and the meta-communication achieved may allow us a critical self-analysis. We could then become—as supervisors—*less preoccupied with formulating what we should do and more receptive to an exploration of what we actually do and undergo*, which may not be always dictated by our theoretical rationales and goals as we once believed.

A psychoanalytic supervision that allows this meta-communication may contribute more to the deep personal growth process at which psychoanalytic training aims. On the other hand, a lack of meta-communication runs the risk of inhibiting this process at times. In such a purely "content-orientated" (or patient-focused) supervision, psychoanalysis may be underutilized.

We might think of supervision as *the cross-roads of a matrix of object relations of at least three persons* (Berman, 1997b) each bringing her or his psychic reality into the bargain, creating a joint intersubjective milieu. In spite of the risks involved in introducing clinically derived terms into the study of supervision (Ekstein and Wallerstein, 1972), it may be helpful to speak of the juxtaposition and interaction of several simultaneous transference/countertransference trends in each analytic-supervisory combination.

I am aware of the hopelessness of fully deciphering all these nuances within the limited time-span of one supervisory process and of natural differences between supervisors (and supervisees) regarding aspects they prefer to focus upon. I am arguing, however, that all these levels should at least be acknowledged and allowed as potential legitimate contents in the supervisory discourse. If this is not achieved, some components (most typically the supervisor's subjective contribution) may be defensively denied or rationalised away and consequently *supervision may become stilted or even oppressive*, not allowing the potential transitional space to evolve within it.

The supervisor–supervisee relationship, I suggest, is always a rich and complex transference/countertransference combination, even if supervision is utterly impersonal; teachers are always a major focus of transference feelings. Naturally, the more personal approach I advocate may add complexity and intensity to the process. It may undermine some of the more defensive modes of avoiding anxiety in the situation and increase the fear of intrusion and humiliation. On the other hand, as a partial remedy, it may allow greater awareness and better resolution of supervisory conflicts and crises, by encouraging the joint exploration of the supervisory relationship itself (Berman, 1988). The supervisor's fuller awareness of moments in which he or she was experienced as intrusive or insensitive, for example, may make reparation possible and serve as a springboard for more tactful work, taking better into account the supervisee's sensitivities, once these were more openly articulated.

While the wishes of both supervisee and supervisor to make their work together instructive and fruitful are usually quite sincere, there are many factors that make their relationship potentially conflictual. Epstein

(1986) thoroughly discusses the possible negative impact of supervision upon supervisees.

The analytic encounter is a very intimate dyadic situation and a third partner in it may be a burdensome intrusion, a chaperone on a honeymoon. This may become noticeable when the analyst's spontaneity is inhibited by a preoccupation with remembering the session, sometimes to the point of taking notes during the session so "nothing gets lost" when reported in supervision.

Analysts often experience rescue fantasies towards their patients (Berman, 1993, 1997a), projecting their own vulnerability on to them; whereas the involvement of a supervisor unavoidably reintroduces the analyst's own vulnerability and neediness into the picture. The supervisor may be experienced as a potentially superior rescuer. "I am sure you would have done it much better" is a common candidate's fantasy. It may sometimes be untrue (with difficult cases a beginner's enthusiasm and optimism may be potentially more helpful than a seasoned professional's sober apprehension), but would the supervisor help in dismantling the fantasy?

Idealisation has a broad range of outcomes in psychoanalytic supervision. It may become a fruitful spur for learning, when related to an experience of being deeply understood, influenced and inspired. At the other end of the spectrum, in a collusively maintained over-idealisation, oedipal and narcissistic dynamics may at times combine in producing in the younger analyst a painful sense of inferiority. An image of supervisor and supervisee as fundamentally differing in their therapeutic potential may become part of *"a myth of the supervisory situation"* (Berman, 1988), equivalent to "the myth of the analytic situation" as involving an interaction between a sick person and a healthy one (Racker, 1968, p. 132).

While in my past work I tended to emphasise sources of conflict that are unique to super-visors and others that are unique to supervisees, I gradually came to see their common features. Within supervision too we may speak of basic mutuality and joint vulnerability (Slavin, 1998), though they are experienced in the context of unavoidable asymmetry and inequality, which should not be denied.

A major source of difficulty for supervisees, for example, is that the learning of new skills requires acknowledgement of their lack and such an acknowledgement arouses shame. But in good supervision the supervisor also needs to learn and change and at times to become aware of blind spots, or to admit not having satisfactory answers to the challenge posed by a troublesome analysand. And while we often discuss the evaluation of candidates by supervisors, actually *mutual evaluation* is going on, even if the evaluation of the supervisor by the candidate is often silent or muted within super-vision and only articulated outside, informally, by word of mouth. This reality turns both partners into threatening judges of each other, both being a potential source of embarrassing exposure and rejection.

Narcissistic needs of supervisors, a possible competitiveness with younger colleagues and fear of being displaced by them, all add to supervisors' vulnerability and to their anxiety about the way supervisees describe them to their peers, to their analyst or to other supervisors. Just as in analysis the direct countertransference to one's analysand may be supplemented by indirect countertransferences (Racker, 1968) involving the reactions of third parties (such as a supervisor), in supervision the direct countertransference to the supervisee may be supplemented by indirect countertransferences as well (e.g. concerns about the opinion of the candidate's analyst). Disregarding this aspect of the supervisory reality implies denying the paradoxical and mutual aspects of the supervisory dyad, just as Etchegoyen (1991) oversimplifies the complexity of the analytic encounter by interpreting indirect countertransference involving the supervisor as merely a displacement of direct countertransference to the patient (Berman, 1994). Such indirect countertransference reactions may be too burdensome to share with a supervisee, but the supervisor's awareness of them may be crucial for them to be worked through.

The Conflict-Generating Triadic Structure of the Analytic-Supervisory Situation

The triadic structure of the analytic-supervisory situation leads to a possible *conflict of loyalties within each participant*. For the candidate analyst such a conflict may appear if the analyst experiences a discrepancy between what appear to be the emotional needs of the analysand and the supervisor's views as to the preferred analytic technique. From the supervisor's end, an inherent conflict of identifications, with the supervisee and with the analysand, may also be a source of difficulty. Being "a servant of two masters," the supervisor experiences two ethical commitments ("I was well aware of feeling in a quandary as to which desperate young woman to help, the patient or the supervisee"; Stimmel, 1995, p. 613).

The dilemma surfaces when the supervisor is unhappy with the supervisee's work and becomes torn between loyalty to the candidate's needs (to develop gradually at the individual pace needed by him or her, without feeling too criticised and threatened) and a sense of responsibility for the analysand's well being. The supervisor may feel quite helpless in dangerous situations (e.g. where there is a risk of suicide or psychosis), while being tempted to assume a more directive position (to put words in the supervisee's mouth, turning into a Cyrano de Bergerac) leads to the risk of an authoritarian disruption of the younger analyst's growth.

An equivalent issue, I should add parenthetically, appears within analysis itself: the analyst may experience a conflict between "concordant identifications" with the analysand and "complementary identifications" with the analysand's inner objects, as personalised through other individuals in the analysand's life (Racker, 1968, p. 134). However, once we realise that these other individuals (e.g. spouse, children etc.) also represent unacknowledged aspects of the analysand, an integration of the conflicting identifications becomes conceivable and both kinds of identifications become the basis of potential empathy towards the analysand. This point is made by Tansey and Burke (1989) and is an important advance over Racker's original view that only concordant identifications can be sublimated into empathy.

Similar understanding may be relevant at times in supervision as well (e.g. a resistant patient may represent a side of the supervisee, just as a rebellious adolescent may represent a side of the parent), but not as consistently. After all, the analyst has not raised the patient from infancy and often has not chosen the patient (as we choose friends, lovers or spouses on the basis of unconscious identifications). Therefore, the conflict of identifications of the supervisor is harder to resolve.

To fully understand the triadic dynamics of analysis/supervision, we should also recognise the evolving relationship between the supervisor and the analysand discussed in supervision. This relationship may develop in fantasy and ultimately gain a powerful real impact, both of the two related parties on each other (even though in a mediated manner), as well as on the "mediator," the analyst.

Many analysands are aware of possible supervision, especially those who are them-selves mental health professionals. Some analysands may find out who the supervisor is, or develop their—wishful or anxious—hypotheses about it. Many more develop a mental image of the supervisor and a transference reaction to this imagined person.

In this context too we discover splits and conflicts. I will mention briefly a few divergent themes as examples: "You are too young and inexperienced to understand me, but your supervisor will help you out." "I feel that our relationship is very close, but it's hard for me to be open because you talk about me to a stranger." "You and your supervisor must have a field day, laughing about my stupidity." "Bring this dream to supervision, I feel we are stuck with it." "Were you in supervision today? This interpretation did not sound like your own." "You probably raised my fee because you were told in supervision you allow yourself to be exploited." "As a man you cannot understand menstruation, but hopefully you have a female supervisor." Brendan MacCarthy (personal communication) describes an applicant for an analysis who refused to go to a fully qualified analyst, preferring to wait for a candidate, saying he would feel safer with someone outside the analysis in control.

Luber (1991) suggests that split transferences to analyst and supervisor may belong to two main categories: attempts to split off one side of an ambivalent transference from the analyst to the supervisor and cases in which the transference is primarily triadic, based on the patient's past involvement with two related figures. In my view, these categories are not mutually exclusive: the initial split in the patient's history may have also been related to splitting off, as in Fairbairn's (1954) analysis of the Oedipus complex as an externalization of the initial ambivalence regarding the mother.

Naturally, the analysand's transference to the supervisor may influence both the analyst's countertransference (e.g. feeling put down, or else seduced into an exclusive alliance) and the supervisor's countertransference to the analyst (e.g. seeing the analyst as weak because the patient yearns for reinforcement) or to the analysand (feeling like a guardian angel, or—at the other extreme—an unwelcome intruder). Consequently, it may influence the supervisory relationship and its impact is another potential focus of an intersubjective exploration in supervision.

In addition, each supervisor may develop an autonomous, unique countertransference to any analysand being discussed: affection, curiosity, annoyance and so on. This affective response also becomes interconnected with the supervisory relationship and various (counter) transferential triadic patterns evolve (Winokur, 1982).

Let me mention three potential basic patterns, each of which creates a different supervisory climate, the latter two being particularly destructive for growth in supervision: (1) supervisor and analyst form a close alliance as the concerned and mutually supportive parents of a problematic child; (2) analyst and analysand form a close and secretive involvement; analyst withholds in supervision part of what goes on (self-disclosures, affective expressions, active interventions; see Yerushalmi, 1992; Mayer, 1996), reporting sessions in a guarded form, as a result of which the excluded supervisor becomes bored and uninvested in both supervisee and analysand; (3) supervisor is deeply interested in the appealing analysand, is critical of the analyst's unempathic work and develops a fantasy of rescuing the analysand from the analyst; the result may be a harsh critical attitude leading to a crisis in supervision and a report to the training committee that the candidate is unsuitable.

When Greenson (1967, pp. 220–221) discusses a supervisee who failed to express interest in the health of his analysand's sick child, he is very attentive to the analysand's hurt, but not empathic to any potential vulnerability at the bottom of the supervisee's guarded inhibition, or to the supervisee's possible hurt when scolded and sent for more analysis (Teitelbaum, 1990). In my reading, an opportunity for change within supervision itself may have been missed, on the basis of a triadic trans-ferential entanglement.

The role of supervisors in supervisory dynamics and difficulties receives scant attention in our professional literature. The literature is written mostly by supervisors, just as analysis is usually reported by the analyst, while written reports by analysands are rare. The other side of the coin, as mentioned before, is often thoroughly explored in informal discussions of candidates about their analysts and supervisors (Fraser, 1996), but these are never recorded or published, a fact that deprives us of a major source of insight about success and failure in analysis and in its supervision. An ideal forum for exploring intersubjective aspects in supervision would therefore involve both supervisor and supervisee, as was attempted at the training analysts' conference in Barcelona in 1997 (Szecsödy, 1999).

Difficulties in Supervision as a Topic of Supervisory Discourse

An intersubjective focus should turn difficulties in the supervisory rela-tionship into a legitimate topic within the supervisory discourse. Their avoidance may pose a bad role model, undermining the supervisor's encouragement of constant attention to affective nuances in the analytic relationship and of their bold verbalisation. Empathy towards the analysand that is unaccompanied by empathy toward the supervisee is a confusing mixed message (Sloane, 1986). Acknowledgment of the supervisor's possible role in difficulties (Sarnat, 1992) is not only crucial in creating a nonthreatening atmosphere, but is also vital for a rich truthful understanding of the dyadic process. *The hope is that both supervisor and supervisee will learn a lot from understanding the repeated gaps between their conscious wishes and the actual outcome of their encounter.*

As an example of the interrelatedness of the two levels of discourse, I am thinking of a supervision in which dealing with the seductive behaviour of a male analysand emerged as a major source of difficulty for the woman analyst. Our open and fruitful work on this issue was enhanced by a prior discussion in our first supervisory session, which took place before that analysis started. As I usually do, I encouraged the supervisee to tell me of any past interactions we have had, which might influence her feeling in supervision. She brought up an interaction from years back, when we were acquainted professionally in another setting, in which she experienced a compliment I gave her as seductive. Our straightforward conversation about that episode turned out to be a valuable springboard for our subsequent work on erotised transference issues, because the possible resonances between sexual currents in analysis and supervision (e.g. the erotic atmosphere that might evolve in supervision when sexual fantasies of the analysand about the analyst are discussed) became less threatening to both of us, as a result of the effective working through of such themes in our own relationship.

The exploration of the supervisory relationship was historically introduced and legitimized through the idea of a parallel process (Arlow, 1963; Searles, 1955, 1962; Doehrman, 1976), in which there are direct influences of the patient–therapist relationship on the supervisory dyad. This was a valuable starting point, but today we can better recognize the risks involved in that conceptual framework (Lesser, 1984). Talking about parallel processes may offer an outlet for the expression of difficulties in supervision, but may also limit this expression through a dogmatic expectation of finding exact parallels, or of sidetracking it through the too easy attribution of supervisory conflicts to the analysand, while avoiding more direct sources within the supervisory dyad itself. ("Parallel process . . . may be used also as a resistance to awareness of transference phenomena within the supervisor in relation to the supervisee" [Stimmel, 1995, p. 609].) Parallel processes should be understood as one *potential* aspect of the complex network of cross-identifications within the supervisor–analyst–analysand triad (Gediman and Wolkenfeld, 1980; Wolkenfeld, 1990; Baudry, 1993). Some supervisory stalemates may develop irrespective of the identity of the analysand supervised; these problems require full attention despite being "unparalleled."

Let me give an example of a supervisory process that ran into difficulty: The supervisory session starts with my supervisee telling me she met outside my building another candidate, whose supervisory session precedes hers. She told him she would blame him for her coming late and he laughed at her for taking things too severely.

She then describes two sessions she had with her analysand after their break. In the first one he smiled at her warmly when entering and told her later he wanted to give her a good feeling. He missed her, but did not feel shaken up as in the previous break. He almost got into his customary acting out, but he thought of her and avoided it. Unlike before, he was less prone to assume she went skiing abroad, a change that for him implied seeing the two of them as less distant (skiing signifies for him that she is an upper-class "lady"). He apologized for still not being in the mood for work and said serious analysis would start in the subsequent session. He expressed a wish to sit up and mentioned that he almost did assume this position when he came in to start the session.

The analyst then made an interpretation that today the analysand came to the "absent her." He (the analysand) could not understand. I admit to my supervisee that I, too, am not sure I understand what she meant by "absent her." (In retrospect I see that "I don't understand" may have been a euphemism for "I disagree.") She apologises that she was in a holiday mood herself and was happy that work would resume only gradually. I suggest that they both too easily agree that "no work is going on," while in my experience this is a very valuable session: the analysand describes an important transition in the transference, a feeling of intimacy rather than of awe, a greater capacity to use her as a protective internalized object and a deeper capacity to experience gratitude, much less of his customary depreciatory self-blaming.

The supervisee now attributes her own reaction in the session to her need to give "deep" interpretations. She relates it to the difficulty between us that came up recently, around her disappointment that I do not help her to develop such deeper interpretations. Her comment coincides with a feeling I have and share with her: that she experiences me (as she sees the candidate who came before her?) as too "light," as belittling the severity of her analysand's condition. She disagrees with "belittling," but feels "making light of" indeed describes her experience. She and her analysand, she comments, have in common a "heavy" superego. I tell her I feel a bit clearer as to the source of the difficulty between us.

In the second session, she now reports, the analysand came late and felt very guilty. She tried to reflect his harshness in judging himself (he works enormously hard and has to schedule his sessions at peak-traffic morning times so as not to neglect his work) and his attempt to turn her into a scolding boss. He responded by expressing disbelief that she really wasn't shocked by his coming late. I ask her whether she pursued his disbelief further and when she says she did not, I wonder about it. (While writing, I think I may have been influenced by the way our session started with her own fear of being late, but this did not come up directly in our session.) I also share a thought I have: she makes many efforts to confront his rigidity, but something in the atmosphere of the sessions does not supply an alternative pole to it, an option of "playing" and not only "working." She comments that her patients rarely laugh in the sessions, though there are individual differences.

These related issues, in the analytic dyad and in our own relationship, were further explored in the following sessions. A few months later my supervisee told me she wanted to switch to another supervisor. We discussed her wish for several weeks, exploring her expectations from supervision and the way they diverged from our actual work and in general our mutual experiences of each other. I supported the legitimacy of a switch, seeing this option as an expression of the freer atmosphere in our institute (Berman, 1998). At the same time, I told her I was sad that we were apparently not able to fully resolve our difficulties, in spite of repeated efforts.

I also found myself concerned as to whether her leaving might deter other candidates from seeking supervision with me, but I felt such concerns should not be shared at that time with the supervisee. (Naturally, self-disclosure by the supervisor is an option to be contemplated with full attention to both possible benefits and potential risks, such as unduly burdening the supervisee.)

In retrospect, I feel her decision indicated that I may not have been sufficiently empathic and patient in my attempts to encourage this talented trainee to allow herself to become a "lighter," more playful analyst. Possibly, I failed to understand fully the appeal of being "heavy" for her, her apparent equation between depth, seriousness and severity. Was I "a bull in a china shop?"

When discussing the issue with this supervisee some years later, after she read a draft of the present paper, she suggested that we did not give sufficient attention to the impact of the theoretical differences between her mostly British sources of inspiration (particularly Klein, Bion, Meltzer) and the relational American emphases in my own work. This, she felt, may explain our difficulties better than the more personal level I emphasised.

Personally, I believe that while our discussions did not stop her from switching supervisors and although we never reached full agreement about the nature of our differences, their frank open exploration contributed to the non-traumatic outcome of the supervisory crisis and to our capacity to maintain a good relationship.

The Triad in the Context of Institutional Dynamics

We should remember that the triad does not exist in a vacuum. An intersubjective understanding, for me, also requires attention to the influences of broader organizational, cultural, and historical currents on the subjective experiences of all individuals involved. (This may be described as moving from a two-person psychology towards a multiple-person psychology.) The supervisory relationship is often colored by its institutional context and by its atmosphere (Shane and Shane, 1995; Fraser, 1996) and by the transferential feelings both supervisor and candidate develop toward their institute: identification, reservations, idealization, rebellion and so on (Berman, 1997b).

A major influence of the institute is in the area of evaluation. The joint exploration of the impact of the supervisor's evaluative role may become vital, as this role may potentially sabotage supervision as a meaningful mutual learning process.

There are inherent critical-evaluative elements in any honest supervisory intervention: enthusiasm or concern, attention to blind spots, suggested changes. Within the live relationship in the dyad, narcissistic vulnerability to criticism can be contained and worked through; possible insults can be discussed and ideally resolved. This is easier when the supervisor avoids assuming an omniscient position and is willing to examine her or his role in difficulties, putting evaluation too in an intersubjective context. Such openness and basic trust in the candidate's capacity for future growth, create a *background of safety*, which makes it possible for the supervisor to express criticism honestly. The exploration of personal aspects of countertransference, some of which may be experienced as arousing guilt or shame, is also naturally easier in a more egalitarian and friendlier atmosphere.

In contrast to straightforward face-to-face criticism within an intimate dyad, reports to institutional committees *take evaluation out of its intersubjective context*, give it the pretense of selfless objective judgment and cut it off from the setting in which criticism can promote change (Berman, 2000). Committees may spend long hours in discussing the personality of trainees, in what borders on a clinical case conference or degenerates into gossip, but they can do very little to help the development of a troubled younger colleague. Moreover, the existence of an elaborate evaluation system may allow the supervisor to "pass the buck" and avoid the stressful moment of expressing criticism within supervision. Anonymous institutional feedback often leads to a defensive anxious confrontation, while reducing the chance for effective learning within the supervisory dyad. Effective learning, I suggest, is most enhanced by a supervisor who is openly critical but also self-critical and willing to explore openly the way in which this criticism is experienced, reducing as much as possible any reporting to external authorities and discussing any such reporting openly within supervision (Sarnat, 1992; Caruth, 1990).

The Boundaries Between Supervision and Analysis

My focus on exploring personal experiences in supervision (counter-transference to patient, kernels of truth encountered in patient's view of analyst's personality, transference to supervisor and to institution) naturally raises the old issue of the boundaries between analysis and supervision. In a way, my approach could bring me closer to the view of the Budapest school (Balint, 1948) that the ideal supervisor is the trainee's analyst. Nevertheless, I disapprove of this suggestion. Such a combination (either simultaneously, or even if supervision is planned to start after analysis) may undermine the depth of the analysis, discourage the expression of negative transference, dilute work on termination and introduce an unanalysable collusion (Berman, 1995). It may lead to an exaggerated identification with *the* analyst-supervisor-mentor as a single parental figure, not allowing the painful but fruitful conflict of competing identifications in moulding one's unique and autonomous analytic self (Berman, 1999). Moreover, the analysis of future analysts benefits from being a very private affair, not directly mobilised for training goals, therefore not regulated or interfered with by training settings (Berman, 1997d, 1998).

My image of good analytic training thus maintains the coexistence—and, at times, the troublesome split—between a personal analyst (preferably more than one along the way) and several supervisors; a degree of *overlap between the contents of analysis and supervision* (Lester and Robertson, 1995); and a continuous *exploration of their complex interaction*, within analysis and at times within supervision as well. Each candidate-analyst-supervisor triangle may arouse new meaningful issues and the significance given to the different figures may not match their declared functions.[1]

The total milieu of the institute creates a complex transferential network, in which various transferential roles are played by different figures (a phenomenon often observed in group analysis). The planned division of labour between analysis and supervision may become partial and secondary for the candidate, in this context. Supervisors may be experienced as auxiliary analysts and the analyst as an auxiliary supervisor. The following example, coming from an analysis, clarifies the way in which supervision may become—in the candidate's inner reality—an extension of analysis:

---

[1] At the Israel Psychoanalytic Institute, candidates typically continue their analysis throughout most of their training, but in some cases (when analysis has started long before the candidate's admission, or when training is prolonged by various circumstances) analysis may be terminated while supervision still goes on.

The analysand describes a dilemma he experiences with one of his psychotherapy patients (a case not in supervision). This young woman is now enraged with her mother, with whom she lives, for not pampering her enough, not buying her the cinnamon rolls which she loves eating in the morning. He is torn between two different inner voices as to the way to react to her rage. One voice challenges her to explore how she could pamper herself more, encourages her to grow out of her prolonged dependency. This voice he identifies with me. (He told me in the past that he feels at times that I don't encourage regression in his analysis, which is both a relief and a disappointment.) The other voice conveys full empathy with the patient's regressive yearnings. This voice he identifies with one of his analytic supervisors, a woman analyst who sees regression as a major curative element.

In principle he knows that the dialogue between these two voices— and maybe also the voices of his former analyst and of other supervisors— could be enriching and productive in gradually fostering his own individual integration. But, emotionally, he feels torn. He is reminded of a period during his army service, when he had two commanding officers. He recalls how one would often shout, "faster, faster!" while the other would say, "calm down, slow down." The combination makes him anxious.

He is reminded of a crisis period he went through with another patient, where he also felt a gap between what emerged from his work with me and with that supervisor. Then he found recently an effective interpretive direction which drew upon both voices, taking from each of us what suits him. He says he realises this was easier to achieve because of his awareness that this supervisor and I are good friends.

When his parents divorced, in his childhood, the break-up was total. They lived utterly different lifestyles, in two different cities. His home, he once joked, was in the bus in between. He identified totally with one parent, maintained emotional distance from the other, in spite of regular visits. The spouse of one parent frequently criticized the other parent in his presence. To avoid conflict, he never talked about one parent with the other. There was no hope of integration.

He now comes to realize how new for him is the present situation. He speaks with his supervisor about his analysis and he speaks with me about his supervision. Our different views, which we both appear very committed to, do not stop me and his supervisor from being friends and he does not feel either of us demands total loyalty of him. Still, handling the differences is not easy.

This analysand "borrows" the analytic experience with me as an indirect supervision (making me a potential role model), while "borrowing" the supervisory work with my colleague as a partial analytic experience. He gets in that supervision legitimization for regressive needs, which he finds are less gratified with me. Does he want to encourage me, I wonder, to allow more space for his own yearning for his version of a cinnamon roll?

Although the analytic setting offers ideal conditions for a full exploration of such a process, I also experienced fruitful discussions of similar dynamics with some supervisees and this exploration aided in improving supervisory work.

Telling trainees "bring it up in your analysis" is of no use, in my experience, for many reasons: it is intrusive and unrealistic (a genuine analytic process cannot follow assignments); it deprives supervision of the understanding of crucial issues, without which we cannot figure out what goes on in the treatment discussed and in the supervisory relationship itself; and it may be experienced as conveying a rule-dominated (or role-dominated) avoidance rather than involvement and openness to full analytic learning.

When I am totally unaware of my supervisee's private life and major personal concerns, I may be grappling in the dark in my attempt to understand many issues in this supervisee's work with analysands. Communicating with the supervisee's analyst (DeBell, 1963) would be a violation of confidentiality on both sides; such paternalistic informal conversations often turn out to be detrimental to both analysis and supervision (Berman, 1995; Langs, 1979). The ethical option is to create in supervision a tolerant and attentive atmosphere, which will make it easier for trainees—only if they wish, of course—to share personal associations and feelings whenever they appear to be potentially relevant to the task at hand, or when their relevance may be intuitively sensed.

A situation in which my own personal example facilitated such an exploration comes to mind. I could sense that my supervisee responded intolerantly to her analysand's cancellation of some sessions, which happened on the background of progress in the analysand's vocational and personal life. I shared with my supervisee a spontaneous association that crossed my mind, to my own feelings of frustration and jealousy when my daughter had less time to spend with me, as a result of her expanding involvement with her peers. The supervisee then recalled similar themes with her own children and related them to her countertransference towards her analysand.

In principle, no personal topic is, for me, out of place in supervision. A supervisee's impending divorce may be a major influence on countertransference to analysands; a childhood event may be the source of identification with a particular patient; a dream may offer the key to the stalemate in a certain case. Naturally, the extent, direction and style of exploration are very different in analysis and in supervision and I do not advocate turning supervision into a "mini-analysis."

The personal analyst attempts to reach the deepest and broadest understanding, proceeding open-mindedly with no immediate goals; the supervisor is much more selective and goal-orientated, focusing on the aspects of the personal theme that can be directly related to visible consequences and dilemmas in the trainee's work with analysands and within supervision itself.

Likewise, the supervisor wishes to identify the supervisee's transference towards her or him, but without searching for its deeper historical roots and at times simply relying on the trainee's account as a summary of analytic work already done. The more crucial focus within supervision is rather on possible reality influences, such as the impact of the supervisor's personality, as well as on the effective resolution of troublesome consequences of transference-countertransference entanglements in supervision, such as anxiety, inhibition, antagonism or estrangement.

Transitional Space Evolving in Supervision

If this work is effective, an open personal atmosphere can develop in supervision and such an atmosphere may facilitate a much fuller creative use of the supervisory situation. This use, aided by attention to immediate affective nuances and to reverie, may become close to what Ogden describes when he speaks of "the analytic third" (see Ogden, 1995, especially part III). The inner freedom achieved may allow a supervision with an intersubjective focus to *evolve into a transitional space, within which the dyad generates new meanings* not accessible by the intrapsychic work of each partner in isolation.

Consider the following session with a supervisee:

He starts our hour by telling me of his difficulty with writing down the sessions with the woman analysand whose analysis I supervise. The sessions themselves, however, he experiences as quite good. She comes at times five minutes early and he enjoys meeting her need and starting early, which he rarely does with other patients. During the sessions this past week he found himself in a drowsy state. His analysand praised him for his soft, gentle side, which "enables her things."

I raise my thoughts about two possible meanings of his difficulty with writing: is it deeply related to an early, primary, pre-verbal side of his analysand, which is hard to put into words? Or is it an avoidance motivated by anxiety?

He recalls that she said about some topic that he should discuss it with his woman supervisor (in Hebrew, one cannot say supervisor without specifying gender). His other analysand, a man with whom he feels much more on his guard, refers to a male supervisor, while he is actually supervised on his work with him by a woman analyst.

Drawing on conversations we have had in the past, I comment on how issues of masculinity and femininity come up here in a complex manner. He conveys to me that in the other analysis he is constantly threatened and attacked by his critical male analysand. He is relaxed, drowsy, more in a "being" state which inhibits "doing" (writing), between his female analysand and me, whom he appears to experience as feminine/motherly.

I remind him, however, of recent episodes in which his woman analysand criticized him for not being strong (maybe manly?) enough. In one case, when she felt he did not do enough to stop some noise which irritated her, she went at the end of the session to protest to the noisy person herself, as if telling her analyst, "if you have no balls, I'll take command." This phallic side of her, I recall, aroused anxiety and embarrassment in him.

He now discusses the sessions. The analysand spoke of anxiety she experienced when she heard an alarm in the house of a bereaved neighbor, a woman who had lost her child in a terrorist attack. She had a fantasy that her neighbor may have committed suicide. Then she suddenly made a comment, that from the place where her analyst sits he sees bodies. They were both perplexed by this comment and I tell him I am too. The word she used implies a dead body (*gufa*), though it is close to the word for a live body (*guf*). He says that as a result of her comment he became more attentive to her *gufa* and when I ask if this was a slip of tongue, he tells me of a slang expression (which I did not know) in which a woman's body is referred to this way. I speak of the defensive significance of this slang usage and relate it to common jokes based on the multiple significance of another Hebrew word, *shahav* (lay down), which has both a strong sexual meaning (roughly equivalent to "slept with") and a connotation of death (the biblical "lay down with his forefathers").

The analysand then spoke of her tendency to buy ornamental items for her house and my supervisee says he felt reserved, experiencing her as too ornate. She specifically talked of an unidentified item she called *tomba*, saying it could seem as a coffin. She commented she was building a little temple in her house.

This material brings to my mind a recent visit to Egypt. I tell my supervisee of a comment a guide made about how little the ancient Egyptians invested in their lifetime houses in comparison to their enormous investment in their "death houses," their tombs. My supervisee relates this to the Jewish traditional view, that life is but a corridor to the parlour of afterlife.

I now recall that this analysand sought treatment right after her neighbor's child was killed and suggest that only now have the emotional reverberations of that event come to the surface. Saying "from the place you sit you see bodies" attributes to the analyst an awesome perspective of an eternal observer, who sees generations come and go, babies grow up, become children and then adults, grow old and die. Her "little temple" is a representation of her preoccupation with death, which she has difficulty in integrating with other sides of herself as a practical and goal-directed woman.

The analyst now recalls that in the sessions following the one discussed the analysand had difficulty in lying down on the couch. Our time is up.

We started from the analyst's difficulty in writing sessions. This was not defined as necessarily a resistance or an obstacle to our work, Indeed, it proved to be a springboard for further understanding, which itself shifted focuses during the session, from issues of gender identity and affective states to issues of life and death, sexuality and annihilation anxiety.

This supervisory session is for me a rich example of the way in which a transitional space can evolve in the supervisory dyad, allowing the generation of meaning in a way that is equivalent to, resonant with and supplementary to the analytic dyad. While no purely personal details concerning my supervisee or myself were discussed, the atmosphere of the session was personal and close and I believe this helped make it more creative.

The combined analytic-supervisory team may allow intersubjective trends to develop and be consciously experienced, promoting their verbalisation and elaboration in a way which is at times more difficult to achieve in the isolation of the unsupervised analytic dyad alone.

A Broad Range of Options

This paper does not strive towards crystallizing a new general technique of supervision. Not believing in a standard analytic technique, I certainly do not advocate a standardization of supervision. I wish to highlight certain dynamic processes and to legitimize their open exploration; but undoubtedly the specific focus and style of each supervisory dyad will always depend on the unique personalities of both partners. It will also be influenced by the analysand, by the candidate's analyst, by the institute and by contemporary values and national culture.

Supervision benefits from evolution through a flexible mutual adaptation, in which the needs of both partners play a role, as each is recognized as a subject by the other (Slavin, 1998). Supervisors are different as individuals and as analysts. Some may utilize their awareness of nuances in the supervisory relationship as a basis for improving supervision without ever discussing the relationship directly, while others may be more prone to bring it up as a topic. Supervision requires making constant choices, as what comes up in each session can be understood on numerous different levels. These choices may be wiser when based on analytic understanding of the intrapsychic and intersubjective dynamics involved; routine solutions of any kind may endanger the freshness and depth of the needed scrutiny.

In my own supervisory work, I find myself quite different with various supervisees. The degree to which personal issues come up and the nature of boundaries, in general, vary considerably. The variance appears to be influenced both by the conscious wishes of supervisees and by more subtle transference–countertransference patterns in each relationship. In some supervisory dyads the process itself is explored in joint curiosity; in others it remains quietly in the background. Imposing one's values and preferences (e.g., insisting that the supervisee share his or her life story, or deeper transferential reactions toward the supervisor, with the supervisor) is counterproductive. Enforced egalitarianism (possibly based on a fantasy of "rescuing the victim," e.g., the underprivileged candidate; see Berman, 1993, 1997a) could be as aggressive as authoritarian paternalism and even more confusing.

Moreover, in the course of one supervisory process there may be different stages and unique moments, which require new creative approaches.

In my earlier work on supervision (Berman, 1988) the issue of resistance to supervision played a central role. While I still believe that in some instances supervisees resist supervision per se (through fear of change, negativism, envy and other individual dynamics that block any new learning, or any learning that is not autodidactic), my guess is that the more common source of difficulty is a specific—and often unarticulated—conflict between supervisor and supervisee, who do not manage to work out together a supervisory agenda that suits both of them.

In conclusion, my hope is not to offer any universal methods, but rather to outline a broad range of options, which supervisors and trainees alike can take advantage of, in moulding and enriching their personal ways of learning.

References

Arlow, J. (1963). The supervisory situation. *J. Amer. Psychoanal. Assn.*, 11:576–94.
Aron, L. (1996). *A Meeting of Minds. Mutuality in Psychoanalysis*. Hillsdale, NJ: The Analytic Press.
Balint, M. (1948). On the psycho-analytic training system. *Internat J. Psychoanal*, 29: 16–73.
Baudry, F. D. (1993). The personal dimension and management of the supervisory situation with a special note on the parallel process. *Psychoanal. Q.*, 62:588–614.
Berman, E. (1988). The joint exploration of the supervisory relationship as an aspect of psychoanalytic supervision. In *New Concepts in Psychoanalytic Psychotherapy*, ed. J. M. Ross & W. Myers. Washington, DC: American Psychiatric Press, pp. 150–166.
———— (1993). Psychoanalysis, rescue and utopia. *Utopian Studies*, 4:44–56.
———— (1994). Review essay on Etchegoyen's *The Fundamentals of Psycho-Analytic Technique*. *Psychoanal. Dialogues*, 4:129–38.
———— (1995). On analyzing colleagues. *Contemp. Psychoanal*, 31:521–539.
———— (1996). The Ferenczi renaissance. *Psychoanal. Dialogues*, 6:391–411.
———— (1997a). Hitchcock's "Vertigo": the collapse of a rescue fantasy. *Internat. J. Psychoanal.*, 78:975–96.
———— (1997b). Psychoanalytic supervision as the crossroads of a relational matrix. In *Psychodynamic Supervision*, ed. M. Rock. Northvale, NJ: Aronson, pp. 160–86.
———— (1997c). Relational psychoanalysis: a historical perspective. *Amer. J. Psychother.*, 51:185–203.
———— (1997d). Letter to the editor. *Psychoanal. in Europe*, 49:95–100.
———— (1998). Structure and individuality in psychoanalytic training: the Israeli controversial discussions. *Amer. J. Psychoanal.*, 58:117–33.
———— (1999). Sandor Ferenczi today: Reviving the broken dialectic. *Amer. J. Psychoanal.*, 59:303–13.
———— (2000). The utopian fantasy of a new person and the danger of a false analytic self. *Psychoanal. Psychol.*, 17:38–60.
Bollas, C. (1987). Expressive uses of the counter-transference. In: *The Shadow of the Object*. New York: Columbia University Press, pp. 200–235.
Caruth, E. G. (1990). Interpersonal and intrapsychic complexities and vulnerabilities in the psychoanalytic supervisory process. In *Psychoanalytic Approaches to Supervision*, ed. R. C. Lane. New York: Brunner/Mazel, pp. 181–93.
DeBell, D. E. (1963). A critical digest of the literature on psychoanalytic supervision. *J. Amer. Psychoanal. Assn.*, 11:546–75.
Doehrman, M. J. (1976). Parallel processes in supervision and psychotherapy. *Bull. Menninger Clinic*, 40:3–104.
Ekstein, R. & Wallerstein, R. S. (1972). *The Teaching and Learning of Psychotherapy*. New York: International Universities Press.
Epstein, L. (1986). Collusive selective inattention to the negative impact of the supervisory interaction. *Contemp. Psychoanal.*, 22:389–409.
Etchegoyen, H. (1991). *The Fundamentals of Psychoanalytic Technique*. London: Karnac.

Fairbairn, W. R. D. (1954). *An Object Relations Theory of the Personality.* New York: Basic Books.

Fraser, K. (1996). What goes on in supervision and isn't talked about: beyond the didactic to the dyadic. Paper in panel, Supervision as an intersubjective process. American Psychoanalytic Association fall meeting.

Gediman, H. K. & Wolkenfeld, F. (1980). The parallelism phenomenon in psychoanalysis and supervision: its reconsideration as a triadic system. *Psychoanal. Q.*, 49:234–55.

Gill, M. M. (1982). *The Analysis of Transference.* New York: International Universities Press.

Greenson, R. (1967). *The Technique and Practice of Psychoanalysis.* New York: International Universities Press.

Grinberg, L. (1979). Countertransference and projective counteridentification. *Contemp. Psychoanal.*, 15:226–247.

Haynal, A. (1993). Ferenczi and the origins of psychoanalytic technique. In *The Legacy of Sandor Ferenczi*, ed. L. Aron & A. Harris. Hillsdale, NJ: The Analytic Press, pp. 53–74.

Langs, R. (1979). *The Supervisory Experience.* New York: Aronson.

Lesser, R. (1984). Supervision: illusions, anxieties and questions. In *Clinical Perspectives on the Supervision of Psychoanalysis and Psychotherapy*, ed. L. Caligor et al. New York: Plenum, pp. 143–152.

Lester, E. & Robertson, B. (1995). Multiple interactive processes in psychoanalytic supervision. *Psychoanal. Inq.*, 15:211–225.

Luber, M. P. (1991). A patient's transference to the analyst's supervisor: effect of the setting on the analytic process. *J. Amer. Psychoanal. Assn.*, 39:705–725.

Mayer, E. L. (1996). Introductory remarks to panel "Supervision as an intersubjective process." American Psychoanalytic Association fall meeting.

Ogden, T. H. (1995). Analysing forms of aliveness and deadness of the transference-countertransference. *Int. J. Psychoanal.*, 76:695–709.

Racker, H. (1968). *Transference and Countertransference.* New York: International Universities Press.

Sandler, J. (1976). Countertransference and role-responsiveness. *Int. Rev. Psychoanal.*, 3:43–48.

Sarnat, J. (1992). Supervision in relationship. *Psychoanal. Psychol.*, 9:387–403.

Searles, H. (1955). The informational value of the supervisor's emotional experience. In *Collected Papers on Schizophrenia.* New York: International Universities Press, 1965.

——— (1962). Problems of psychoanalytic supervision. *Collected Papers on Schizophrenia.* New York: International Universities Press, 1965.

Shane, M. & Shane, E. (1995). Un-American activities and other dilemmas experienced in the supervision of candidates. *Psychoanal. Inq.*, 15:226–39.

Slavin, J. (1998). Influence and vulnerability in psychoanalytic supervision and treatment. *Psychoanal. Psychol.*, 15:230–44.

Sloane, J. (1986). The empathic vantage point in supervision. *Progress in Self Psychology*, 2:188–211. Hillsdale, NJ: The Analytic Press.

Springmann, R. R. (1986). Countertransference clarification in supervision. *Contemp. Psychoanal.*, 22:252–77.

Stimmel, B. (1995). Resistance to the awareness of the supervisor's transference with special reference to parallel process. *Int. J. Psychoanal.*, 76:609–18.

Szecsödy, I. (1999). Report on the follow-up responses received from the presenting supervisors/supervisees at the 8th IPA conference of training analysts. *Int. Psychoanal.*, 8:20–23.

Tansey, M. & Burke, W. (1989). *Understanding Countertransference*. Hillsdale, NJ: Analytic Press.

Teitelbaum, S. H. (1990). Supertransference: The role of the supervisor's blind spots. *Psychoanal. Psychol.*, 7:243–58.

Winokur, M. (1982). A family systems model for supervision of psychotherapy. *Bulln. Menninger Clinic*, 46:125–38.

Wolkenfeld, F. (1990). The parallel process phenomenon revisited: some additional thoughts about the supervisory process. In *Psychoanalytic Approaches to Supervision*, ed. R. C. Lane. New York: Brunner/Mazel, pp. 95–109.

Yerushalmi, H. (1992). On the concealment of the interpersonal therapeutic reality in the course of supervision. *Psychother.*, 29:438–46.

Afterword

My development as a relational analyst has its roots in my first analytic training at the NYU Postdoctoral Program in the 1970s, when I took both Freudian and interpersonal seminars, and where my first supervisor was Emmanuel Ghent (the other two were Ruth-Jean Eisenbud and Mark Grunes, Freudians with a strong interest in object relations and in countertransference). During the same years I worked at the Bronx Psychiatric Center, affiliated with the Albert Einstein College of Medicine, where I was trained in psychoanalytic group therapy and in family therapy, both with a strong emphasis on analyzing relationship patterns. My interest in the work of Ferenczi, Balint, Fairbairn, and Winnicott followed me through my second analytic training, at the Israel Psychoanalytic Institute.

This background can be sensed in my first paper on supervision (Berman, 1988), dedicated to the value of the supervisor–supervisee dialogue about their relationship. In the following decade, however, I came to realize that my understanding of that relationship had emphasized each partner's unique conflicts, without sufficient attention to the common anxieties and to their mutual impact. Also, the focus on resistance and on crises expressing negative therapeutic reactions suited me less as time went on, even though the way I conceptualized the negative supervisory reaction was inspired all along by "two-person psychology" models, such as the notion of an "interactional negative therapeutic reaction" (Langs, 1976) and the understanding of a negative therapeutic reaction as a result of "prolonged, unrecognized transference-countertransference disjunctions" (Stolorow, Brandchaft, and Atwood, 1983, p. 120).

My involvement during the 1990s with the new relational orientation at NYU (where I teach on sabbaticals) and with *Psychoanalytic Dialogues*, helped to crystalize my more systematic thinking about the intersubjective dimension of supervision, and about its nature as the "crossroads of a relational matrix" (Berman, 1997).

The growing interest in relational supervisory processes in the international community allowed me also to help initiate a setting for their live exploration. Such a forum was successfully created at the International Psychoanalytic Association's training analysts' conference in Barcelona in 1997 (Szecsödy, 1999), when dyads of supervisor and supervisee brought up their respective experiences in supervision for discussion in small groups of analysts. The two-sided account often allowed much better understanding of the supervisory process and its dilemmas than could ever have been achieved by hearing the supervisor alone, as usual. This innovative format was established over the objections of numerous analysts, particularly from France and from Britain, who were concerned about boundaries being eroded, complained that the candidates asked to present became overexcited, and expressed a fear that the joint presentation would destroy the psychic process of supervision (Brenman-Pick, 1997).

The paper included here was initially prepared for the next meeting of the IPA, in Santiago in 1999. Building on the theoretical foundation of the 1997 paper, it introduced new, richer, and fuller examples. It can be considered a twin to another paper published simultaneously, dealing with the broader social and emotional dilemmas of analytic training (Berman, 2000). There I attempt to pinpoint the idealizations that contribute to persecutory and infantilizing trends in training and trace their potential contribution to a strengthening of "analytic false-self" components in the analyst's professional identity.

The discussion of these issues, as well as of intersubjectivity in supervision, is considerably expanded in my book *Impossible Training* (Berman, 2004), in which the complex interrelations of the dynamics of analytic and other clinical training settings, of the broader social and cultural milieu, of the trainees' personal analysis, and of supervision are explored. As I demonstrate in that book, the conflictual dynamics of two "generative dyads"—Freud-Ferenczi (a relationship that combined analysis, friendship, and occasional supervision) and Klein-Winnicott (a relationship that started as supervision)—can be seen as the springboard for Ferenczi's and Winnicott's profound relational intuitions.

The literature on the intersubjective dimension of supervision has been expanding quickly in the last few years. Thinking of supervisory relationships has become characterized by an ambience of self-disclosure (Coburn, 1997). Frawley-O'Dea and Sarnat (2001), developing a typology of supervisory models, differentiate between a patient-centered model (classical); three therapist-centered models, emphasizing learning problems (ego-psychological), empathy (self-psychological) and anxiety (object relations); and a supervisory-matrix-centered model (relational). In the relational model further explored by Frawley-O'Dea (2003), patient, therapist, and supervisor are "viewed as co-creators of two mutually influential dyads" (p. 356). She writes, "The more fully and freely supervisor and supervisee represent the intricacies of their own relationship . . . the more completely and effectively the supervisee can engage with the patient in identifying and speaking about the relational paradigms operating within the treatment" (p. 360).

An alternative formulation is offered by Brown and Miller (2002), who speak not of two dyads, but rather of a triadic intersubjective matrix that can be seen (to paraphase Ogden) as creating "a supervisory fourth." Their work, including mutual disclosure of dreams by supervisor and supervisee, attempts to uncover "the confluence of the interlocking unconscious processes of the patient, analyst and supervisor" (p. 814).

Kantrowitz (2002) reports a study of four analysand-candidate-supervisor triads based on detailed interviews with both candidate and supervisor. She chose to study only triads having a beneficial impact, but, because one of her cases involved switching supervisors, the experience of mismatch comes up too. When the basic supervisory relationship is well understood, she demonstrates, it is also possible to notice how the analyst's encounter with the analysand influences it.[1] A major issue Kantrowitz raises is the delicate balance between comfort and challenge: "When candidates feel more confident, they are less prone to fear criticism or experience shame, and are more receptive to learning something new" (p. 960).

I am sure that by the time this book appears there will be additional interesting contributions. We seem to be moving away from a didactic emphasis on what should be done in supervision (by the domi-

---

[1] There is, however, no expectation that this influence will be fundamental as the older parallel process literature suggests.

nant supervisor) to an observational, introspective, and empathic emphasis on what actually happens in the supervisory process, often beyond the conscious intentions of its participants. I believe this new trend is more deeply loyal to a psychoanalytic view of emotional life. It can help in training analysts and therapists who are freer to be in touch with themselves and therefore can meet more creatively and more flexibly the challenges of future patients and future society.

References

Berman, E. (1988), The joint exploration of the supervisory relationship as an aspect of psychoanalytic supervision. In: *New Concepts in Psychoanalytic Psychotherapy*, ed. J. Ross & W. Myers. Washington, DC: American Psychiatric Press, pp. 150–166.

———— (1997), Psychoanalytic supervision as the crossroads of a relational matrix. In: *Psychodynamic Supervision*, ed. M. Rock. Northvale, NJ: Aronson, pp. 160–186.

———— (2000), The utopian fantasy of a new person and the danger of a false analytic self. *Psychoanal. Psychol.*, 17:38–60.

———— (2004), *Impossible Training: A Relational Psychoanalytic View of Clinical Training and Supervision*. Hillsdale, NJ: The Analytic Press.

Brenman-Pick, I. (1997), Letter to Dan H. Buie. *Internat. Psychoanal.*, 6:32–33.

Brown, L. & Miller, M. (2002), The triadic intersubjective matrix in supervision. *Internat. J. Psycho-Anal.*, 83:811–823.

Coburn, W. (1997), The vision in supervision: Transference-countertransference dynamics and disclosure in the supervision relationship. *Bull. Menninger Clin.*, 61:481–494.

Frawley-O'Dea, M. G. (2003), Supervision is a relationship too. *Psychoanal. Dial.*, 13:355–366.

———— & Sarnat, J. E. (2001), *The Supervisory Relationship: A Contemporary Psychodynamic Approach*. New York: Guilford Press.

Kantrowitz, J. L. (2002), The triadic match: The interactive effect of supervisor, candidate and patient. *J. Amer. Psychoanal. Assn.*, 50:939–968.

Langs, R. (1976), *The Therapeutic Interaction*. New York: Aronson.

Stolorow, R., Brandchaft, B. & Atwood, G. E. (1983), Intersubjectivity in psychoanalytic treatment. *Bull. Menninger Clin.*, 47:117–128.

Szecsödy, I. (1999), Report on the follow-up responses received from the presenting supervisors/supervisees at the 8th IPA conference of training analysts. *Internat. Psychoanal.*, 8:20–23.

On Misreading and Misleading Patients: Some Reflections on Communications, Miscommunications, and Countertransference Enactments

(2001)

Theodore Jacobs

▼　▼　▼　▼　▼

Editors' Introduction

The relational turn has transcended any single "school" of psycho-analysis. Perhaps no contemporary analyst has done more than Theodore Jacobs to expand the scope of classical psychoanalytic tech-nique. Over the course of his career and in his masterful book, *The Use of the Self* (1991IUP,). Jacobs has demonstrated how one can maintain the classical psychoanalytic situation while valuing and uti-lizing the analyst's emotional responses to patients. While tracing his own analytic influences to such classic thinkers as Isakower, Arlow, and Loewald, he has expanded their notions of "the analytic instru-ment" and the importance of unconscious fantasy to emphasize how much an analyst personally brings to the process. Jacobs was among the first to introduce the idea of enactment into the psychoanalytic literature. Since its introduction, enactment has become among the central clinical concepts in the relational tradition.

The term enactment is so frequently used that its meaning has been broadened, extended, and stretched beyond recognizable bounds. By enactment, Jacobs was trying to convey the idea that there are behaviors on the part of patient, analyst, or both that arise as a response to conflicts and fantasies aroused in each by the ongoing therapeutic work. While linked to the interplay of transference and countertransference, these behaviors are also connected, through memory, to associated thoughts, fantasies, and experiences of childhood or adolescence. Thus, for Jacobs, the idea of enactment contains within it the notion of reenactment, the reliving of bits and pieces of our psychological past.

Examining a variety of styles of analytic interaction, in 1997 Stephen Mitchell wrote that "Jacobs's clinical descriptions are enormously rich in their detailing of the evocation in the analyst of memories, affects, and self-states, generally from the analyst's own distant past, that are mirror images of the patient's central relational configurations" (p. 146). He referred to Jacobs's genius for making available past self-states to deepen his affective understanding of his patient's struggles by finding "resonating parallels" between the patient's and the analyst's life histories.

Jacobs's own personally revealing, yet nonexhibitionistic, writing style facilitates the exposition of his groundbreaking ideas. Jacobs points to our narcissistic vulnerability as analysts and to how our "petty faults" get in the way of our analytic work. He writes here of "our moments of meanness, of spiteful retaliation, of boastfulness, of greed, of inattention, or self-justification and of small-minded competitiveness with colleagues." Jacobs demonstrates, by revealing to us his own foibles, how the analyst's personal shortcomings exert a powerful influence on an analysis that may ordinarily go unacknowledged and unexamined.

In his recent work, Jacobs has developed his understanding of enactment to examine more closely how even ordinary analytic technique may be used at times for unconscious communication within the transference–countertransference interaction to serve as covert enactments. He has sensitized analysts to the significance of the nonverbal sphere, in which gesture, movement, and posture may express the feelings and fantasies of both patient and analyst. In the article that follows, Jacobs uses his characteristically vivid, personally revealing, and witty clinical writing style to illustrate how covert enactments may take the form of accurate and technically correct psychoanalytic interventions.

On Misreading and Misleading Patients:
Some Reflections on Communications, Miscommunications, and Countertransference Enactments*

As contrasted with the earlier conceptualization of countertransference as an obstacle to analytic work (Reich, 1951), contemporary views of countertransference (McLaughlin, 1981, 1987; Schwaber, 1992; Renik, 1993; Ehrenberg, 1997; Levine, 1997; Smith, 1999), emphasize its central role as a pathway to the unconscious of both patient and analyst.

While this perspective has been invaluable both in correcting the one-sided and limited view of countertransference that prevailed for many years and in underscoring the importance of the analyst's subjectivity as a means of understanding the patient, the current focus on this aspect of countertransference has led to some diminution in contributions that explore aspects of its other face; its problematic side.

Some contemporary authors, extending Brenner's view of countertransference as a compromise formation, maintain not only that countertransference represents the product of multiple, conflicting forces operating in the mind of the analyst, but that every instance of countertransference simultaneously facilitates and interferes with the analytic work (Smith, 1999).

While a theoretically plausible and an understandable extension of the contemporary view of countertransference as a multiply determined entity that can exert a number of effects on the analytic process, the idea that every countertransference response functions in this dual way has yet to be convincingly demonstrated.

Moreover, although this view may be theoretically correct, unless one can demonstrate how a piece of countertransference behavior both facilitates and retards the analytic work and the extent to which each effect operates in a session, such a perspective is, clinically, of limited value. In fact, by not making clear that the obstructing and facilitating effects of countertransference are rarely of equal importance and that in a given session, one of these forces may have a far greater impact on the process than the other, such a view of the clinical manifestations of countertransference can be misleading.

* Originally published in *International Journal of Psychoanalysis*, 82:653–669.
© 2000 International Psychoanalytic Association. Reprinted by permission.

Clearly there are instances in which the analyst's countertransference behavior is so disruptive—even destructive—and so derails the process that whatever facilitating effect it may also have, is, for all intent and purposes, a negligible factor in what is taking place in the clinical moment. The same is true on the positive side. At times the analyst's subjectivity, including particular countertransference responses, may have the effect of advancing the treatment. In such situations the positive effect of the countertransference is the central clinical fact that requires exploration and interpretation. At that moment any other effects that the countertransference may have induced, including the possibility that it covertly increases resistance in some manner, while not unimportant, are, from a clinical vantage point, secondary to the change that has taken place in the analytic process.

To determine the actual effect of countertransference on analytic work, as opposed to theoretical considerations, it is important not to confuse theory with the realities of the clinical encounter. Pragmatically, it is also important to assess the extent to which a countertransference response has actually enhanced or has retarded the analytic process. Failure to make these distinctions and assessments has the effect of clouding, rather than clarifying, the clinical picture.

In this paper, my focus will be on the clinical situation and on one facet of countertransference, its troublesome side; on an aspect of countertransference, in fact, that is easily overlooked. I am referring to situations in which particular needs, conflicts and biases of the analyst, not infrequently rooted in narcissistic conflicts, lie embedded within, and are concealed by, his quite proper and correct interventions; interventions which are derived from well-accepted theory and long-established techniques.

To illustrate these matters, I will offer several clinical examples in which issues of this kind led me to carry out troublesome countertransference enactments. In two instances these enactments were quite unconscious, and were it not for the patients' responses to them—in one case by confronting me with my behavior, in another by developing a symptom closely related to it—in all likelihood I would not have become aware of the impact of my actions.

In the third example, my behavior was also carried out spontaneously and, initially, outside of conscious awareness. Soon thereafter, however, I realized that the intervention that I had just offered was itself an enactment which misled the patient by deflecting her attention from behavior of mine which I did not wish to confront. Despite this understanding and the opportunity it gave me to make an immediate correction of my error, for reasons that I will discuss, I did not do so.

My purpose in describing these clinical vignettes is not solely to illustrate the way in which countertransference elements may be woven into the fabric of the analyst's interventions. I will also discuss several controversial issues raised by the clinical material.

One such issue concerns the analyst's countertransference reactions and whether or not they are inevitably enacted in sessions. That is, whether, as Renik (1993) maintains, such responses can neither be identified nor contained by the analyst prior to their being expressed in action.

On the basis of my clinical material, I will discuss this question from the standpoint of two pathways that countertransference reactions can take. While these means of communicating countertransference responses are not mutually exclusive and, in practice, regularly exist in some combination, at any given time, for reasons that have largely to do with forces operating in the mind of the analyst, one pathway may become the predominate one.

One form of countertransference, enacted outside of conscious awareness, is expressed primarily through nonverbal means. The other, which can be enacted through a variety of channels, initially registers in consciousness as an affect, thought, fantasy or memory. As I will discuss presently, it is the latter form of countertransference expression that the analyst may, through self-monitoring, be better able to contain rather than enact, while the former type, nonverbal reactions, expressed unconsciously in quite automatic fashion, conforms more closely to Renik's description of countertransference responses which can neither be identified nor controlled prior to being enacted in sessions. I will also comment on the relationship that not infrequently exists between the two types of countertransference reactions and the way in which the handling of one may affect the extent to which the other is enacted in sessions.

In connection with one of the cases that I will report, I will also touch on the thorny question of the handling of certain types of countertransference reactions; those in which, to avoid issues that cause him pain or embarrassment, including, and most especially, errors that he has made, the analyst intervenes in a way that misleads the patient by deflecting her attention away from the issue at hand. While for the most part such countertransference enactments are carried out spontaneously, only to be discovered later—if, in fact, the analyst recognizes them at all—they may also be consciously, and quite deliberately, performed. When troublesome countertransference behavior of this kind occurs, the question arises as to whether frank acknowledgment by the analyst of his actions and open discussion of the impact that his error has had on the patient advances the analytic work or, as some colleagues hold, unnecessarily burdens the patient and the treatment with the analyst's own issues. In connection with a case example, I will offer some thoughts about this difficult problem in technique.

Current thinking in psychoanalysis, supported by child observational research studies, Fonagy and Target (1996), Stern (1985), Emde (1988), has clarified the central role played by perception of the other, both in the development of self and object representations and in ongoing psychological functioning of the adult. In the analytic situation, through the work of such colleagues as Gill (1982), Ehrenberg (1992), McLaughlin (1981), Renik (1993), Schwaber (1992), Hoffman (1983), Poland (1992), Levine (1997), Stolorow and Atwood (1992), Aron (1996), Natterson (1991) and others in the U.S., and Casement (1985), Sandler (1987), Joseph (1985), Steiner (1993) and Feldman (1993) in England, we have come to recognize that the patient's experience of the analyst, often registered outside of awareness, regularly influences the emerging material and the developing analytic process.

It goes without saying that as perception is strongly colored by transferences and projective identifications, the patient's view of the analyst requires thorough exploration. Our entirely correct—and indispensable—efforts to utilize this analyst centered material (Steiner, 1993) as a pathway to the unconscious of the patient, however, may, at times, cause us to overlook something else of importance: the way in which the patient's conscious responses to, and thoughts about, the analyst are defensively utilized to screen out and suppress certain accurate, but anxiety-provoking, perceptions of him and the covert countertransference elements contained in the analyst's communications.

While active questioning of the patient about her perceptions of the analyst or other active means of searching out this information—a technique favored by a number of colleagues (Aron, 1996; Ehrenberg, 1997; Renik, 1993)—can be effective in eliciting those perceptions which are conscious, or can be readily made so, others which have registered subliminally or have undergone repression are ordinarily not accessible in this way. Often it is only through dreams, daydreams, or hints embedded in the patient's associations that such perceptions can be uncovered. To accomplish this it is necessary for the analyst to employ the kind of receptive, open-ended technique involving much quiet listening that fosters regressive movements in the minds of both participants and favors the emergence of such material.

In addition to certain correctly perceived countertransference reactions, not infrequently defended against by patients are their perceptions of particular traits, attitudes and values of the analyst which are inevitably transmitted in the course of analytic work. When, as often happens, such perceptions evoke anxiety or other troubling conflicts in patients, they are repressed or otherwise excluded from consciousness.

It is not the patient alone, however, who defends against the emergence of these perceptions. For reasons of his own, the analyst, too, often wishes to avoid the patient's conscious recognition of, and comments on, certain of his personal qualities as well as those countertransference reactions that he regards as constituting lapses of control or other embarrassing errors.

Often overlooked, too, in the process of exploring the transferences and projective identifications contained within the patient's experience of the analyst is material that may be exerting an important effect on the treatment; material transmitted by both parties that refers to unconsciously established rules and agreements about their relationship and about what may, and may not, happen in the analysis. Like the unconscious collusions that often lie concealed behind the patient's suppression of his accurate perceptions of the analyst, the failure to identify and confront these tacit agreements often represents the living out of mutually shared needs of patient and analyst; needs that, not infrequently, center for each about the avoidance of anxiety and the maintenance of emotionally important self representations.

In what follows I will try to illustrate how such unconscious communications may, at times, operate in the clinical situation. Some years ago I began the analysis of an intelligent and verbal but quite inhibited young woman. My work with her illustrated some of the difficulties inherent in our ideas about what constitutes confirmation of an interpretation.

Raised in a joyless atmosphere by anxious and depressed parents, Ms. C was herself a bundle of fears. Extremely cautious in everything she did, she was convinced that any venture that she undertook would end in disaster. In analysis she risked little and months would go by without her daring to express a thought about me. Her life, too, was bound and constricted by her anxious expectations. Without enthusiasm, she carried out a daily round of routine activities unleavened by the slightest pleasure.

Ms. C's resistance to change was such that the smallest movement in treatment met with powerful opposition. This fact, together with an absence of much in the way of dream or fantasy material, gave the analysis a weighty, plodding quality. After a time I found that I did not look forward to sessions with Ms. C. In fact, in the middle of an hour, I would sometimes become aware that my musculature was tense and that I was sitting with my body rotated away from her. Aware of these reactions, I would try to attend more closely to what my patient was saying, hoping to catch a whisper of the unconscious in the reports from the field that characterized her sessions.

In our sessions Ms. C would appear not only depressed, but defeated. She gave the impression that for her life was an unending burden. In presenting herself in this way, Ms. C was not only giving expression to her state of mind but was also transmitting a complex communication about our relationship and about the role in her life that she hoped I would play.

Ms. C's childhood experiences had convinced her that the only way to obtain help from her parents was to be in trouble; that is, to be sick, miserable or otherwise incapacitated. It was the only approach that elicited even a hint of a caring response. Thus, in Ms. C's tone, manner, affect and posture, she was communicating to me a mute appeal for help and nurturance.

By presenting herself as she did, however, Ms. C was also warding me off; protecting herself against the emergence of threatening erotic feelings and insuring that I would not find her a sexually appealing woman. Although it became clear that Ms. C very much wanted me to be attracted to her and, at times, unconsciously carried out seductive movements on the couch as an expression of that wish, the sexual stirrings that she experienced in sessions terrified her. Thus by feeling and appearing continually miserable and unhappy, Ms. C was not only making certain that she would not act on her sexual feelings, but unconsciously, was bringing on punishment both for her sexual wishes and for the envy, competitive feelings and resentment that she also harbored toward me. A number of these elements, and my response to them, were contained in the hours that I will describe.

One day as Ms. C was speaking of her limited life and despairing of ever breaking out of her shell—a feeling that more frequently than I cared to acknowledge I found myself sharing—an unexpected image appeared in my mind. I envisioned a small oval object, grayish-brown in color and rather delicate looking, with something alive inside. At first I could not identify this object, but after a moment or two I recognized that it was a cocoon. Then it occurred to me that this image must have arisen in response to the material of the hour. Taken with this idea—and using it, as I later realized, to screen out certain anxiety provoking feelings of my own—I recognized no other source of this fantasy.

In fact, without actually using the word, cocoon, Ms. C had been representing herself as living within such a protective shell. With sadness and little hope that she could actually do so, she had also expressed a yearning to emerge from this self-created prison.

Utilizing the material of the hour and the fantasy I'd had in association to it, I offered the interpretation that Ms. C seemed to be expressing the idea that she lived in a cocoon that she was struggling to break out of. This notion of herself, I added, seemed not only to be a long-standing one that had helped shape many of her experiences in life, but was her way of expressing feelings that she was having right now with me in this session. It was also a view of herself, I said, that she seemed to want me to share.

In response, Ms. C was silent for several minutes. Then she curled into herself, pulled up her legs, and lowered her head. The thought occurred to me then that with these movements she was pantomiming being wrapped into a cocoon. While this may, in fact, have been true, I failed at that time to recognize the aversive nature of Ms. C's movements. Feeling hurt by what I had said, she was retreating into a protective shell.

Ms. C then spoke about how trapped she felt in sessions. She needed me, she said, but she felt all bound up by fear of me and of my disapproval. She wished to express herself, to tell me how she really felt in sessions, to let herself go and to break the bonds that encased her, but she was too afraid of me and her feelings about me to do so. This is the way it was in her family. Terrified of making waves and especially of incurring the wrath of her father, for years she sat on her feelings and felt totally squelched. Then Ms. C told me of her childhood interest in butterflies and how she had wished that she could be such a free and beautiful creature. In reality, however, she said, she knew that she was nothing but a dingy moth trapped in the cocoon of this treatment and the cocoon of her family. But while the cocoons of nature eventually fall away, hers had become rigidified and hardened; in essence, it was a tomb from which there was no escape.

I recall being pleased with this piece of work and with an intervention which had not only elicited a confirming response, but had put the patient in touch both with an immediate experience with me and with a long-standing, ongoing fantasy. What I did not recognize at that time was that in addition to the meaning that I had suggested, Ms. C's actions, as well as her words, expressed a defensive wish to retreat from feelings of hurt and anger that she experienced at my remark, one that she took to be a put down of her as a woman. In retrospect, I thought that in her movements, she was also conveying a wish for me to comfort her and, by positioning her legs in the way that she did, unconsciously attempting to interest me sexually.

The scene now shifts to a session that took place a week later. Due to a family obligation that conflicted with one of her analytic hours, Ms.

C had announced earlier in the week that she would have to miss that session. Later in the hour in which she made this announcement, I pointed out what I thought to be a significant omission based on aspects of Ms. C's character; her fear of asking for anything for herself and of my disapproval and rejection if she did so. I mentioned that she had not brought up the possibility of a change of appointment. She acknowledged that this was so, and after exploring her underlying feelings of guilt and unworthiness, as well as the shameful fantasies of entitlement that give rise to her fears, she summoned up her courage and asked me if I had another time available. In fact, I did, and Ms. C gratefully accepted the new appointment. Both she and I, I believe, recognized that in addition to confronting her avoidance, my intervention constituted the offer of a gift. It was, in short, an enactment on my part that had to do both with my wish to reach out to Ms. C and, unconsciously I suspect, make amends for the opposite wish; the desire to flee the situation and not have to contend with someone who, all too often, could make me—and unconsciously was seeking to make me—feel as inadequate and despairing as she herself felt.

Emboldened by my offer of a substitute appointment, which meant to her that I found her to be a person of some value, Ms. C became braver in the next session. That hour, in fact, was unlike any that had occurred before. In it Ms. C spoke with surprising openness.

"I appreciate what you did today," she began, "you did not have to change the appointment. You didn't even have to bring up the subject. I wouldn't have. You could have used the free hour for yourself, to read the paper or to sleep late. I appreciate the consideration you showed. It makes me think that maybe you like me after all. Maybe I'm not just a pill and a bore." Ms. C paused, then went on.

"There is something I've been meaning to say to you but I haven't been able to until now. It's about something that has upset me. I don't know if you realize it, but sometimes you get irritated with me. Not that I blame you. If I were you, I'd be bored out of my mind. But when you feel that way you can be critical. Then you are liable to put me down, not in a big way, but in a subtle, analytic way. Like when you said I exist in a cocoon. I was upset by that. I felt like saying don't we all live in cocoons? Don't you live in a cocoon with your practice and your nice house and your professional associations? I don't notice you going out to state hospitals to deal with really troubled patients. You have your own little life—we all do. I guess you are right in one way, though. Your cocoon is of your choosing. Mine is part of my illness. It is true that as a kid I used to imagine being as lovely as a butterfly, but I know now that I never will. One day, though, I am going to break out of my cocoon, and maybe one day you'll break out of yours."

What had happened was clear. On one level, Ms. C understood and confirmed the interpretation I made. And her associations demonstrated, as I had imagined, that we had indeed shared an unconscious fantasy. But on another level, she was wounded by the interpretation which she experienced as a subtle attack on her. For some time I was puzzled by her response. Then I thought about her words. I had been impatient with her, she said, impatient and annoyed. In my mind I reviewed the session and tried to recapture my mood of that day and what it was that I was feeling. The session, I remembered, had begun on a heavy note. Ms. C had looked morose and she was silent for quite a while. I recalled sitting quietly and patiently but also experiencing a familiar kind of weighty feeling. Ms. C had begun several recent sessions in this way and they had not been very productive. Use of my own feelings of heaviness, boredom, and growing helplessness as a guide to understanding and interpreting certain inner states that Ms. C was experiencing and, through projection, was invoking in me, while useful in helping her gain insights that she did not have before, did not result in any discernible movement in my patient. Ms. C recognized the truth of these observations, but this understanding was not accompanied by much alteration either in her mood or in the sustained silences that emanated from it.

The hour I spoke of was heading in the same direction, and although I was not consciously aware of experiencing annoyance or irritation at the time, I have no doubt that such feelings—which were never far from the surface and had been growing in recent weeks—came through in my interpretation.

On reflection, I recalled that some weeks earlier Ms. C had spoken with self-contempt of feeling like an insect or, worse, a larva waiting to hatch. Thus, on one level my use of the cocoon imagery unconsciously echoed my patient's negative view of herself. In using this imagery I was, I believe, not only unconsciously retaliating for the feelings of inadequacy that Ms. C was able to evoke in me, but playing into her defensive need to keep me at a distance and to cause me to experience her as an unattractive woman.

This is not to say that this intervention was not reasonably accurate and useful. I think that it was and Ms. C's response indicated that this was so. But equally important, I believe, is that my intervention also concealed an inner response of mine that was related to covert communications taking place in the hour. This interplay between patient and analyst involved Ms. C's silences and her largely uncommunicative behavior on the one hand and my frustration at her tenacious resistances and inability to make greater progress on the other. Ms. C heard that aspect of my message that spoke to my feelings of frustration and anger as well as the one that addressed her long-standing fantasy. Because she was afraid of her aggression, afraid of any confrontation with me, she suppressed her reaction to the critical message and gave voice only to the one that, although useful in its own right, was also less threatening. What is of interest also is that it was only after I had agreed to change her hour, an act that to Ms. C served as evidence that I cared about her, that she was able to discuss that part of her reaction to my interpretation that had gone underground. Had she not done so, I would have had no reason to question my belief that on the basis of an unconscious communication I had done nothing other than offer an interpretation that had provided a piece of insight and had advanced the analytic process.

On reviewing the transactions that had taken place between Ms. C and myself, I realized that my focus had been almost exclusively on our verbal exchanges. I had paid comparatively little attention to the array of messages that were being transmitted nonverbally as accompaniments to, commentaries on, and sometimes contradictions of the verbal material.

Now in order to better understand what had transpired, and was continuing to transpire, between Ms. C and myself, I began to pay close attention, not only to the covert meanings contained within our words, but to these nonverbal messages. Conveyed through posture, gesture and movement, in facial expressions, in the tone, syntax and rhythm of speech, and in the pauses and silences that punctuated the hours, these unconscious communications anticipated both subsequent conscious recognition in patient and analyst of the affects and fantasies to which they referred and the later verbalization of this material.

As I observed Ms. C and myself in interaction, I became aware of certain patterns in our movements. Often reciprocal and cueing off one another, these movements were enacted in a repetitive manner, almost like a familiar dance.

It became clear, for instance, that in connection with the mobilization of certain emotions Ms. C and I engaged in predictable behavior. Thus, in sessions if we began to feel negatively toward one another—not a rare occurrence in light of Ms. C's tenacious resistances and the feelings of frustration that they evoked in me—each of us unconsciously and automatically would carry out particular movements.

Typically, for instance, during periods of silence Ms. C would rotate her body slightly to the left, fold her arms across her chest, and turn her head toward the wall.

On my side, I became aware at such times that I would turn my body slightly to the right, away from Ms. C and in a direction opposite to her movement. I would also lean back in my chair and, for brief intervals, would close my eyes when listening.

After a period of time ranging from several minutes to a half-hour or more, not infrequently Ms. C would again reposition herself. She would draw up her legs, flex her knees, and let her arms fall to the side. At the same time, she would roll onto her back so that she was no longer facing the wall. Then she would begin to speak in a quiet, modulated voice and in a tone that seemed placating or appeasing. At these times, there was about her a muted, but definite, seductive quality.

In response, I would find myself turning back toward Ms. C. I would lean forward in my chair and when offering an intervention would speak in a tone that came close to matching hers.

In addition to my effort to communicate understanding and empathy in this way, there was in my action, I believe, a resonant response to Ms. C's seductive behavior.

Although at the time I did not appreciate the significance of these nonverbal enactments, which conveyed negative emotions, efforts at repair, and a covert sexuality between Ms. C and myself, later, upon reflection, I realized that they anticipated the conscious registration of emerging feelings in both patient and analyst. They operated, in other words, as an early signal system for affects that were approaching but had not yet reached consciousness. Many years ago, Felix Deutsch (1952) demonstrated that certain nonverbal behaviors regularly predicted and anticipated the appearance of particular themes in the patient's subsequent material.

If, as happened later in the analysis, I was able to observe these non-verbal communications in Ms. C and myself and decipher their meaning, it often became possible to gain access to the underlying affects and fantasies. Gaining conscious awareness of these responses, in turn, helped me both to better contain them and to utilize them interpretatively.

When, on the other hand, I overlooked the nonverbal interactions taking place in sessions, the related affects often grew in intensity with the result that the increased feeling of pressure from within not infrequently led to the kind of troublesome countertransference enactments that I have described.

Awareness of the kinds of covert messages that may be concealed within our so-called correct interpretations may throw some light on another familiar clinical entity: the negative therapeutic reaction. While it is well known that both unconscious guilt and the need to maintain an object tie with a masochistic parent may contribute to the development of this reaction, other factors that play a role in its formation are often overlooked. I will illustrate what I mean with this brief example.

Ms. A was an angry woman who, when she began analytic psychotherapy with me, announced that she was simultaneously taking on her third husband and third analyst. Her two previous marriages and two previous tries at analysis had all ended in failure. Weary and battle-scarred, her husbands and analysts had all thrown in the towel.

Ms. A's anger began in childhood and for understandable reasons. Her mother died suddenly when she was four and, unable to care for her, her father had sent her to live with an aunt. This woman had little interest in, or tolerance for, children and she openly resented the burden that had been placed on her. Feeling deeply rejected by this aunt and unwanted in her home, the child thought repeatedly of running away. This she never did, however, because, among other reasons, there was no other place for her to go.

In our work together, Ms. A was difficult and provocative. Endlessly critical of me, she also repeatedly threatened to break off treatment. For the most part I was able to maintain my composure in the face of these attacks, but there were times when her behavior got under my skin.

One day when my patient was particularly angry, had accused me of being antagonistic to her, and once again threatened to leave treatment, I offered a transference interpretation which attempted to link past and present. Because I did not provide what she felt she needed, I said, Ms. A was experiencing me as the mean-spirited aunt of her youth whom she deeply resented. And it seemed to me, I added, that to pay me back she was trying to induce in me the very same feelings of frustration and anger that she had experienced at her aunt's hands. Then I went on. Just as she threatened to leave her aunt but never did because she was the only mother Ms. A had, she repeatedly threatened to leave me but had not done so because of her conviction that there was no one else she could rely on; that I was the only therapist in the city who could work with her.

Ms. A's reaction lingers in memory. She broke down, cried bitterly, and remained depressed for several days thereafter. It took neither of us long to understand what had happened. Ms. A had responded, not to my transference interpretation which on one level was correct enough, but to the true meaning of my message. Tired of the battle, and with my patience[1] worn thin, I had unconsciously sent Ms. A a familiar message;

---

[1] At this point in an earlier version of this paper I committed the parapraxis of writing the word *patient* instead of *patience*, a clear illustration of how endur-

the same message, in fact, sent by her husbands, her previous analysts and her aunt and father before them. I had invited her to leave.

As in the case of Ms. C, nonverbal communication played out in posture, gesture and movement in this treatment offered early clues to nascent affects in both patient and therapist, affects that , on my side, were eventually enacted in this unhelpful way. Whenever, for instance, Ms. A launched one of her typically veiled attacks on me, her words would be accompanied by particular actions. As she spoke, Ms. A would move toward the edge of her chair, her upper body would be thrust out and angled forward, and her head, with chin leading, would follow suit. The posture was one of belligerence, but curiously mixed with a kind of provocativeness that at times I experienced as covertly sexual.

I, on the other hand, would sit leaning back in my chair; leaning as far back, in fact, as I possibly could in what clearly was an involuntary retreat from Ms. A's poorly concealed aggression and provocative behavior.

After she had given vent to her feelings, in this way, Ms. A would straighten up, slide backwards in her seat, and appearing drained, would remain quiet for several minutes.

In response, I would move forward, my body no longer angled backwards and I would resume my usual listening posture. These see-saw movements, backwards and forward, advance and retreat, communicating anger, a breach between Ms. A and myself, and efforts to heal that breach, punctuated the sessions and were reliable markers for what at any given time was transpiring between my patient and myself.

Had I been able at the time to understand the importance of such movements, it would have been possible, I believe, for me, early on, to identify and explore the underlying feelings of irritation and rising anger experienced by both patient and therapist before they spilled over into the kind of verbal enactment that was the cause of much trouble in this treatment.

If, in fact, such nonverbal elements can be identified and explored as they appear, it is often possible for the analyst, through introspection and attunement to what is rising from within, to monitor, better contain, and early on make interpretive use of some of his countertransference responses rather than unconsciously enacting them and attempting, after the fact, to grasp the meaning and significance of such enactments. Increasing the scope of his awareness, then, to include the movement patterns of patient and analyst as they engage in the analytic hour is, I

---

ing countertransference feelings, stimulated by memories, can infiltrate and affect the operations of the ego even years after treatment was ended.

believe, a valuable tool in the analyst's ongoing effects to turn his subjective reactions into useful insights rather than automatic actions.

This example and others like it raise a question about our patients' negative reactions to interpretations that seem correct. How often, one wonders, do such reactions represent accurate readings of the analyst's unconscious meaning?

I would like now to describe another clinical example, one in which my need to protect my self-esteem at a particular moment in an analysis led to a skewing of the analytic dialogue, to the development of a tacit agreement not to broach a potentially painful and embarrassing issue, and to make use of an analytic intervention as a decoy aimed at shifting the focus of the patient's attention. As I've mentioned, this kind of enactment, which involves a collusion with the patient, serves protective functions for both participants in analysis and may exert a profound, and even decisive, influence on the course of outcome of the analytic work.

Some years ago, in the early days of the women's movement, when most male analysts wore their chauvinism like a comfortable old cardigan, a militant young feminist came to see me. She did so quite warily and reluctantly, accepting the recommendation of a teacher who had been in treatment with me only when a valued friendship ended because of her poorly controlled aggressive behavior. That she did so for target practice, however, soon became evident, for from the moment Ms. N stepped foot in my office she unleashed a blistering attack on Freud and his testosterone-heavy theories, on analysis as male propaganda, and on me as one of its sexist practitioners. Finally, leaning forward in her chair and looking for all the world like a bull about to charge, she hurled a challenge at me.

"I'm into consciousness-raising," she announced. "What are you into?" Taken aback, I did not know what to say. For several seconds I stared at her blankly. Then a response popped into mind.

"Unconsciousness-raising," I replied.

That exchange pretty much summed up the situation between Ms. N and myself. From the outset a major disagreement divided us. For Ms. N, the pain and suffering that she experienced and the unhappiness in her life for which she sought relief stemmed from a single source; society's discriminating attitude towards women. I, on the other hand, was interested in promoting the idea that in addition to this harsh reality the inner world of fantasies and beliefs that Ms. N developed as a consequence of her unique psychological experiences played a role in her troubles.

It was a standoff, and as the result of this non-meeting of the minds for some months progress in the analysis could be measured by the thimble-full. In time, however, things began to change. Largely, I think, because we came to understand one another, Ms. N and I finally reached an accommodation. I learned to listen to and appreciate her realities, external as well as psychological, and to convey that appreciation to her, and she, grudgingly, allowed that the particular way in which she put things together in her mind might have influenced her thinking about herself and others.

We still had our troubles, though, and one problem centered around the feeling of boredom which I sometimes experienced during Ms. N's sessions. Although her capacity for self-reflection gradually improved, Ms. N was given to much externalization. It was not rare for her to focus on the shortcomings of others and to complain at length about the way that she was treated by friends and family. Leaving no detail to the imagination, she would cite every fault, foible and blemish of the miscreants who had used her badly. A particular target of hers was her father, a vain, bigoted, and devious man who fancied himself a scholar and a gentleman and who sought, through lies and rationalizations, to induce others to believe in this deluded self-image.

While the material relating to Ms. N's father and other family members was assuredly important, after a while it became so familiar, the same complaints and stories so oft repeated, that I found myself experiencing fatigue in sessions. Recognizing that strong emotions must be lurking behind this reaction of mine, I undertook what self-reflection I could and came into touch with the feelings of anger and annoyance that Ms. N's clearly defense behavior was evoking in me. While useful in providing some insight into what was transpiring beneath the analytic surface, this approach had little effect on my responses to Ms. N.

I felt a clear sense of relief, then, when, in the second year of treatment some new and rather dramatic material made its appearance in Ms. N's sessions. This material had to do with the strong possibility that my patient, as a young child, had been sexually fondled by a male teenage cousin who occasionally baby-sat for her. Although, generally speaking, I am wary of the idea that such experiences are the key to neuroses, I was interested in exploring the sequelae of this episode. I thought that the fantasies it had evoked and the transformations in memory it had undergone over the years might help account for Ms. N's persistent and irrational anxiety over physical contact with men; a symptom for which I did not, at that point, have an entirely satisfactory explanation.

Keenly interested in this newly emerging material and eager to hear more about it, I was frustrated and disappointed when, soon after making a transient appearance in Ms. N's associations, it disappeared from view. It was as if the repressive forces that had originally overtaken it had, once again, driven it underground. And although I worked as actively as I could with the defenses that I thought were keeping the relevant affects and memories out of conscious awareness, they remained undercover.

Instead of speaking of the material that was new and possibly of great significance in her development, Ms. N returned to the old complaints, wrapping herself in them as though they were a suit of used clothing.

Once again I found it difficult to keep attuned to her; once again I experienced tedium. During one early morning hour following a night in which I had had little sleep, I was particularly restless. As often happens when I am tired, I moved about more than usual in my chair. I twisted, I fidgeted, I shifted positions, all no doubt in an effort to stay alert. Finally, as Ms. N was droning on about one of her tight-fisted relatives, I found myself reaching for the notebook that I keep at my side to record an occasional dream, an intriguing sequence of associations, or other material that I may wish to review. There was nothing in what Ms. N was saying, however, that I really wished to record. Nonetheless, I had reached for the book and fingered its binding. Then I opened it to the section reserved for Ms. N and glanced at an old note that I had written. All this I did as a distraction. I was bored and tired and I wanted some stimulation, some relief from the feelings of dullness and vague uneasiness that I was experiencing. And in the process of thumbing through the notebook and glancing at the previous note, I had tuned my patient out and had missed a few sentences of what she was saying. I had managed to blank them out.

Although my movements were carried out quietly, they were not so quiet that Ms. N did not hear them. At first she said nothing and simply carried on with her dissection of the penny-pinching relative. There was something different in her voice, however. She was speaking in a routinized way, like an actor reciting his lines while thinking of an unpaid rent bill.

Then, suddenly, Ms. N was silent. For several minutes she did not speak.

"Something's happened," I said. "Something seems to be blocking you."

"I didn't think that you were interested in what I was saying," Ms. N replied. "I thought that you were distracted. I heard noises."

"And what did you make of what you heard?"

"I don't know. There were odd sounds, like you were stroking something or fingering something. Then it sounded as though you were opening a book and turning pages."

As Ms. N spoke, I recalled something that she had told me sometime before; that as he read her a goodnight story her cousin's fingers would begin to play over the pages of the book. Then, slowly, he would reach out, touch her thigh, and move his hand toward her genital area.

"I thought that you had no interest in what I was saying," Ms. N went on; "that I was totally boring and that you had picked up a book and were leafing through it. Either that or you were just playing with it to amuse yourself."

"'Stroking it,' you said before."

"Yes, that, too. I heard rubbing noises. Maybe that's the way shrinks get off in sessions when they are bored. They rub their books instead of their dicks. That's their perversion." After a moment of silence, I spoke.

"Such sounds are familiar to you," I said.

Then Ms. N fell silent again. When she resumed speaking her voice contained a note of resignation.

"Okay. I get it. You think I thought that you were like my cousin, George; ready to make a move, ready to reach for my crotch. I wasn't aware of that, but maybe I did. Actually I wouldn't put it past any shrink. Most of them end up screwing their patients one way or another. You guys are a pious lot, but sneaky. Patients get abused in therapy all the time."

Ms. N went on to speak at some length of her distrust of analysts, especially males, and of her suspicion that I might turn out to be as devious as most men who, one way or another, use women. Then towards the end of the session she spoke once more of the night time scene with her cousin, repeating what she had told me and recalling for the first time that she had a crush on him and felt very excited in his presence. Then she added that there was probably something to the fact that she had come to believe that all men, basically, were like George; charming, exciting, but not to be trusted. And rising from the couch she added a final note.

"It's true," she said, "that lying down scares me. I don't see you and I don't know what you are about. When you start moving around I get jittery. I don't know what might happen next. In that sense I've probably gotten you and George all mixed up in my mind. But what bugs me, what really makes me crazy, is when I begin to think that you are like my father. Not only that I *imagine* that you are like him, but that you *really are* like him."

After that session, Ms. N's distrust of me increased. Her resistances hardened and silences dominated the sessions. When she did speak, what she said was mostly reportage; dispatches consisting largely of descriptions of other people and accounts of events at work. She had gone into hiding and the reason for this was clear. In some part of her Ms. N knew that I had deceived her with a piece of psychoanalytic slight of hand. Out of boredom, anger, and a wish to escape from those feelings, I had turned away from Ms. N and tuned her out. I had not been doing my job, the job she was paying me to do and for which I had signed on. And, seeking distraction from inner tensions, I had been caught out. Ms. N sensed what was happening. Rather than acknowledging the truth of her perceptions, however, and thereby experiencing the feelings of shame and guilt that would accompany such an acknowledgment, I had led Ms. N down another path. And for reasons of her own which had much to do with her fear of a threatening confrontation, she went along with me.

It so happens that the path on which I set her needed to be explored and both of us knew it. And that exploration had its own value, for significant memories concerning a traumatic and influential childhood experience were, in fact, triggered by my behavior in making covert noises. Moreover, although I had not recognized it at the time, my behavior was part of a pattern of interaction taking place between Ms. N and myself.

Through the quality of her verbalizations; repetitious, reality-oriented, focused on details, Ms. N was not only employing powerful resistances against the emergence of threatening affects, particularly sexual feelings towards her analyst, but with concealed aggression, was causing me to experience the kind of frustration and disappointment that characterized her experiences with her father, with George, her cousin, and with other important men in her life. And with some concealed anger of my own, I had responded to her behavior by turning away from her and shutting her out. Only later did I realize that my anger had much to do with Ms. N's teasing behavior and that a sexually tinged and sadomasochistic interaction had been taking place between us.

In addition, outside of conscious awareness, both of us, I believe, were enacting a scenario that had to do with the George episode. Ms. N had set the stage by bringing up sexual material, holding it out, as it were, in front of me, and then withdrawing it. Then, in an unconscious effort to evoke the now submerged material, I, in essence, became George; that is, a male sitting behind Ms. N, holding a book and, like a reader, slowly turning pages. In this way—perhaps both in response to a fantasy of Ms. N's that was communicated to me and out of some anger and frustration of my own—I was recreating a threatening scene from my patient's childhood. All of this—and more—needed to be, and eventually was, interpreted and usefully explored. But as important as these factors were, it is also true that both patient and analyst made use of them to avoid confronting what, for each, was a more anxiety-provoking issue.

By moving rapidly to the past we entered into a collusion in which the apparent analytic investigation of an important childhood experience was used in the service of mutual avoidance. Utilizing a particular kind of body English, I had turned Ms. N away from the truth. In doing so I had, in fact, become what she feared most that I would be; an untrustworthy person. Ms. N's remark at the end of the hour summed up the situation succinctly. As a consequence of the deception that I had initiated I had become not only the father in the transference but a man who, in actuality, had behaved like Ms. N's father. And until I could return to this incident, replay it with my patient, and help her understand what had truly happened, she could not trust me.

It was necessary to look again at what had occurred, and through an appropriate intervention, let Ms. N know that her perceptions had been correct.

When in a subsequent session, I detected a reference to the incident in question in Ms. N's associations, I drew her attention to her ongoing concern with it and sought to continue exploration of her thoughts about what had happened. This approach yielded little, however, nor did interpretations of anxiety about speaking frankly about the episode.

Recognizing the untenable position in which Ms. N had been put— she had, in reality, been gaslighted—and realizing that meaningful work in analysis could not take place under these circumstances, I felt it important to address the issue more directly. I therefore asked Ms. N if she had any awareness of the fact that her perceptions had been accurate and that she had correctly identified the sounds she heard as my thumbing through a notebook. I also said that I had become distracted, that my attention had wandered, and that, embarrassed by my behavior, I focused Ms. N's attention on the childhood experience with George rather than deal with the affects of my own actions. Ms. N replied that she had sensed what had happened but had quickly dismissed that thought from her mind when I moved away from the present situation and alluded to the George episode. The whole experience, she said, was too frightening. She felt I was evading something but could not confront me with my evasion. She was too afraid of the consequences; too afraid that I would become furious and send her away.

By offering this intervention, I not only raised the question of how Ms. N had dealt with her original perception, but I confirmed that it had been accurate. I am well aware that not all analysts would have dealt with the matter in this way. Many colleagues would have been content to work exclusively with the patient's defenses, fantasies and projections and to leave the reality of what occurred ambiguous.

In fact, not a few analysts contend that to acknowledge a mistake to a patient rather than simply exploring the patient's perception of what occurred in an hour is a serious error. Maintaining that such self-disclosures are often motivated by feelings of guilt, by a need to confess, by the hope of obtaining forgiveness from the patient, or by a wish to undo the error made, these colleagues hold that disclosures of this kind essentially serve the analyst's needs and unnecessarily burden the patient with the analyst's issues.

There is much truth to this argument and to the corollary idea that it is the analyst's responsibility, to the extent possible, to monitor his countertransference responses and to utilize them in the service of understanding. It is true, too, that the danger of using the patient to serve the analyst's needs, always present, is increased in situations in which the analyst experiences distress over an error that he has made and, unconsciously, may seek relief by revealing his mistake to the patient. There is also the possibility that the analyst's actions in disclosing his mistake may have the effect of limiting or foreclosing the patient's exploration of her perceptions of what occurred in the hour.

While these considerations are clearly important and must be taken into account whenever the analyst is faced with the question of disclosing a mistake that he has made, there are times, I believe, when not to disclose an error which has been perceived by the patient and which has had an adverse effect on the treatment is itself a mistake and creates a serious—and sometimes insuperable—problem in the treatment; one that, in fact, places a heavy burden on the patient.

Such behavior on the part of the analyst compounds the error already made and puts the patient in an impossible, and often destructive, bind. Realizing that the analyst does not want her to know the truth, she has to suppress or deny what, in fact, some part of her knows to be true. She is being asked, in other words, to enter into a collusion with the analyst and, along with him, to be the bearer of a secret that can have a deforming effect on the analytic process. Moreover, the patient may, and often does, experience the analyst as being unwilling, or unable, to face up to his own errors, seeking instead, to conceal that fact behind the protective cover of proper and quite correct analytic technique. Such a situation, I believe, cannot foster growth. It can only lead to deception, collusions and increased distrust, both of the analyst, and of the patient's own perceptions.

Once the air was cleared and Ms. N and I had dealt with what had actually happened between us, we could do what we should have been doing all along; exploring more fully the transactions and covert communications taking place between us that had led, on the one hand, to my experiencing boredom and fatigue during Ms. N's hours and, on the other, to her need to present herself in a way that contributed to the evocation of such reactions.

Later on we had a chance to explore other relevant issues; Ms. N's reaction to my evasion, her own need to evade the truth and not confront me with her perceptions, and the response she had to my finally acknowledging what had happened. Each of these reactions was important as they contained views of me, initially as weak and vulnerable, then as more hardy and able to face harsh realities, that were meaningfully connected with long-standing self and object representations. Of particular importance in this regard was Ms. N's shifting perception of her father, a talented and effective, but thoroughly devious, businessman with whom she was unconsciously identified.

On Mr. N's part, then, this enactment constituted a re-employment of an important mode of defense; the unconscious denial of an accurate perception whose conscious recognition would have led to the mobilization of rage and to consequent inner turmoil based on the fear that to reveal her feelings would result in the loss of a person that she both loved and needed. It was this conflict, involving me at the moment, but related in the past both to her father and to her beloved cousin, George, that Ms. N handled through a familiar enactment, one whose interpretation proved to be a very significant experience in her analysis. Its effectiveness came, I believe, from the immediacy of the experience with me and from Ms. N's recognition of how, out of fear, she had denied what she knew to be true.

What I have wished to illustrate in this example, then, is the way that, as analysts, we often manage to sidestep issues that cause us pain, embarrassment or anxiety. Not infrequently concealed within our well-accepted analytic techniques and timely interventions are subtle expressions of envy, rivalry and aggression towards our patients. Hidden, too, in our interpretations, and often well rationalized, may be our needs to maintain our position of authority and superiority. Even more troublesome at times are the unrecognized sexual feelings that may be stimulated in sessions as well as feelings of love and dependency that we commonly experience in the course of our work. We are somewhat better, in fact, at recognizing and confronting negative feelings than positive ones. The vast majority of papers on countertransference deal with conflicts over aggression. Very few touch on the vicissitudes of loving and sexuality in an analytic treatment.

Other potential sources of tension and anxiety in the analyst, too, may be avoided. Often overlooked and not confronted as important influences on our work are our attitudes towards money and its importance to us; the effect on us of growing older; the impact of our personal losses and disappointments on our approach to patients; and the role that our status in our institutes and in the profession plays in affecting our sense of ourselves and the way we function in the clinical situation.

It is our petty faults, too, that we have trouble acknowledging and integrating into our clinical work; our moments of meanness, of spiteful retaliation, of boastfulness, of greed, of inattention, of self-justification, and of small-minded competitiveness with colleagues. Often we shut out recognition of these traits in ourselves and effectively manage not to be aware of them. And when we are unable to do that, we may find ways to ignore them, to set them aside, and to avoid the hard task of confronting the impact that they have on our patients. Instead we may find ourselves focusing on the patient's material. As that pathway is so readily available, so integral a part of analytic work, we may not be aware of how we can pick up themes and trends in what patients say that are relevant to their conflicts, interpret them accurately and with insight, and to all appearances do a useful piece of analysis. What we are doing in those situations, however, is not only useful (which on its own terms, it clearly is); we are also utilizing what might be called an analytic screen; that is, using our skills and insights, in part, to avoid an uncomfortable truth; that our personal shortcomings, whether they take the form of a lapse of attention, an unnecessarily critical comment, a failure to recognize the truth of a patient's perception, or a momentary need to upstage him, exert a powerful influence on all that occurs at any given time in the treatment situation.

In short, it is our natural and normal self-esteem needs operating as ever-present forces in analysis as they do in life that may, at times, constitute a significant source of difficulty for the analyst. While contending with such personal responses is an inevitable, even necessary, part of doing analytic work, our ongoing efforts to understand and explore not only our conflicts but also issues of self-esteem as they may be subtly conveyed both in our interventions and in our omissions can be a valuable source of fresh insights. Unrecognized or not confronted, however, such problems may lead to the kinds of unconscious collusions and avoidances that I have attempted to describe in this paper.

On my side, my enactment clearly served defensive purposes. It spared my self-esteem, for I was deeply ashamed of my behavior, and helped stave off the intense self-criticism that was on the verge of being released. Thus, it served as a rationalized effort to avoid a narcissistic injury, a maneuver not unknown to analysts as well as their patients.

But there was also a less conscious determinant of my behavior, a factor that I became aware of only later, when, at home, I reflected on what had happened. As an adolescent, I had experienced seductive behavior on the part of a female relative who, in her own way, had acted in a manner not unlike Ms. N's. After some time in this situation, I found myself responding in kind. When this girl would try to engage me, I would ignore her; pretending to listen, but, in fact, tuning her out.

It was this old response, among others, that was activated, I believe, in my work with Ms. N and that I enacted in the session I've mentioned. Clearly, I was more frustrated with, and annoyed by, her behavior than I knew, a reaction that, in part, was linked to a piece of my own history. As I have mentioned, Ms. N had, unconsciously been teasing me by dangling intriguing sexual material in front of me and then withdrawing it. It turned out that she had often acted in this way with boyfriends and with her father, a pattern of behavior that represented an identification both with his teasing behavior and that of her cousin, George. Interpretation of this aspect of her behavior opened up channels of memory and Ms. N recalled a number of incidents in which she attempted to turn the tables on others, teasing and mocking playmates and siblings as she had been teased and mocked by men whom she loved.

In summary, what I have tried to present in this paper are some thoughts about the way in which the two people in the analytic situation, often acting in concert, may selectively screen out certain realities having to do with aspects of the analyst's person, his attitudes and his behavior. Unrecognized and unacknowledged, these subtly and often unconsciously expressed qualities are not infrequently embedded within our quite proper and correct theories and techniques. It is there that we must look for and uncover them for left to do their work they can undermine our best efforts. Fostering the kinds of errors and collusions that I have described in this communication, they can have a profound effect on the course and outcome of the analytic work.

References

Arlow, J. (1993), Discussion: The mind of the analyst. *Int. J. Psychoanal.* 74: 1147–1154.

Aron, L. (1996), *A Meeting of Minds: Mutuality in Psychoanalysis*. Hillsdale, NJ: The Analytic Press.

Calef, V. & Weinshel, E. (1981), Some clinical consequences of introjection: Gaslighting. *Psa. Q.* 50:44–65.

Casement, P. (1985), *Learning From the Patient*. New York/London: Guilford Press.

Deutsch, F. (1952), Analytic posturology. *Psa. Q.* 20:196–214.

Ehrenberg, D. (1997), *The Intimate Edge: Extending the Reach of Psychoanalytic Interaction*. New York/London: Norton.

Emde, R. (1988), Development terminable and interminable: Recent psychoanalytic theory and therapeutic consideration. *Int. J. Psychoanal.* 69:283–296.

Feldman, M. (1993), The dynamics of reassurance. *Int. J. Psychoanal.* 74:275–285.

Fonagy, P. & Target, M. (1996), Playing with reality I: Theory of mind and the normal development of psychic reality. *Int. J. Psychoanal.* 77:217–233.

Gill, M. M. (1982), *Analysis of Transference. Psychological Issues.* Monograph 53. New York: International Universities Press.

Hoffman, I. (1983), The patient as interpreter of the analyst's experience. *Contemp. Psychoanalysis.* 19:388–422.

Joseph, B. (1985), Transference: The total situation. *Int. J. Psychoanal.* 66:447–454.

Kestenberg, J. (1972), How children remember and parents forget. *Int. J. Psychoanal. Psychother.* 1:103–123.

Levine, H. (1997), The capacity for countertransference. *Psychoanal. Inq.* 17:44–68.

McLaughlin, J. (1981), Transference, psychic reality and countertransference. *Psa. Q.* 50:639–660.

——— (1987), The play of transference: Some reflections. *J. Amer. Psychoanal. Assoc.* 39:595–611.

Milne, A. A. (1924), The doctor and the dormouse. In *When We Were Very Young.* New York: Dutton, 1961.

Natterson, J. (1991), *Beyond Countertransference.* Northvale, NJ: Aronson.

Ogden, T. H. (1994), The concept of interpretive action. *Psa. Q.* 63:219–245.

Poland, W. (1992), Transference: An original creation. *Psa. Q.* 61:185–205.

Reich, A. (1951), On countertransference. *Internat. J. Psychoanal.* 32:25–31.

Renik, O. (1993), Analytic interaction. Conceptualizing technique in light of the analyst's irreducible subjectivity. *Psa. Q.* 62:553–571.

Sandler, J. (1985), On internal object relationships. *J. Amer. Psychoanal. Assoc.* 38:859–880.

Schwaber, E. (1992), Countertransference: The analyst's retreat from the patient's vantage point. *Int. J. Psychoanal.* 73:349–361.

Smith, H. (1999), Countertransference, conflictual listening and the analytic object relationship. *J. Amer. Psychoanal. Assoc.* 48/1:95–126.

Steiner, J. (1993), Problems of psychoanalytic technique: Patient-centered and analyst-centered interpretations. In *Psychic Retreats: Pathological Organizations in Psychotic, Neurotic and Borderline Patients.* London: Routledge.

Stern, D. N. (1985), *The Interpersonal World of the Infant.* New York: Basic Books.

Stolorow, R. & Atwood, G. (1992), *Contexts of Being: The Intersubjective Foundation of Psychological Life.* Hillsdale, NJ: The Analytic Press.

Afterword

A central issue that I wished to raise in this paper concerns the question of the analyst's handling of those countertransference reactions that are misleading or hurtful or otherwise contribute to blocks and impasses in treatment.

This issue came up for discussion—and sharp disagreement—when, at the British Psychoanalytic Society, I presented the case of a young woman who had overheard me turning the pages of a notebook. Several Kleinian analysts, and some other colleagues as well, objected to my acknowledgment to the patient of the correctness of her perceptions. They maintained that it was an error to make such an acknowledgment and that it is far preferable to analyze the patient's fantasies about the event.

While I certainly agree that it is essential to investigate and analyze the patient's fantasies, I believe it is just as important not to double-bind, or gaslight, patients by casting doubt on the accuracy of their perceptions. Silence and avoidance by the analyst in these situations is not being neutral. It conveys the message that the analyst cannot, or will not, acknowledge his or her error or troublesome reaction. Such a response cannot build trust. It communicates the analyst's unwillingness to recognize his or her contribution to an ongoing problem in the analysis and conveys the message that the analyst is neither honest enough nor secure enough to do so. This also is not a useful message to send to patients. It is much better, I believe, in such situations, for the analyst to confirm the accuracy of the patient's perception and then to explore the patient's reactions, fantasies, and defenses in response to the event. It is also important, however, then to explore the patient's reactions to the analyst's confirmation of his or her perceptions. Such an approach opens pathways to communication and, ultimately, to fruitful exploration of the inner world of the patient.

Part II

Relational Perspectives on Development

Developmental concerns have not always or consistently been at the forefront of relational theory. Mitchell's early writing included an argument against what he termed "the developmental tilt" in psychoanalytic theory, a tendency to include relational factors within traditional theory by slipping them in as developmentally earlier, while keeping drive-related and oedipal issues later along the developmental axis. Mitchell, very much a product of his interpersonal training and tradition, feared that too much focus on childhood development would lead the analyst to deemphasize the presence and participation of the adult in the clinical dyad.

A refocus on development is perhaps one of the most dramatic areas of change in relational theory, including changes in Mitchell's own interests. His penultimate book, *Relationality* (2000), was his engaged encounter with attachment theory and accounts of early development. He was working with the fascinating accounts, including the work of the authors in this section, of the way early experience leaves profound gestalts and procedural forms of being and doing on any adult character. Relational analysts have begun to attend to the developmental origins of other relational phenomena, for example, Jessica Benjamin has been particularly concerned with constructing a developmental line tracing the origins of intersubjectivity.

It is in this section of this volume that one can see the powerful interrelations of different theoretical traditions. Mitchell's interests were meeting up with a body of work situated both in empirical developmental psychology and psychoanalytic work that had its own ambivalent connections to the work of John Bowlby in the post-war period in England. All the authors in this section live comfortably and creatively in the world of empirical research and the world of the clinic. Theoretical antecedents and influences include Bion and Winnicott, self psychology, contemporary infancy research, and the groundbreaking research program of Ainsworth and her colleagues, work that links Bowlby to contemporary child psychology.

The research wing of this group of authors itself merits some comment. Carefully and precisely empirical, possessed of a very labor-intensive methodology, the "baby watchers" combine acute observation with experimental rigor. We have now, through the work of these authors and their colleagues, a kind of "thick description" of infant life and mother–infant interaction. In the work of the four authors in this section, we can watch the fascinating insights that this empirical tradition has provoked come into play in the clinical dyad.

Representation and Internalization in Infancy:
Three Principles of Salience

(1994)

Beatrice Beebe
Frank M. Lachmann

▼ ▼ ▼ ▼ ▼

Editors' Introduction

Beebe and Lachmann, over two decades of creative, inspired collaboration, have worked to keep two domains firmly in view and firmly in tension and interdependence. Looking at the subtle, nonverbal, vocal, and bodily dances of mother and child over unfolding time is one domain. Tracking the presence and power of archaic and transforming patterns of relational engagement in the analytic work with adults is the other domain. The trick, if you like, and one that Beebe and Lachmann negotiate beautifully, is to see both the power of the procedural, preverbal levels of experience and the endless permutations and transformations in psychic functioning, to see emergent change and trenchant pattern. This balancing act yields both developmental theorizing and theories of treatment.

Beebe and Lachmann's theoretical and clinical work depends on an absorption in and mastery of the vast literature on mother–infant interaction and on the empirical, hands-on research program of Beebe and her colleagues. We must note that what appears in this essay (and in much of their other work) as clear, simple summaries of empirical study is a set of ideas, concepts, and hypotheses that draw on data sets that often take a decade to collect, arrange and analyze. Baby-watching is labor-intensive work.

In this influential essay, Beebe and Lachmann draw out three principles of what they term "salience," principles that guide developmental theorizing and clinical attention. In the decade since this article appeared, each of these principles has emerged into clearer and clearer focus as a matter of striking clinical implication. The core principle of mutual and self-regulation lies at the heart of relational understanding of coconstruction and intersubjectivity. Attention to rupture and repair alters one's clinical stance and allows attention to mismatching and misreading and finding ways back to mutual and self-regulation. Attention to affect attunement anticipates one of the broad directions psychoanalytic work has taken toward understanding affect attunement as a dyadic phenomenon as well as an intrapsychic one.

Representation and Internalization in Infancy: Three Principles of Salience*

▼   ▼   ▼   ▼   ▼

What is central in the infant's experience? What organizing principles determine the salience of events to the infant? What does the infant expect from his or her interactive encounters?

We reviewed current work on the organization of infant experience and derived three principles of salience with which to describe interaction structures in the first year of life. These principles constitute hypotheses about how social interactions between caretaker and infant become patterned and salient. Although researchers and clinicians tend to favor one of these principles over others, an integration of all three is necessary for a more differentiated view of how representations of social relatedness are formed in infancy. We focus narrowly on purely social interactions and omit consideration of related issues such as the regulation of sleep and wake states, feeding and alone states.

Of the three principles, the overarching one is *ongoing regulations*, based on the expected and characteristic ways in which an interaction

---

    * Originally published in *Psychoanalytic Psychology*, 11:127–166. © 1994 Lawrence Erlbaum Associates.

unfolds. The other principles are *disruption and repair* of expected interactions, and *heightened affective moments*. These principles are variations on the ways in which expectancies of social interactions are organized.

The principle of ongoing regulations captures the characteristic pattern of repeated interactions. Disruption and repair captures a specific sequence broken out of the broad pattern. In heightened affective moments, one dramatic instance stands out in time. Thus the three principles provide a hierarchical definition of interaction structures, temporally organized at three levels: the broad pattern, a sequence, and a moment. These three levels of organization should be seen as a nested series in which each level constitutes a context for the next.

Each of our three principles of salience provides a different perspective of the organization of presymbolic representations and on the origins of internalization in the first year. Self- and object representations can be seen as based on early perceptual capacities; interaction structures; and emerging capacities for category formation, abstraction, and later, symbol formation (Beebe, 1986; Beebe and Lachmann, 1988a; Beebe and Stern, 1977; Stern, 1985b). Interaction structures are characteristic patterns of mutual and self-regulations that the infant comes to recognize, remember, and expect. Whereas in our previous work we used only the principle of ongoing regulations, we now conceptualize interaction structures and representations as organized by all three principles.

This description of representations as organize by the three principles of salience can simultaneously illuminate the origins of internalization. Interactive regulation is a central concept in both the empirical infant literature and discussions of internalization (Schafer, 1968). However, in our view, interactive regulations do not *become* inner regulations. Rather, interactive regulations have always been inner, in the sense that they always occur in tandem with self-regulations. We suggest a view of internalization in the first year in which both partners jointly construct modes of regulation that include interactive as well as self regulations. The expectation and representation of the dyadic modes of regulation, as organized by the three principles of salience, constitute the inner organization.

Why Three Principles?

In considering the question of what principles determine the centrality of events for the infant, is it the infant's recognition of what is regular, predictable and "invariant" in his interactions that becomes salient? Stern (1985b) held this view in his discussion of the invariance of sequence causality, affect, and memory. Similarly, we also argued (Beebe and Lachmann, 1988a, 1988b) that the predictable ongoing regulations in mother-infant interactions create expectancies that organize the infant's experience. Wilson and Malatesta (1989) also argued that repetitive interactive experiences influence what is subject to repetition in adult life. We term this principle *ongoing regulations*.

Or, is it the infant's recognition that something changes, or disrupts his interactions, or violates his expectancies, and is it the subsequent effort to repair the disruption that organizes his experience? Behrends and Blatt (1985), Horner (1985), Stechler and Kaplan (1980), and Tronick (1989; Gianino and Tronick, 1988) noted the formative impact of these interactions of disruption and repair. Kohut (1984), in the analyses of adults, emphasized this sequence in his discussion of structure formation through empathic ruptures and transmuting internalizations. We term this principle of salience *disruption and repair*.

Or, is it the power of heightened affective moments, both positive and negative, that "colors" and thus organizes experience? Demos (1983, 1984), Emde (1981), Socarides and Stolorow (1984/1985), and especially Pine (1981, 1986), in his concept of heightened moments, proposed this point of view. We term this principle of salience *heightened affective moments*. Wilson and Malatesta (1989) noted that it is still an unresolved empirical question whether chronicity of exposure—or intensity of exposure, or an interaction of the two—most contribute to later dispositions.

Rather than viewing each of these principles as operating separately, they need to be conceptualized together. For example, an ongoing pattern of regulation must first exist before a disruption may itself become an expected interaction pattern. A heightened affective moment may function either as a disruption or as a repair. All three principles must be brought to bear on any particular interaction to fully explicate its organizing potential. The three principles constitute different angles of the camera. In a particular instance, however, one may be more compelling than the others. For heuristic purposes, we are pulling them apart. However, it is important to note that the three principles potentially interact. Following our presentation of the three principles separately, we describe their integration.

Stern's (1985b) theory of representations of interactions generalized (RIGs) implicitly uses the principle of ongoing regulations to explain how RIGs are organized. That is, the RIG is based on a generalized abstraction of a typical sequence. In adding the principles of disruption and repair and of heightened affective moments, we define other critical aspects of interactions that organize experience. There may well be additional salient principles yet to be explicated that will further broaden our understanding of how representations may be organized in the first year.

In addressing the question of what attributes of the infant's experience are dominant in the formation of representations, Stern (1988a) argued that affect does not have a privileged role. He suggested that all attributes of experience (perceptual, cognitive, motoric, sensory, affective) organize representations and that any one may play a central role for a particular event. Instead, we propose that there *are* privileged routes—salient organizing principles—that partake of but cut across Stern's wide range of factors. That is, perception, cognition, action, affect, and arousal are all organized by each of our three principles. Although we agree that affect is not necessarily the central organizer, we suggest that heightened affect is one salient route, along with ongoing regulations and disruption and repair. Although affect is a component of all three principles, intense affect is a sufficiently unique dimension of the creation of expectancies to justify its consideration as a third principle of organization.

Although the affect and arousal are linked, they are distinguishable. We reserve the term *affect* for facial display and vocal pattern (such as contour, pitch and volume). We define *arousal* as the pattern of physiological indices such as EEG, heart rate, and respiration. Nevertheless, in experience, a particular facial or vocal pattern is always associated with a particular arousal state (Ekman, 1983). Although numerous categorical approaches to affect (Izard, 1979; Malatesta, Culver, Tesman & Shepard, 1989; Tomkins, 1980) have been useful in studying infants, our approach lays equal emphasis on the gradient and display fluctuations within any particular affect category (Beebe, 1973; Oster & Ekman, 1977; Stern, 1985b; Tobach, 1970; Werner, 1948). Affect is a component of all three principles.

Self- and Object Representations Are Rooted in Interaction Structures

Interest in the formative role of interaction has a history within psychoanalysis in which the representation of relationships has been emphasized. Interactions with the object world have been viewed as constituting an inner regulation as well as an interactive regulation (see Behrends & Blatt, 1984, for a review; Hartmann, 1939; Jacobson, 1964; Loewald, 1960; Schafer, 1968; Spitz, 1983). Loewald (1960), in discussing psychic structure formation, proposed that the internalization of the interactional processes of the individual with his objects is an essential constitutive factor.

Other current conceptualizations view early experience as organized through dyadic interactions. The dyadically forged mind (Wilson & Malatesta, 1989), the interpersonal self (Kegan, 1982; Stern 1983, 1985b, 1989), the intersubjective matrix (Benjamin, 1988; Stolorow, Brandchaft & Atwood, 1987), and the relational mind (Fast, 1988; Mitchell, 1988) all conceptualize self and object and their representations as rooted in interaction structures (see Zelnick & Bucholz, 1990, for a review). In our view, both mutual and self-regulation organize interaction structure. This view is consonant with the work of Demos (1983, 1984), Lichtenberg (1983, 1989), Sander (1977), Stern (1985b), Stolorow et al. (1987), and Tronick (1989). Thus the influence of dyadic regulation is integrated with the critical contribution of self-regulations.

The Principles of Salience and Self- and Object Representations

We confine our discussion to representations of self and object. Traditionally the terms *self-representations* and *object representations* have conveyed encapsulated and atomistic images (Modell, 1984, 1992). In our view, representations result from interactions. We hold a dynamic process model of representations in which a schema is constructed of the expected moment-to-moment interplay of the two partners. What is represented is the dynamic interactive process itself (Beebe & Lachmann, 1988a, 1988b; Beebe & Stern, 1977; Lachmann & Beebe, 1992; Stern, 1977).

Representations are relatively persistent, organized classifications of information about an expected interactive sequence. They are formed by the active process of constructing incoming information. Representations can be reorganized and transformed as incoming information is reinterpreted and reordered based on both past experience and current expectations. In this transformational model, development proceeds through a process of regular restructurings of the relations within and between the person and the environment (Reese & Overton, 1970; Sameroff & Chandler, 1976; Sameroff, 1983). Predictability in development is found not in the child, not in the environment, but rather in the transactions between the child and the environment and in their regular transformations (Sameroff & Chandler, 1976; Zeanah, Anders, Seifer & Stern, 1989).

Basic to representation is the capacity to order and recognize patterns, to expect what is predictable and invariant, and to create categories of these invariants. The ability to categorize experiences provides the organizational framework for memory, language and the symbolic function (Basch, 1988; Bornstein, 1985; Shields & Rovee-Collier, 1992;

Stern, 1985b; Strauss, 1979; Younger & Cohen, 1985). A category is formed as the infant perceives regularities, and forms a summary or central tendency of the features that vary within the category. This ability develops between 3 and 12 months (Cohen & Gelber, 1975; Sherman, 1985; Shields & Rovee-Collier, 1992; Stern, 1985b; Strauss, 1979; Younger & Gotlieb, 1988).

For example, infants categorize colors (Bornstein, 1985), faces (Cohen, DeLoache & Strauss, 1979), and shapes (Ruff, 1980; Younger & Cohen, 1985). Shields and Rovee-Collier (1992) suggested that infant categorization "is ubiquitous across ages and should not be regarded as an emergent, higher-order cognitive ability. Rather, it appears to be a natural by-product of the normal, ongoing process of memory encoding and retrieval" (p. 257). The category is a representation of the common elements of a set of distinctive experiences that the infant discriminates (Sherman, 1985; Strauss, 1979; Younger & Gottlieb, 1988). For the infant, this "representation" is presymbolic (see Beebe & Lachmann, 1988b; Meltzoff, 1985; Stern, 1985b). In elaborating on this presymbolic representation, Mandler (1988) argued that a primitive form of representation ability exists in the early months of life which links the infant's sensory-motor schemata to a later symbolic form of representation (see Werner & Kaplan, 1963).

We propose that over the course of the first year and beyond, the three principles constitute criteria by which interactions will be categorized and ultimately represented. In the same way that infants categorize faces, shapes, colors, or animals, they will also form schemas or categories of interpersonal interactions (see Beebe & Lachmann, 1988b; Beebe & Stern, 1977; Stern, 1985b).

After the first year and beyond, as representations become increasingly symbolic, using the principle of ongoing regulations, the eventual representation if ever translated into verbal form may be something like, "I can expect that things will usually go like this." Using the principle of disruption and repair, the representation will be, "This is what happens when things are off. I can expect that they will get fixed, and this is how we fix them." Using the principle of heightened affect, the representation may be "What a wonderful (terrible, awesome) moment." If these interactions are verbalized and labeled, this process may transform the original representation (Stern 1985b).

We assume that representations in the first year are encoded in a nonverbal, imagistic, acoustic, visceral, or temporal mode of information and that they may not necessarily be translated into linguistic form. Bucci (1985) suggested that verbal and nonverbal information each have separate specialized systems for representation. Whereas verbal information is stored in linguistic form, nonverbal information is stored in perceptual channels through, for example, images, sounds, smells, touch and temperature. Both systems are potentially accessible to consciousness. Nonverbal imagistic schemata may be under certain circumstances inaccessible to attention or language but may nevertheless continue to operate and affect how we act and feel (Bucci, 1985). The nonverbal representational system begins in the first year of life, and the three principles of salience provide hypotheses about how such perceptual information will be organized.

The Principle of Ongoing Regulations

Ongoing regulations provides the most basic principle organizing representations. Numerous authors from widely divergent vantage points implicitly use it to infer what organizes experience (e.g. Bretherton, 1985; Demos, 1984; Lichtenberg, 1989; Loewald, 1960; Malatesta et al. 1989; Sander, 1977; J. Sandler & A. Sandler, 1978; Stern, 1985b; Wilson & Malatesta, 1989).

The principle of ongoing regulations refers to those characteristic, predictable and expected ways in which an interaction unfolds. A shared system of rules for the regulation of the actions of the two partners develops. In a well-ordered interaction, each partner's communicative behavior conforms to the other's expectations (Tronick, 1980).

The principle of ongoing regulations derives from a regulatory systems perspective (Beebe et al., 1993; Sander, 1977, 1983). Organization is evaluated as a property of the infant-caretaker system, as well as a property of an individual. It is not well established that there are many such shared systems of rules for the regulation of joint action in the first year of life, well before language develops (see e.g. Bakeman & Brown, 1977; Beebe, Jaffe, Feldstein, Mays & Alson, 1985; Bruner, 1977, 1983; Cohn & Tronick, 1988; Field, 1981; Stern, 1977, 1985b; Tronick, 1989).

There is extensive experimental evidence that babies form expectations of predictable events from birth and even before (DeCasper & Carstens, 1980; DeCasper & Fifer, 1980; DeCasper & Spence, 1986; Fagen, Morrongiello, Rovee-Collier, & Gekoski, 1984; Fagen, Ohr, Fleckenstein & Ribner, 1985; Greco, Rovee-Collier, Hayne, Griesier & Early, 1986). Haith's (Haith, Hazan, & Goodman, 1988; see also Emde, 1988) work on visual activity in the early months suggests that the infant is biologically prepared to detect regularity, generate expectancies, and act on these expectations.

The fact that expectancies operate so pervasively, so early, accounts for the enormous influence they have in organizing experience (Fagen,

Ohr, Singer & Klein, 1989). Neurophysiological evidence also suggests that familiarity, repetition and expectancy provide the most powerful organizing principle of neural functioning (Cormier, 1981; Gazzaniga & LeDoux, 1978; Hadley, 1983, 1989).

The infant's perception of ongoing regulations is thus based on this capacity to notice and predict what is expectable in the environment and the critical ability to detect that the behavior produces consequences. The neonate detects *contingencies*—predictable relationships between his own behavior and the environment's response (DeCasper & Carstens, 1980; DeCasper & Fifer, 1980; H. Papousek & M. Papousek, 1979; Watson, 1985). The infant develops an expectation of when events will occur and an expectation that his behavior produces consequences. Whether the environment provides contingent and expectable responses for the infant will affect his attention, memory, emotions and the very capacity to learn (DeCasper & Carstens, 1980). Reciprocally, the infant perceives predictable relations between environmental events and his own behavior. The infant develops an expectation that the environment affects him. Thus, both partners develop expectations that they affect and are affected by the other in predictable ways.

The principle of ongoing regulations encompasses any characteristic pattern with which the two partners regulate their communicative behavior. Successful as well as unsuccessful patterns are encompassed by this principle. The principle of ongoing regulations includes both mutual regulation and self-regulation. We first explicate mutual regulation and then address the interdependence of mutual and self-regulation.

Ongoing Regulations: Mutual Regulation

A mutual regulation model is central to the principle of ongoing regulations. It has emerged over the past two decades in reaction to much previous work that focused on one-way influences in child development. The parent's influence on the child was primarily studied to the relative exclusion of the child's influence on the parent (Bell, 1968; Capella, 1981; Gianino & Tronick, 1988; Lewis & Lee-Painter, 1974; Lewis & Rosenblum, 1974). Interest in patterns of mutual regulation paralleled increasing recognition of infants' social capacities (Lewis & Rosenblum, 1974). Although each partner does not influence the other in equal measure or necessarily in like manner, both actively contribute to the regulation of the exchange. The mother obviously has greater range and flexibility in this process. By *mutual regulation*, we mean that each partner's behavioral stream can be predicted from the other's.

In previous publications (Beebe, 1986; Beebe & Lachmann, 1988a, 1988b; Beebe & Stern, 1977), we proposed a central role for early interaction structures in the organization of infant experience. Using the principle of ongoing regulations, interaction structures are characteristic patterns of mutual and self-regulation. The dynamic interplay between the actions (including perceptions, affects and proprioceptions) of infant and caretaker, as each influences the other, creates a variety of mutual regulatory patterns. In the following sections, interaction structures are also defined by the principles of disruption and repair and heightened affective moments.

The study of the regulation of mother-infant interaction has been occupied to a considerable degree with detailing the various influences of each partner on the other's behavior. Numerous patterns of mutual regulation have been variously termed synchronization (Stern, 1971, 1977), behavioral dialogue (Bakeman & Brown, 1977), protoconversation (Beebe, Alson, Jaffe, Feldstein & Crown, 1988; Beebe, Stern & Jaffe, 1979), tracking (Kronen, 1982), accommodation (Jasnow & Feldstein, 1986), mutual dialogues (Tronick, 1980, 1982, 1989), reciprocal and compensatory mutual influence (Capella, 1981), and coordinated interpersonal timing (Beebe & Jaffe, 1992a, 1992b; Beebe et al., 1985; Jaffe et al., 1991). Patterns of mutual regulation have been demonstrated across various modalities such as gaze, vocalization, facial expression, timing and general affective involvement, at numerous ages across the first year, using diverse methods of coding and statistical procedures (see Beebe et al., 1993, for a review). Although bi-directional influences are preponderant in the literature (see e.g. Beebe & Jaffe, 1992a; Cohn & Tronick, 1998; Jaffe et al., 1991; Stern, 1971, 1988, 1985), one-way influences—where one partner influences the other, but without reciprocation—can also be found (e.g. Gottman & Ringland, 1981; Thomas & Martin, 1976; Zelner, 1982).

Using a definition of early representation as the storage of distinctive features, we proposed that the distinctive features of ongoing mutual regulations will be presented (Beebe & Lachmann, 1988b). This proposal depends on the crucial assumption that the patterns of mutual regulations that have been demonstrated by researchers are also perceived as salient by the infant. The distinctive features of these patterns can be described as the organization of the interaction along temporal, spatial, affective and proprioceptive dimensions. For example, the infant will represent the temporal pattern, such as rate, rhythm and serial order of both partners; the presence or absence of interpersonal contingencies and mutual influences; the pattern of the movement of the two partners in space such as approach-approach or approach-withdrawal; and the interactive regulation of facial and vocal affective patterns. The accompanying proprioceptive stimulation and pattern of arousal will also be represented. Thus, ongoing patterns of regulation as they are organized by time, space, affect and arousal will organize the infant's experience and will be represented.

Illustration of Interactions Organized by Ongoing Regulations

Facial mirroring. In previous publications (Beebe & Lachmann, 1988a, 1988b) we described two patterns of ongoing mutual regulation that illustrate qualitative differences in the patterns of regulation that may be represented. One pattern, facial mirroring, illustrates moment-by-moment matching of affective direction, in which both partners may increase together, or decrease together their degree of engagement and level of positive affect. This responsivity has been shown to occur well within ½ sec for both mother and infant (Cohn & Beebe, 1990). We suggest that the infant will represent the expectation of being matched by, and being able to match, the partner. This matching provides each partner with a behavioral basis for knowing and entering into the other's changing feeling state.

Derailment. Also termed *chase and dodge*, derailment illustrates the organization of the interaction primarily along the spatial dimension. In this interaction, the mother repeatedly attempts to engage the infant, and the infant displays a virtuoso range of avoidance maneuvers. For example, the infant may move the head back, duck the head down, avert the head fully to a ninety degree position away from the partner, or go limp and collapse his body tonus. Each partner's behavior continues to influence the other's on a moment-by-moment basis. This interaction illustrates the possibility that a mutual regulation structure may be intact, and yet the pair may be "misattuned," in the sense that the infant's attention, affect and arousal are not optimally regulated. We suggested that when such interactions are characteristic, they are represented as expectancies of misregulation.

Interpersonal timing. The regulation of the mother-infant interaction along the temporal dimension was described in a series of articles on kinesic rhythm (Beebe et al., 1979), coactive and alternating vocal exchanges (Stern, Jaffe, Beebe & Bennett, 1975), vocal congruence (Beebe et al., 1988; Jasnow & Feldstein, 1986) and the interpersonal timing of vocal interaction (Beebe & Jaffe, 1992a; Jaffe et al., 1991). These studies documented a remarkable temporal sensitivity on the part of both partners to the ongoing durations of their own and the partner's behavior. These behaviors last on the order of approximately 1 second or less.

Each monitors and matches the durations of the other's behavior on a second-by-second basis.

Curvilinear prediction of attachment. There is a further group of recent studies that documented effects into toddlerhood, predicted from interaction structures in the early months of life. These effects are based on the attachment paradigm (Ainsworth, Blehar, Waters & Wall, 1978; Bowlby, 1969; Sroufe, 1979; Sroufe & Fellson, 1986) that classifies toddlers as securely attached versus insecurely attached. Insecure attachment has two forms: avoidant and angry-resistant. Following a brief separation from mother in a laboratory setting, insecure-avoidant toddlers avoid the mother at reunion. In contrast, insecure-resistant toddlers both seek the mother and resist the contact, failing to be comforted. Secure toddlers seek and maintain contact during reunion, are easily comforted and can resume exploration of the environment.

A number of studies (Belsky, Rovine & Taylor, 1984; Isabel & Belsky 1991; Malatesta et al., 1989) now converge on a curvilinear regulation between maternal behavior in the first year and toddler attachment outcomes in 1 to 2 years of age. Infants who later become securely attached have mothers who stimulate with a midlevel range of intensity, contingency and reciprocity. Infants who will later become insecure-avoidant have mothers who are overstimulating, intrusive, high intensity, noncontingent or overly contingent. Infants who will later become insecure-resistant have mothers who are underinvolved, detached or inconsistent, who fail to respond, or who attempt to interact when the infant is not available.

A specific example of this group of studies is the work of Malatesta et al. (1989), who evaluated maternal contingent responsiveness at $2\frac{1}{2}$, 5 and $7\frac{1}{2}$ months and toddler attachment outcome at 2 years. Maternal contingency was measured by a maternal facial expression change within 1 sec of the onset of an infant facial expression change. Mothers who show moderate levels of facial contingency to their infants have toddlers at 2 years of age who look at them more and show the most positive affect. Moderate levels of maternal facial contingency at $7\frac{1}{2}$ months predicted secure attachment at age 2, whereas high maternal contingency at $7\frac{1}{2}$ months predicted insecure-avoidant attachment at 2 years of age. There were no insecure-resistant toddlers in the sample.

Whereas the foregoing studies focus exclusively on the nature of the mother's behavior, a study by Jaffe et al. (1991; see also Beebe & Jaffe, 1992a) predicted infant attachment at 1 years from 4-month maternal and infant contingent responsiveness. Using time series regression analysis, contingent responsiveness was measured by the degree to which increases in the durations of one partner's vocalizations and pauses were systematically followed by increases (or decreases) in the duration of the other partner's vocal behavior. The findings were again largely curvilinear. Midrange values of contingent vocal responsiveness at 4 months predicted secure attachment at 1 year. Very high or very low values of infant contingent responsiveness predicted secure attachment at 1 year.

This series of studies illustrates the principle that ongoing regulations of interactions organize the infant's experience of relatedness over the first 2 years of life. Particular kinds of interactions are facilitative or disruptive of the infant's attachment. Evidence from different laboratories is converging on the powerful curvilinear finding that optimal interactions are mid-range in intensity and contingency, both on the mother's part and the infant's. Extremes of responsiveness at the very high or very low end, by either partner, predict compromised infant attachment.

Ongoing Regulations: Integration of Mutual and Self-Regulation

In the infant literature on the development of psychic structure and the self, some authors emphasize self-regulation as the key organizing principle (see e.g. Emde, 1981; Stechler & Kaplan, 1980), other authors emphasize mutual interactive regulation (see e.g. Beebe & Lachmann, 1988a; 1988b; Stern, 1971, 1977) and others emphasize an integration (see e.g. Beebe et al., 1993; Demos, 1983; Gianino & Tronick, 1988; Lichtenberg, 1989; Sander, 1977). Sander's (1983, 1985) view that organization is an emergent property of the dyadic system, rather than solely of the individual, integrated the simultaneous influences of self-regulation and mutual regulation. Because both processes are organized at birth and play a crucial role in the development of social relatedness from birth, we hold that they must be integrated in conceptualizing the development of representations.

The Brazelton Neonatal Behavioral Assessment Scale (Brazelton, 1973) is designed to evaluate the joint contribution of infant self-regulation capacity and the mutual regulation between infant and partner. For example, it assesses the infant's capacity to dampen his state in response to aversive stimuli. At the same time it assesses how much help from the partner is required and can be utilized by the infant to stabilize his state after stress and to maintain engagement with the environment.

The infant's capacity to respond and be socially engaged depends not only on the nature of the caretaker's stimulation and responsivity, and on the nature of the infant's response to the specific stimulation, but also on the infant's regulation of his internal state of arousal. Babies differ from birth constitutionally and temperamentally in this crucial capacity to modulate their arousal, shift their state and in general to organize their behavior in predictable ways (Als & Brazelton, 1981; Brazelton, 1973). The importance of the initial intactness of the capacity of the organism to tolerate and use stimulation alerts us to the enormous contribution of normal self-regulatory capacities that we usually take for granted. These capacities are prerequisite for engaging with the environment (Resch, 1988).

Self-regulation can be demonstrated in the fetus (Brazelton, 1992). The fetus can change his state, dampen his arousal, and eventually put himself to sleep to cope with aversive stimulation. When the stimulation becomes more than moderate, the infant again changes state and shows patterns of information processing. Thus, even the fetus can regulate the level of arousal and responsivity as a function of nature of the stimulation provided.

Although the infant has the capacity to organize states, Sander (1977, 1983) showed that this system is successfully established only by an adequate mutual regulation between infant and caretaker. In the normal caregiving environment, babies who room-in with their own mothers establish day-night differentiation within 4 to 6 days. Organizing states so that sleep occurs more at night and wakefulness more during the day is a crucial accomplishment of the infant in the first week of life. Maternal care is a mutually regulated process such that the mother is sensitive to the infant's cues of state change and the infant is responsive to the mother's attempts to activate or dampen arousal.

Sander (1976) studied babies who were to be adopted and showed that the development of self-regulation is dependent on mutual regulation. For the first 10 days of life these babies were placed in the normal hospital nursery with a set schedule and many nurses. Caretaking in this environment was not a mutually regulated process. During these 10 days, the infants did not establish any day-night differentiation or stable sleep-wake patterns. For the second 10 days of life, each baby was transferred to his own special nurse where caretaking was mutually regulated. Within 10 days, these babies all established day-night differentiation and stable sleep-wake cycles. The quality of mutual regulation affects the infant's internal regulation, sleep-wake cycle and biorhythms. Only where adequate mutual regulation occurred did adequate self-regulation occur. Although Sander does not specifically address the converse in this study, the intactness of the infant's self-regulation will affect the ease and quality of the mutual regulation as well. Sander's conclusions provide support for our position that ongoing regulations are based on an integration of self- and mutual regulations.

In her studies of heart rate and looking patterns, Field (1981) also illustrated how self regulation and mutual regulation form an inter-dependent system. During face-to-face social play at 2 to 6 months of age, the infant briefly looks away from the mother and then quickly returns to look at her. Looking away is one of the infant's major methods of dosing the level of stimulation and regulating arousal (Brazelton, Kozlowski & Main, 1974; Stern, 1971, 1977). The infant's regulation of arousal is evaluated by examining heart rate patterns. In the five seconds just before the infant looks away, the heart rate shoots up, indicative of a protective process in which information shoots down again, indicative of a receptive process in which information intake is facilitated. The infant then looks back at the mother.

Field's (1981) study illustrated the infant's use of looking away to perform a self-regulation. At the same time, a mutual regulation process will proceed. If the mother can use the infant's gaze away to lower her level of stimulation while the infant if re-regulating his arousal, and if the infant can likewise use the mother's lowering of stimulation so that he then looks back at her, adequate mutual regulation will be established. If, on the other hand, the mother "chases" when the infant looks away, and increases her level of stimulation, both self-regulation and mutual regulation will be interfered with for the infant. If the mother chases and increases her stimulation, the infant will look away for a longer period and will withdraw more severely (Beebe & Stern, 1977; Brazelton et al., 1974; Hirschfield & Beebe, 1987; Stern, 1977).

Optimal mutual regulation is also interfered with if the mother chases, because the infant is then deprived of the capacity to influence the mother's behavior toward a more moderate range. If the mutual regulation is optimal, the infant simultaneously can influence his own level of arousal and the mother's level of stimulation. The very same behaviors through which the infant regulates arousal (e.g. looking away) function at the same time as interactive regulations. If the mutual regulation is optimal, the mother's lowering of her stimulation also influences the infant to return to the vis-à-vis more quickly.

Gianino and Tronick (1988) made the integration of mutual and self-regulation central to their work. They described the infant's repertoire of self-regulatory skills in detail. Their position is that self-regulation and interactive regulation occur at the same time. The same interactive repertoire with which the infant initiates, maintains and modifies well-regulated interactions and repairs, avoids and terminates disrupted interactions simultaneously performs self-regulatory functions.

Tronick (1989) offered experimental evidence that the nature of the mutual regulation is associated with the adaptiveness of the self-regulation. Infants are subjected to the stress of the "still-face" experiment, where the mother remains oriented and looking but becomes completely immobile and unresponsive. In those dyads where the mutual regulation is going well, the infant's self regulation capacity as measured in the still-face situation is more adaptive, and vice versa. In the still-face experiment, these infants continue to signal the mother rather than turn to self-comforting, withdrawal or disorganized scanning.

The integration of mutual and self-regulation has direct bearing on current conceptualizations of the development of representations as organized through the dyad. The current concept that self and object and their representations are rooted in interactions holds true only so long as interactions are broadly construed to include an integration of self-regulation with mutual regulation. To focus on dyadic interaction alone omits the equally crucial contribution of the organism's own self-regulatory capacities.

The Principle of Disruption and Repair

In contrast to the principle of ongoing regulations, which emphasizes what is expectable in the interaction using the principle of disruption and repair, interactions are organized by violations of expectancy and ensuing efforts to resolve these breaches (Behrends & Blatt, 1985; Gianino & Tronick, 1988; Horner, 1985; Klein, 1967; Kohut, 1984; Piaget, 1954, 1957; Stechler & Kaplan, 1980; Tronick & Cohn, 1989; Tronick & Gianino, 1986).

Infants notice and are powerfully affected by the confirmation and violation of expectancies. DeCasper and Carstens (1980) demonstrated that the confirmation of the infant's expectancies is associated with positive affect, and the violation of expectancies is associated with negative affect. Stern's (1985a) work on affect attunement in 10-month-olds also provides evidence of the infants' capacities to notice the disruption of an ongoing sequence and to notice if the disruption is repaired.

The concept of disruption has been used to cover phenomena of varying degrees of severity. The terms *mismatch* or *violation of expectancy* are less severe than the term *disruption*. In addition, various phenomena of normal development do not fit the definition of disruption as violation of expectancy, but nevertheless do elucidate the disruption and repaid model. In particular, Tronick and Cohn's (1989) data on sequences of match-mismatch-rematch fit this category. Disruptions can be mild and expectable. Therefore we propose the following distinctions.

We retain the metaphor of disruption and repair to refer to a broad array of phenomena from mild to severe. Whereas violation of expectancy occurs in many disruptions, we consider it too narrow a concept to cover the full range. We introduce the concept of *disjunction* as a particular sub-type of disruption to describe instances of nonmatch, or mismatch, that occur frequently in normal interactions. They may or may not involve violations of expectancy, and they are relatively easily rerighted. Not all violations of expectancy are experienced as disruptive. Slight variations on expected themes are necessary to prevent habituation. Mild violations of expectancy are incorporated into playful exchanges and can produce positive excitement, such as the "I'm gonna getcha" game (Stern, 1982). We exclude these positive violations of expectancy from this discussion.

Three kinds of data illustrate the principle of disruption and repair. First, the consequences of actual experimental disruptions of the normal ongoing interactions come closest to operationalizing the concept of violations of expectancy. Second, in the study of normal interactions, disruptions are translated into the concept of mismatch of states of engagement, which we term *disjunctions*. These two sources of data are later discussed in more detail.

The study of clinically disturbed situations provides the third kind of data. Although a survey of the literature on clinically disturbed interactions is beyond our scope, several studies serve to illustrate the organization of expectancies of misregulation. For example, depressed mothers are described as angry, poking, intrusive and disengaged, and their infants are primarily protesting and disengaged (Cohn, Campbell, Matias & Hopkins, 1990; Cohn & Tronick, 1989b; Field, Goldstein & Guthertz, 1990). These infants develop expectancies of interaction structures characterized by chronic infant distress and protest, with maternal intrusion and withdrawal. Field et al. (1988) showed that infants of depressed mothers show depressed behaviors seen with nondepressed adults. Thus the infant develops expectancies of misregulation, which carry over into interactions with normally responsive new partners.

In this clinical example, the definition of disruption as violation of expectancy must shift. These infants experience disruption in the sense that their interactions are atypical, but we have no evidence that these disruptions actually violate infant expectations. It is more parsimonious to assume that chronic disruptions or misregulations come to be expected by the infant. These expectancies are sufficiently organized to continue to hold in the face an optimally responsive new adult partner.

Within the interaction structure of expected disruption, the infant also develops an associated self-regulatory style. Thus the infant learns to expect chronic disruption and to expect certain consequences from self-regulatory efforts. What is being organized is both the expectable interactive misregulation and an associated self-regulatory style (E. Tronick, personal communication, May 18, 1993).

The eventual longitudinal follow-up of such infants will enable us to describe the formation of representations where disruptions cannot be easily repaired. When there are unresolvable mismatches and disruptions without repair, which is characteristic of interactions of depressed mothers and their babies, the balance between self-regulation and mutual regulation is disturbed. The infants become preoccupied with self-regulation and the management of negative affect (Tronick, 1989). As Tronick argued, if self-regulation becomes the predominant goal, it sets the stage for psychopathology. In addition, the expectation of misregulation colors interactions with an unfamiliar adult, so that all interactions for such an infant are likely to be more negative (Field et al., 1988; Tronick, 1989). In this case, chronic disruption becomes the expectation of disruption and nonrepair, and this expectation organizes new interactions.

Disruption and repair: Disjunctions. The concept of disjunctions comes from research findings that mothers and infants do not necessarily match their states of engagement during normal successful play encounters (Kronen, 1982; Malatesta & Haviland, 1983; Tronick & Cohn, 1989). For example, Kronen (1982) found that at 4 months, mothers and infants significantly do not exactly match expression. Malatesta and Haviland (1983) found that only approximately 35% of mothers' contingent facial responses to infant facial changes are exact matches. Tronick and Cohn (1989) described mothers and infants at play at 3, 6 and 9 months as continuously shifting back and forth between matched and nonmatched states, spending approximately only one third of their time in matched states.

In a state of nonmatch, a mother might be engaged in social play, looking and smiling at her infant, but the infant might be a social attend, looking at the mother with a neutral face without smiling. Such nonmatched states are prevalent in normal, successful interactions. They cannot be considered to be actual violations of what is expected. Thus we have termed them *normative disjunctions*. Likewise, matchers are not considered a "repair," but a special state of coordination against a background of slight disjunctions. Matching constitutes too limited a model of the nature of facial-visual communication.

Tronick and Cohn's (1989) data on match and nonmatch are central to the disruption and repair metaphor. They found that when two partners enter an unmatched state, within 2 sec, 70% of the unmatched states return to a match. Furthermore, an analysis of who influences the interaction (e.g. which partner is responsible for the repair) shows that both mothers and infants influence the repair sequence (Cohn & Tronick, 1989a; Tronick & Cohn, 1989). The repair of disruption is a mutually regulated achievement.

Disjunctions and the organization of representation. Mother-infant interactions can be described as continuously shifting back and forth between greater and lesser degrees of coordination, matches and disjunctions, with a flexibility to span the range. When lesser coordinated states occur, there is a powerful tendency to reright the interaction by return to a more coordinated state within 2 sec. Thus, repairing disjunctions is a pervasive interactive skill for infants. Tronick (1989; Tronick & Gianino, 1986) suggested that the experience of repair increases the infant's effectance, elaborates the coping capacity, and contributes to an expectation of being able to repair, which he can bring to other partners. These capacities provide one definition of what is being organized in the infant's expectancies of interaction structures of disjunction and re-righting.

The reparative function is a mutually regulated achievement. As usually described (Kohut, 1984; Stechler & Kaplan, 1980), it is the *infant's* efforts to resolve disruptions that contribute to structure formation. We suggest that an interaction where the mother did not also contribute to the repair might interfere with the infant's experience of rerighting. The infant operates in a dyadic system to which both partners actively contribute.

Disjunctions and the ensuing search for rerighting is an important organizing principle to its own right. Although we include it in the metaphor of disruption and repair, it is somewhat different because it describes an ongoing characteristic process of regulating lesser and greater degrees or coordination. Disjunctions thus approach the ongoing regulations model as the resolution of minor mismatches becomes an expected sequence. The powerful tendency to search for coordination following mismatch establishes the expectancy that non-matches return to matches and thus constitutes an ongoing regulation. The expectancy is established that repair is possible (Tronick, 1989).

Experimental studies of disruption and repair. Experimental disruptions of infant social expectancies were studies by Tronick and his colleagues (Gianino & Tronick, 1988; Tronick, 1989; Weinberg, 1991). In the still-face experiment, the mother presents a completely still, unsmiling face to the infant (Tronick, Als, Adamson, Wise & Brazelton, 1978). The situation can be seen as drastically violating the infant's expectations of a contingently responsive partner. It thus fits the usual definition of disruption as violation of expectancy. The infant first attempts to elicit the normal interaction by greeting the mother with smiles. As the mother continues to be nonresponsive, the infant repeats a sequence of looking at mother with animated face, then looking away. After a number of repetitions of this eliciting sequence and still no response from mother, the infant withdraws, head and body averted from mother, often slumping and losing postual tonus. The infant attempts to repair the violation of his expectation of a normally responsive partner. But when the infant cannot, he withdraws, as if giving up.

The infant's performance in the still-face experiment has been compared to the mother and infant's tendency to match, mismatch, and rapidly return to match in a normal interaction (Tronick, 1989; Tronick & Cohn, 1989; Tronick & Gianino, 1985). A coping scale for the still-face situation rates infants from *most adaptive* (attempts to continue signaling the mother, alternative focus on something other than mother, self-comforting behavior) to *increasingly maladaptive* (withdrawal through arching away, giving up postural/motor control, and generally disorganized state). At 4 to 6 months, individual differences in this coping style stabilize, and the infant begins to rely on characteristic ways of coping. Finally, these differences predict developmental outcomes at 1 year. Infants who experience more repairs of nonmatch in the normal situation, and who use more adaptive methods of coping in the still-face, have more secure attachments to their mothers at 1 year (Cohn, Campbell & Ross, 1991; Tronick, 1989).

Representations and the reparative function. These findings have implications for the organization of infant experience. In the face of the drastic violation of the expectation of a responsive partner, infants make repeated efforts to "repair" breaches and elicit expected responsiveness from their mothers. This persistent effort to repair, demonstrated so early in development, gives the concept of repair a more firmly grounded developmental status. An infant of only 2 to 3 months will try to repair a nonresponsive mother. Furthermore, the way disruptions and repairs are managed, both in the still-face experiment and the match-mismatch analysis of ongoing interactions, predicts the future course of the quality of the infant's attachment to his mother. Experience is being organized with discernibly different consequences across the first year. These findings suggest that the reparative function is indeed a crucial force in the organization of the infant's experience. The expectation of the possibility of repair facilities the development of secure attachment.

Evidence for organization and representation can be inferred from these findings. When the mother resumes a normal interaction with her infant following the still-face, the infant continues a negative mood and reduced looking at mother. Tronick (1989) interpreted this finding as evidence that the still-face episode continues to exert an effect on the infant and thus that a representation of the prior interaction has been organized. "This finding suggests that even three-month-old infants are not simply under the control of the immediate stimulus situation but that events have lasting effects, that is, they are internally represented" (p. 114). In addition, particular methods of coping with violations of expectancies become characteristic for the infant by 6 months. This finding attests to how quickly the infant's social capacities become organized in enduring the characteristic ways.

A further source of evidence that expectancies become represented is derived from the Field et al. (1988) study presented previously, that infants of depressed mothers continue to be more negative in interactions with a nondepressed adult stranger. By 6 months, the infant of the depressed mother already has a more rigidly structured expectancy of relatedness. Whereas a normal 6-month-old infant has the capacity to engage positively with a stranger, the infant of the depressed mother brings the misregulated patterns that belong with the depressed mother to a new, potentially responsive partner. The infant seems to expect disruption without repair.

A final source of evidence that interactive behavior is being organized in the first year comes from the work of Weinberg (1991). She examined the stability of behavior across two play sessions at 6 and 6½ months, for 80 infants. The *stability*, or session-to-session consistency, can be constructed as an index of the degree to which behavior is being organized or the degree to which there is a way of doing things that is relatively stable. A sequence of three episodes was videotaped for each dyad: face-to-face play, still-face, and resumption of face-to-face play. Infant interactive behavior (infant looks at mother, looks at object, scans the room, signals to mother with vocalization and gesture) and infant affect (joy, interest, sadness, anger) were coded on a second-by-second basis. Robust episode-to-episode correlation was found. These findings corroborate session-to-session consistencies reported by Tronick (1989), Cohn & Tronick, (1989a) and Zelner (1982). The fact that there is a considerable degree of stability of interactive behavior by 6 months points to a strong, early organizing process.

Ongoing regulations and disruption and repair: An integration of the two principles. The disruption and repair model has had a wide-ranging influence on psychoanalytic theories of internalization and structure formation (Blatt & Behrends, 1987; Freud, 1917; Klein, 1967; Kohut, 1984; Loewald, 1960, 1962; Tolpin 1971). Disruption, breach, loss, incompatibility, frustration and disequilibrium are seen as nodal points around which new organization occurs. The new organization is variously conceptualized as a repair of the breach, as an internalization of the lost object, or as a structuralization within the psyche of functions of the relationship that were disrupted.

Deprivation and frustration have generally been assumed to underlie the disruption and repair model of psychic structure formation. For example, Behrends and Blatt (1985) argued that it is the unavailability of the object that promotes internalization; with a fully available object that would be no motivation to convert the affective tie to an internal function. The most extreme version of this model posits that disruption is a necessary precondition for all psychological development, internalization and structuralization (see e.g. Behrends & Blatt, 1985; Meissner, 1981). In contrast, Loewald (cited in Behrends & Blatt, 1985) argued that internalization can occur without disruption through intimacy or resonance.

We suggest that there is an ongoing organizing process, based on the creation of expectancies of characteristic interaction patterns. Disruption and disequilibrium and efforts to resolve these breaches of integration also undoubtedly generate expectancies and are thus powerful opportunities for organizing experience. However disruption is not a necessary condition for such development. Expectancies of characteristic ongoing regulations are an equally powerful organizing dynamic.

In the ongoing-regulations model, it is unnecessary to posit a deprivation motive. In fact, it is the very availability of the object and the consistency and predictability of responsivity that constitutes the organizing process. In our use of disruption and repair, we also do not assume a deprivation model of motivation. We assume and information-processing model in which the infant's perceptual abilities ensure a capacity for seeking out, perceiving and interacting with social partners (Ainsworth et al., 1978; Basch, 1988; Berlyne, 1966; Haith et al., 1988; Hunt, 1965). The disruption and repair of expected interaction sequences will organize the infant's experience based on the inherent ability to perceive confirmation and violation of expectations of ordered information.

We suggest that the two models, ongoing regulations and disruption and repair, organize different chunks of time and different aspects of experience. To the degree that the ongoing regulations are in the positive range, such as various matching interactions, experience is organized by what is predictable, expectable, coherent and coordinated. In this view, the goal of the system is an optimal range of coordination. In contrast, the principle of disruption and repair points toward experience as organized by contrast, disjunction and difference. The gap between what is expected and what is happening can also be repaired. In this view the goal of the system is optimal management of disjunction and repair. We consider these counterpoints to be simultaneously constituted.

Disruption and repair organizes experiences of coping, effectance, righting and hope (Tronick, 1989). Interactions are represented as reparable. The expectation develops that it is possible to maintain engagement with the partner in the face of strains and mismatches. In contrast, optimally coordinated, ongoing regulations organize experiences of coherence, predictability, fitting together with the partner and being well-related. The expectation develops that it is possible for the coordination to be sustained, the better the infant will be able to tolerate and benefit from experiences of disruption and repair. Horner (1985) and Stechler and Kaplan (1980) similarly proposed the integration of both regularities and discrepancies in organizing the patterns of interaction.

The Principle of Heightened Affective Moments

Having discussed ongoing regulations and their disruption and repair as two basic principles of organization, we now turn to the third principle, heightened affective moments. According to this principle, interaction structures are organized through heightened affective moments, in which the infant experiences a powerful state transformation

Whereas affect is a component of the first two principles, we consider intense affect to be a sufficiently unique dimension in the ongoing creation of expectancies to justify its consideration as a third principle of organization.

Affect. The infant has innate patterns of facial, vocal and bodily expressions of affect that are readily observable (Demos, 1984; Field, Woodson, Greenberg & Cohen, 1982; Malatesta et al., 1989; Oster, 1978; Oster & Ekman, 1977; Stern, 1977, 1985b; Tomkins, 1980). Izard (1979) showed that newborns express interest, joy, distress, disgust and surprise. Ekman (Ekman & Oster, 1979) demonstrated that these affective patterns exist in various cultures and argue for their universality. Numerous studies have shown that a range of affect is regulated in complex and subtle ways in early interactive exchanges (see e.g. Cohn & Beebe, 1990; Cohn & Tronick, 1988; Demos, 1984; Stern, 1977, 1985b; Tronick, 1982).

Tomkins (1980) described the amplifying function of affect: "Affect either makes good things better or bad things worse . . . by adding a special analogic quality that is intensely rewarding or punishing" (p. 148). This amplifying function sets the stage for the power of heightened affect. Stern's (1985a, 1985b) work addressed heightened affect through his discussion of the importance of the "vitality" dimension of affect in the communication of emotion. Affects surge and face, crescendo and decrescendo. Affects vary according to intensity, degree of display, and urgency, as well as by the nature of the category itself such as joy, distress, sadness, or anger (Stern, 1985b; Werner, 1948).

We define a heightened affective moment in infancy as the full display of any facial or vocal pattern, such as a cry face or a fully opened gape smile (Beebe, 1973). The full expressive display of the face or voice will of necessity be accompanied by heightened bodily arousal (Ekman, 1983).

Heightened moments. Pine (1981) described the power of affectively supercharged moments as an avenue toward the accretion of psychic structure. These supercharged moments become central to the organization of an array of percepts and memories and are formative in their effect far out of proportion to their mere temporal duration. Pine gave as examples prototypic moments of merger, such as echoing, cooing voices of mother and infant in unison; the infant falling asleep at the mother's breast; or moments of intense negative arousal in the absence of comfort or gratification.

Although the examples cited by Pine are heightened moments that tend to occur with some frequency in the ongoing daily rhythm of events, this concept also includes those heightened affective moments that are relatively rare and not part of everyday experience. Nevertheless, Pine (1981) noted that these heightened moments are only organizing if they capture the essence of similar though less intense moments. These affectively supercharged moments can thus be conceptualized as prototypes of a category of similar affective experiences. The organizing power of affectively supercharged moments thus derives from both the infant's capacity to categorize and expect similar experiences, as well as from the impact of the heightened affect itself. When expectancies play a role in organizing affectively supercharged moments, an ongoing regulations model is already implicitly within the model of heightened affective moments.

The single event. There is another type of affectively supercharged moment that can be conceptualized as a "one-shot" event, rather than a prototype of a category of similar experiences. This description raises the issue of trauma. There is considerable controversy over theories of trauma and whether an adult's memory of a traumatic event can be based on a single instance or is representative of a range of similar experiences.

It is hard to evaluate whether the concept of one-shot trauma is a viable one in infancy. First, it is difficult to know whether an event indeed happened only once or whether it might not constitute a prototype of a series of similar events. Second, there is a dearth of research evidence addressing the question of whether a single event can organize infant experience. Nevertheless, there is some suggestion from neurophysiological data that certain single experiences can induce brain changes, particularly if they contain certain qualities such as novelty (Spinelli & Jensen, 1979).

There is some experimental work suggesting that the infant's experience may be organized by a single event. Stern (1971) cites Gunther, who reports research on breast occlusion in neonates, in which the infant momentarily cannot breathe during feeding. Only one episode of breast occlusion influences newborn behavior for several feedings afterwards. However, it may be argued that it may be the mother who is traumatized and that her continuing anxiety influences the infant's feeding behavior.

It is also noteworthy that an experimentally induced singular event in 6-month-olds, sufficiently unusual that it would not occur in the normal course of events, is remembered by these infants when they become 1 and 2 years old. In this study of memory (Perris, Myers & Clifton, 1990) infants reached to find an object that was making noise—a rattle. They reached first in the light and then in the dark. When these infants were toddlers, they reached more frequently and were more successful in obtaining the rattle than did the control group, who did not reach without instruction. Thus it is clear from this research that a single event from 6 months can be remembered at 1 and 2 years later. This memory capacity may provide a way of understanding how earlier experiences can be carried forward in development. However the organizing impact of this event was not investigated. Therefore, no statement can be made about whether it organized the infant's experience.

Further support comes from clinical work with adults where a single traumatic event was organizing. Casement (1990) described an adult treatment in which the patient was preoccupied by having been severely burned at 11 months. The singular traumatic event became a major organizing theme in the analysis. Bernstein and Blacher (1967) described an adult treatment in which the patient remembered a traumatic physical sensation which he termed a "stick in the tushie" which was documented to have been a lumbar puncture as the age of 6 months.

Stern also discussed the possibility of a single event organizing the infant's behavior. In Stern's (1985b) theory of RIGs, events that are similar are averaged and represented by a prototype, a central tendency of the category. In the process of forming RIGs, Stern (1988b) discussed two sources of distortion. In the formation of prototypes, the averaging process itself may somewhat distort the event. These distortions err on the conservative side, so those more extreme examples of the category tend toward the central tendency. However, specific memories can also be a source of distortion, when one memory constitutes the category. One event then becomes more influential, because it is not averaged with many similar ones. Stern suggested that a specific memory provides a heightened affect influence as part of its power of distortion and therefore may be more potent than the averaged RIG. In this work Stern does not address the organizing potential of trauma, per se.

Heightened negative moment. There is experimental evidence that heightened negative affective moments may not only organize memory, as Pine (1981) suggested, but may also interfere with memory (Fagen et al., 1985, 1989; Singer & Fagen, 1992). Three to 4 month old infants learned to produce movement in an overhead crib mobile containing 10 identical components. The infants were then switched to a mobile containing only two components. Those infants who cried in response to the switch in mobiles failed to show evidence of retention of learning 1 week later. However, the "forgetting" by the crying infants was subsequently reversed by a brief reexposure to the two-component mobile. Fagen et al. (1985, 1989) concluded that crying affected a retrieval of the memory, but not its storage. The infants who had cried needed the reexposure to facilitate retrieval, but they had not lost the memory. The infant's retrieval of the memory of the training context is subject to modification and elaboration by the intense affect of crying.

These experiments provide evidence for the concept that intense affective experiences provide a unique dimension in the ongoing creation of expectancies. Although affect is a central feature in all three principles, these experiments further justify the inclusion of heightened affect as a separate organizing principle. The infant's retrieval of expectancies and memories can be altered by intense affect. The infant's memory representation of events is more elaborate than previously believed and includes not only the details of the learning cues but also his own emotional state (Ohr, Fleckenstein, Fagen, Klein & Pioli, 1989; Singer & Fagen, 1992).

The organizing impact of heightened affect moments. The data reviewed include consideration of several dimensions: the singular moment, its storage, its heightened affective quality, and its organizing impact. Neurophysiological evidence and the "reaching-in-the-dark" experiment simply illustrate the infant's capacity to store a single event. The remaining studies expand the argument by providing evidence that the singular event stored may include heightened affect and may be organizing. Organizing impact is inferred from the breast occlusion experiment by the observation that the infant's subsequent behavior is disrupted. Organizing impact is inferred from the mobile experiment by the observation that the infant's retrieval facility is altered. Organizing impact is inferred in the adult treatment case from the observation that the patient was preoccupied as an adult by the memories and bodily sensations of the burn. Although the infant data are suggestive and the adult treatment report is supportive, further evidence is necessary to evaluate the extent to which a single heightened event may organize infant and adult experiences.

We argued that the heightened affective moment potentially has an organizing impact. We now address the nature of this impact and propose that, at the moment of heightened affect, there is a state transformation (Lachmann & Beebe, 1993). We use the term *state* broadly to include physiological arousal, affect and cognition.

Following Sander (1983), states of alertness, arousal, activity and sleep are socially negotiated, a product of mutual regulation. Sander suggested that the earliest experiences are organized through the infant's recognition of recurrent, predictable transitions of state, in particular interactive contexts. Thus, early state transformations are related to both self-regulation and the expectation that mutual regulation will facilitate or interfere with these transformations.

In the reaching-in-the-dark experiment, the moment of state transformation occurred when the infants re-encountered the toy in the dark at 2 years. We speculate that the nature of the state transformation was both cognitive and affective: a moment of recognition and accompanying surprise, joy or efficacy. In the breast occlusion study, the state transformation occurred at the moment of difficulty in breathing. The state transformation entailed the experience of less air and an accompanying affective distress. In the mobile experiment, the state transformation occurred at the moment the infant recognized that the second mobile contained fewer components than the first. It was a cognitive transformation, in the sense that an expectancy was violated when the infant recognized that the new mobile was not the same as the old one, and the remembering process was altered. It was also an affective transformation, because the infants became distressed and half of them cried. In the case of the infant who was burned, a state transformation occurred at the moment of the burn. The transformation was a physiological one due to the pain, and an affective one due to the distress. We suggest that heightened moments are organizing because they affect a potentially powerful state of transformation.

Integration of the three principles. The three principles of salience constitute criteria by which events are categorized over the course of the first year and beyond. These categories will be used to represent aspects of experience once the symbolic function is more developed. The infant's early presymbolic representational capacity will be used to store those interaction patterns that are salient by virtue of any of the three principles. Using all three organizing principles, the infant forms prototypes—that is, generalized categories or models—of patterns of interactions, which become represented as the "rules" of the relationship. A self-regulatory style is represented within these prototypes of patterns of interaction.

Because all three principles interact, they need to be conceptualized together. For disruption to occur, an ongoing pattern of regulation must first exist. The particular nature and sequence of disruption and repair in itself becomes an expected interaction pattern. Thus, its potential to organize experience derives both from the power of the repair and the predictable, expected nature of the sequence. Furthermore, as Pine (1981) argued, heightened affective moments have a formative impact irrespective of their frequency or duration. But they do occur within an interactive context and sequence. Thus, their organizing impact derives from both the predictable nature of the sequence as well as from the power of the heightened affective moment itself. Moreover, heightened affective moments, when positive, can function to repair disruptions. When disruptions are sufficiently severe, they lead to heightened negative affective states which cascade and may traumatically disrupt self-regulation (E. Tronick, personal communication, May 18, 1993).

The facial-mirroring interaction illustrates how all three principles interact. It fits an ongoing regulations model, because each partner influences the other to match the direction of affective change. In addition, at various points, both infant and mother hit peak, heightened, positive moments (Beebe, 1973). The notion of disjunction also applies, because at several moments, the baby sobers and looks away without distress. Although in general the mother matches the direction of affective change, occasionally the infant is still looking away. The infant's ability to reregulate arousal, and the dyad's ability to return to the play encounter, will contribute to organizing the infant's experience.

The three principles and affect. The use of all three principles will yield a more differentiated way of conceptualizing qualitative difference in the organization of infant experience. Specifically, affect is regulated within all three principles, but in different ways. Examples of the regulation of affect occurring during heightened affective moments include tantrums or falling asleep at the mother's breast. The predominance of prolonged heightened affect states, either negative or positive, may lead to stimulation beyond the ability to organize and thus the expectation of misregulation of affect. These examples describe more global transformations of affective states.

Quite different are the subtle, moment-by-moment regulations of slight shifts of attention, affect and arousal within the narrower range typically described in the face-to-face encounter. Here affect is a continuously changing, subtle, incremental process. The ongoing misregulation of attention, affect and arousal will organize non-optimal ranges of self- and mutual regulation. For example, over- or underarousal signal that the mutual regulation has not succeeded in contribution to adequate infant self-regulation.

In sequences of disruption and repair, the nature of the affect regulation emphasizes a transformation of affect, from positive to negative and back to positive. When expectancies are grossly violated, the infant may anticipate ruptures. When these ruptures are difficult to repair, the infant may develop an expectancy of nonrepair, such as documented in the infants of depressed mothers, which may contribute to later experiences of helplessness (see also Cohn et al., 1990; Cohn & Tronick, 1989b; Tronick, 1989).

The three principles and bodily experiences. The three principles provide a more differentiated way of conceptualizing how bodily experiences are organized. Broadly defined, the body is the subject of our entire discussion, because perception, cognition, affect and arousal are all bodily experiences. However, more narrowly defined, the regulation of bodily states has been addressed in each of the principles through the dimension of arousal. The infant will represent bodily states as an aspect of all three principles of interaction structures.

In the principle of ongoing regulations, bodily states organize experience insofar as they are repeated and expected. Processes of mutual regulation and self-regulation shift with respect to which is in the foreground and background. Some urgent bodily needs, such as feeding, are of necessity regulated through the partner. Although adequate self-regulation is necessary, these experiences tilt toward mutual regulation. Other experiences, such as the infant's control over elimination, emphasize self-regulation. Nevertheless, even these latter experiences are colored by the nature of the mutual regulation. Does the infant expect the comfort of cleaning or a handling that is rough and constraining? Does the mother have postural, facial and vocal responses of aversion, disgust and withdrawal? What will be organized is the expectation that compelling bodily needs will or will not be adequately regulated, with particular affect and arousal patterns.

The crucial role of the body is self-evident in the principle of heightened affective moments, because heightened affects are simultaneously heightened bodily states. Ekman (1983) showed that patterns of physiological arousal closely correspond to facial-affective patterns (see also Beebe & Lachmann, 1988b).

Using the principle of disruption and repair, bodily experiences of disruption can be defined as those instances where mutual regulation is inadequate to sustain self-regulation. Bodily experiences such as hunger, cold or fatigue then impinge and overwhelm the self-regulatory process. However, when the partner is available for repair, the balance is shifted back toward more adequate mutual regulation. Using this principle, it is the expectation of a disruption of adequate bodily regulation that is organized. Or, with repair, the expectation is organized that a transformation of state will occur toward a more comfortable range.

Evidence that the infant will represent bodily states can be inferred from the treatments of children and adults. Casement's (1990) description of an adult treatment in which the patient was preoccupied by having been severely burned at 11 months has already been cited. Herzog (1983) described a toddler who expressed the wish to be hurt. This child had a history of multiple invasive medical procedures as an infant. The infant's experience in both cases can be seen as organized by transformations into heightened negative bodily states, with the disruption of the expectation of adequate bodily regulation. In addition, the infant's experience in the Herzog case can be seen as organized by the ongoing regulation of the expectation of repetitive painful bodily events and the expectation that mutual regulation fails.

The three principles of salience provide us with criteria to determine what aspects of experience will assume centrality and priority. Individual differences in their course of regulation and emphasis will create different configurations or themes in the representation of the interrelatedness of self and object.

The three principles and internalization. We described the organization of presymbolic representation in the first year. This description can simultaneously illuminate processes of internalization. Although it has been argued that internalization is different from processes that establish the original representations of the internal and external world, we hold that internalization in the first year is not a process distinct from the organization of representations. Both Loewald (1962) and Schafer (1968) pointed out the intimate connection between the first representations and the earliest forms of internalization.

The term *internalization* has generally been applied to processes after the first year, *secondary internalizations* (Loewald, 1962; Schafer, 1968), when symbolic levels of self- and object representations are in place. We are interested in applying the three principles of salience to a reconceptualization of processes in the first year that have been referred to as *primary internalization* (Schafer, 1968). We thus confine our discussion to the presymbolic origins of internalization.

Schafer (1968) defined internalization as "all those processes by which the subject transforms real or imagined regulatory interactions with his environment, and real or imagined characteristics of his environment, into inner regulations and characteristics" (p. 9). Because we are discussing the presymbolic origins of internalization, we are not referring to the "imagined" aspect of Schafer's definition.

Using Schafer's (1968) definition of *inner*, internalization proper cannot be applied to the first year of life. In Schafer's view, "inner" indicates that the stimulation and impact of the regulations does not depend on the actual presence, action or emotional position of the external object" (p. 10). In the first year, the infant is dependent on the actual presence of the object. In this sense, when we conceptualize the origins of internalization in the first year, we substantially change the concept.

Even in the first year, however, Schafer's term *inner regulation* has meaning. Two of the studies we cited, the still-face experiment (Tronick et al, 1978) and the study in which infants of depressed mothers act depressed with a nondepressed adult (Field et al., 1988), provide evidence for inner organization. These experiments suggest that the infant establishes an interactive expectancy, with an associated self-regulatory style, that he can, under certain stressful circumstances, utilize in ways that are not dependent on immediate environmental input (E. Tronick, personal communication, May 18, 1993). In our view, the presymbolic origins of autonomy of inner regulations begin to evolve in the first year. The distinction between primary and secondary internalization thus beings to blur.

Furthermore, we argue that there is continuity between primary and secondary internalization. The presymbolically represented experiences of the first year bias the developmental trajectory in transformational ways (Sameroff, 1983; Sander, 1983; Sroufe & Fleeson, 1986; E. Tronick, personal communication, May 18, 1993). When these experiences are later encoded symbolically, they retain the impact of the first year.

Internalization and Interactive Regulation

There are remarkable parallels between the empirical infant literature, documenting varieties of interactive regulation, and Schafer's (1968) notions of internalization defined as regulatory interactions. Interactive regulation is the central concept in both. For this reason, we confine our discussion to Schafer's (1968) definition.

Schafer (1968) noted that Hartmann and Loewenstein's (1962) revision of Freud's 1938 definition of *internalization* "[shifted] the accent from *reactions* to *interacting regulations* [recognizing] both the importance of the developing organism's activity and the matrix of object relationship within which development takes place . . . [italics added]" (p. 8). Schafer also noted that Loewald (1960, 1962), like Erikson (1950), emphasized that it is relations that are internalized. As Schafer put it, "the regulatory *interaction* has been interiorized" (p. 11). Infant research underlines and richly elaborates this interactive emphasis that was originally in Schafer's definition.

There is a further congruence between the experimental findings of infant research and Schafer's concepts that what is regulated are behavior patterns involved in perceiving, remembering and anticipating.

Experimental infant perception research has by now documented remarkable early capacities for anticipation and memory.

Although Schafer created a fully interactive model, he frequently lost sight of it in various one-way influence concepts. For example, the environment provides the regulations of restraint, guidance and mastery. It is the less well-modulated tendencies of the child or patient that are regulated. Similarly, the environment is seen to influence the child, in the formulation that it is the object's motives that are reproduced by the subject. Thus, there is a tension within this model. On the one hand, it is a truly interactive model, so that internalization is based on what both the organism and the environment construct. On the other hand, various one-way influence concepts are used in which the organism receives the influence of the environment. In clinical practice and much theorizing, the latter version of internalization has dominated our thinking. Only a fully bi-directional model can take into account the complexity of early interactive organization and the origins of internalization processes.

Interactive regulation and self-regulation. There is a second essential difference between Schafer's formulations and our view. In Schafer's definition, inner regulations are assumed to result from the subject's transformation of regulatory interactions with the environment. We prefer the term *self-regulation* to *inner regulation.* In our view, all regulatory interactions with the environment have simultaneous self-regulatory consequences from the beginning of life. Thus, regulatory interaction with the environment does not become inner regulation in any linear fashion.

In our view, regulatory interactions and self-regulation proceed hand in hand and shape each other. Rather than viewing interactive regulations as transformed into self-regulations, existing self-regulations are altered by, as well as alter, interactive regulations, which are simultaneously construct, elaborate, and represent the regulations, which are simultaneously interactive and self-regulatory. In our view, internalization is not an optimal metaphor (see also Goldberg, 1983). It inevitably carries the implication of transporting the outer to the inner and the suggestion that the internal increasingly supplants the external. Likewise, the idea of "taking in the functions of the other" has no place in our model, because the regulatory functions are always jointly constructed.

Whereas Schafer's inner organization is defined by a transformation of the outer, our "inner" organization is always jointly defined by self-regulation and the mutual regulations in which it is embedded. We thus alter the concept of what is inside. We concur with Schafer that what is at stake in the internalization process is the increasing relative autonomy from actual interactions with the environment. Such autonomy can only begin with the advance of symbol formation, when these regulations will be increasingly abstracted and depersonified.

Internalization in the first year. We thus suggest a view of the origins of internalization in the first year in which both partners bring to the interaction organized behavior and mutually construct modes of regulating their joint activity. These dyadic modes include mutual as well as self-regulation. The expectation and representation of the dyadic modes of regulation constitute the internal organization (see also Beebe & Lachmann, 1988b; Benjamin, 1988). With the advance of symbol formation, these modes are increasingly abstracted and depersonified. That is, they become increasingly autonomous. This model puts the bi-directional nature of the regulation center stage. It further articulates the role of the subject in the regulation process, and it emphasizes the dyadic nature of the construction of experience.

Conclusion

We described a different view of how interactions function internally. In the principle of ongoing regulations, the way in which interactions typically proceed is expected and represented and defines the inner regulation. Generating, elaborating, anticipating and representing the regulations that are jointly constructed constitutes the organizing process.

In the principle of disruption and repair, expectancies of a sequence of disequilibrium and rerighting constitute the inner regulation. What is organized is the dyad's management of the transformations back and forth across a range of greater or lesser degrees of coordination. Flexibility to manage the range is a consequence of this organization (Lachmann & Beebe, 1989). In disruption, experiences of contrast, disjunctions and difference are organized. Without repair, experiences of disruption organize expectancies of misregulation. With repair, the experiences of coping, effectance, rerighting and hope are organized. Because disruption and repair are both mutually regulated, the infant represents his capacity to influence and be influenced by the rerighting process.

In the principle of heightened affective moments, powerful affective shifts that transform the infant's state constitute the inner regulation. These shifts may organize the transformation of bodily states where self-regulation is in the foreground. If the regulation is experienced positively, as with a pleasurable bowel movement or falling asleep at the breast, these heightened moments organize experiences of control over one's own body, either active or passive. If the regulation is experienced negatively, as with an intense crying jag, these heightened moments organize experiences of loss of control.

These heightened affective shifts may also accentuate dyadic regulations, in which self-regulation is in the background. If the shift is positive, such as facial-mirroring interactions in which each face crescendos higher and higher, peak experiences of resonance, exhilaration, awe and being on the same wavelength with the partner are organized. If the shift is negative—for example, when the infant arches his back as far away from the mother as possible, as the mother pulls his arm and tries to force a reorientation—state transformations of inundation, overarousal and inability to escape are organized.

In conclusion, the three principles define a hierarchy of inner regulations at different levels of organization in time. Each principle is a distinct mode of organization, but each requires the others to describe the full range of experience. The three principles of salience simultaneously illuminate the origins of representation and internalization in the first year. An integration of all three is necessary for a more differentiated view of how representations and internalizations are formed in infancy.

Acknowledgments

This work was partially supported by National Institute of Mental Health Grant R01MH41675 and the Fund for Psychoanalytic Research of the American Psychoanalytic Association.

The contributions of Joseph Jaffe, Jessica Benjamin, Adrienne Harris, Marvin Hurvich, Kenneth Feiner, Sarah Hahn-Burke, Marina Koulomzin and Nancy Freeman are gratefully acknowledged.

References

Ainsworth, M., Blehar, M., Waters, E. & Wall, S. (1978). *Patterns of attachment.* Hillsdale, NJ: Lawrence Erlbaum Associates.

Als, H. & Brazelton, T. B. (1981). A new model of assessing the behavioral organization in preterm and fullterm infants. *Journal of the American Academy of Child Psychiatry, 20,* 239–263.

Bakeman, R. & Brown, J. (1977). Behavioral dialogues. *Child Development, 28,* 195–203.

Basch, M. (1988) *Understanding psychotherapy: The science behind the art.* New York: Basic.

Beebe, B. (1973). Ontogeny of positive affect in the third and fourth months of life of one infant. (Doctoral dissertation, Columbia University). *Dissertation Abstracts International, 35,* 1014B.

Beebe, B. (1986). Mother-infant mutual influence and precursors of self- and object representations. In J. Masling (Ed), *Empirical studies of psychoanalytic theories* (Vol 2, pp. 27–48). Hillsdale, NJ: The Analytic Press.

Beebe, B.; Alson, D., Jaffe, J., Feldstein, S. & Crown, C. (1988). Vocal congruence in mother-infant play. *Journal of Psycholinguistic Research*, 17(3). 245–259.

Beebe, B. & Jaffe J. (1992a). Mother-infant vocal dialogues. *Infant Behavior and Development*, 15. 48. ICIS Abstracts Issue, May.

Beebe, B. & Jaffe, J. (1992b). The contribution of infant responsivity to the prediction of infant attachment. *Infant Behavior and Development*, 15. 113. ICIS Abstracts Issue, May.

Beebe, B., Jaffe, J., Feldstein, S., Mays, K. & Alson, D. (1985). Interpersonal timing: The application of an adult dialogue model to mother-infant vocal and kinesic interactions. In T. Field & N. Fox (Eds), *Social perception in infants* (pp. 217–240) Norwood, NJ: Ablex.

Beebe, B., Jaffe, J. & Lachmann, F. (1993). A dyadic systems view of communication. In N. Skolnick & S. Warshaw (Eds), *Relational views of psychoanalysis* (pp. 61–81). Hillsdale, NJ: The Analytic Press.

Beebe, B. & Lachmann, F. (1988a). Mother-infant mutual influence and precursors of psychic structure. In A. Goldberg (Ed) *Frontiers in self psychology: Progress in self psychology* (Vol. 3, pp. 3–26). Hillsdale, NJ: The Analytic Press.

Beebe, B. & Lachmann, F. (1988b). The contribution of mother-infant mutual influence to the origins of self and object representations. *Psychoanalytic Psychology*, 5, 305–337.

Beebe, B. & Stern, D. (1977). Engagement disengagement and early object experiences. In N. Freedman & S. Grand (Eds). *Communicative structures and psychic structures* (pp. 35–55). New York: Plenum.

Beebe, B., Stern, D. & Jaffe, J. (1979). The kinesic rhythm of mother-infant interactions. In A. Siegman & S. Feldstein (Eds), *Of speech and time* (pp. 23–34). Hillsdale, NJ: Lawrence Erlbaum Associates, Inc.

Behrends, R. & Blatt, S. (1985). Internalization and psychological development throughout the life cycle. *Psychoanalytic Study of the Child*, 40, 11–39.

Bell, R.Q. (1968). A reinterpretation of the direction of effects in studies of socialization. *Psychological Review*, 75(2), 81–95.

Belsky, J., Rovine, M. & Taylor, D. (1984). The Pennsylvania Infant and Family Development Project III: The origins of individual differences in infant-mother attachment: Maternal and infant contribution. *Child Development*, 55, 718–728.

Benjamin, J. (1988). *The bonds of love*. New York: Pantheon.

Berlyne, D. (1966). Curiosity and exploration. *Science*, 153, 25–33.

Bernstein, A. & Blacher, R. (1967). The recovery of a memory from three months of age. *Psychoanalytic Study of the Child*, 22, 156–161.

Blatt, S. & Behrends, R. (1987). Internalization, separation-individuation, and the nature of therapeutic action. *International Journal of Psycho-Analysis*, 68, 279–297.

Bornstein, M. (1985). Infant into adult: Unity to diversity in the development of visual categorization. In J. Mehler & R. Fox (Eds), *Neonate cognition* (pp. 115–138). Hillsdale, NJ: Lawrence Erlbaum Associates.

Bowlby, J. (1969). *Attachment and loss. Vol 1. Attachment*. New York: Basic Books.

Brazelton, T.B. (1973). *Neonatal behavioral assessment scale*. London: Heinemann. Clinics in Behavioral Medicine, 50; Spastics International Medical Publications.

Brazelton, T.B. (1992, May). *Touch and the fetus*. Paper presented at the Touch Research Institute, Miami.

Brazelton, T.B., Koslowski, B. & Main, M. (1974). The origins of reciprocity. In M. Lewis & L. Rosenblum (Eds), *The effect of the infant on its caregiver* (pp. 49–70). New York: Wiley.

Bretherton, I. (1985). Attachment theory: Retrospect and prospect. In I. Bretherton & E. Waters (Eds), *Growing points in attachment theory and research: Monographs of the Society for Research in Child Development*, 50 (1–2, Serial No. 209)

Bruner, J. (1977). Early social interaction and language acquisition. In H.R. Schaffer (Ed), *Studies in mother-infant interaction* (pp. 271–289). New York: Norton.

Bruner, J. (1983). *Child's take: Learning to use language*. New York: Norton.

Bucci, W. (1985). Dual coding: A cognitive model for psychoanalytic research. *Journal of the American psychoanalytic Association*, 33, 571–608.

Capella, J. (1981). Mutual influence in expressive behavior: Adults and infant-adult dyadic interaction. *Psychological Bulletin*, 89, 101–132

Casement, P. (1990, December). *Case report*. Paper presented at the meeting of the American Psychoanalytic Association, Miami, FL.

Cohen, L., DeLoache, J. & Strauss, M. (1979). Infant visual perception. In J. Osofsky (Ed), *Handbook of infant development* (pp. 393–438). New York: Wiley.

Cohen, L. & Gelber, E. (1975). Infant visual memory. In L. Cohen & P. Salapatek (Eds), *Infant perception: From sensation to cognition* (Vol I, pp. 347–403). New York: Academic.

Cohn, J. & Beebe, B. (1990). Sampling interval affects time-series regression estimates of mother-infant influence. *Infant Behavior and Development*, 13, 317.

Cohn, J., Campbell, S., Matias, R. & Hopkins, J. (1990). Face-to-face interactions of post-partum depressed and nondepressed mother-infant pairs at 2 months. *Developmental Psychology*, 26(1), 15–23.

Cohn, J., Campbell, S., & Ross, S. (1991). Infant response in the still face paradigm at 6 months predicts avoidant and secure attachment at 12 months. *Development and Psychopathology*, 3, 367–376.

Cohn, J. & Tronick, E. (1983). Three month old infants react to simulated maternal depression. *Child Development*, 4, 185–194.

Cohn, J. & Tronick, E. (1988). Mother-infant face-to-face interaction: Influence is bidirectional and unrelated to periodic cycles in either partner's behavior. *Developmental Psychology*, 24(3), 386–392.

Cohn, J. & Tronick, E. (1989a). Mother-infant face-to-face interaction: The sequence of dyadic states at 3, 6, 9 months. *Developmental Psychology*, 23, 68–77.

Cohn, J. & Tronick, E. (1989b). Specificity of infants' response to mothers' affective behavior. *Journal American Academy Child & Adolescent Psychiatry*, 28(2), 242–248.

Cormiert, S. (1981). A match-mismatch theory of limbic system function. *Physiological Psychology*, 9, 3–36.

DeCasper, A. & Carstens, A. (1980). Contingencies of stimulation: Effects on learning and emotion in neonates. *Infant Behavior and Development*, 4, 19–36.

DeCasper, A. & Fifer, W. (1980). Of human bonding: Newborns prefer their mothers' voices. *Science*, 208, 1174.

DeCasper, A. & Spence, M. (1986). Prenatal maternal speech influences newborn's perception of speech sounds. *Infant Behavior & Development*, 9, 133–150.

Demos, V. (1983). Discussion of papers by Drs Sander and Stern. In J. Lichtenberg & S. Kaplan (Eds). *Reflections on self psychology* (pp. 105–112). Hillsdale, NJ. The Analytic Press.

Demos, V. (1984). Empathy and affect: Reflections on infant experience. In J. Lichtenberg, M. Bonnstein & D. Silver (Eds), *Empathy* (Vol 11, pp. 9–34). Hillsdale, NJ: The Analytic Press.

Ekman, P. (1983). Autonomic nervous system activity distinguishes among emotions. *Science*, 221, 1208–1210.

Ekman, P. & Oster, H. (1979). Facial expression of emotion. *Annual Review of Psychology*, 30, 527–554.

Emde, R. (1981). The prerepresentational self and its affective core. *Psychoanalytic Study of the Child*, 36, 165–192.

Emde, R. (1988). Developmental terminable and interminable: Recent psychoanalytic theory and therapeutic considerations. *International Journal of Psycho-Analysis*, 69, 283–296.

Erikson, E. (1950). *Childhood and society*. New York: Norton.

Fagen, J.W., Morrongiello, B.A., Rovee-Collier, C. & Gekoski, M.J. (1984). Expectancies and memory retrieval in three-month-old infants. *Child Development*, 55, 936–943.

Fagen, J., Ohr, P., Fleckenstein, L. & Ribner, D. (1985). The effect of crying on long-term memory in infancy. *Child Development*, 56, 1584–1592.

Fagen, J., Ohr, P. Singer, J. & Klein, S. (1989). Crying and retrograde amnesia in young infants. *Infant Behavior & Development*, 12, 13–24.

Fast, I. (1988). *Interaction schemes in the establishment of psychic structure and therapeutic change*. Unpublished manuscript.

Field, T. (1981). Infant gaze aversion and heart rate during face-to-face interactions. *Infant Behavior and Development*, 4, 307–315.

Field, T., Goldstein, S. & Guthertz, M. (1990). Behavior-state matching and synchrony in mother-infant interactions of depressed and nondepressed dyads. *Developmental Psychology*, 26, 7–14.

Field, T., Healy, B., Goldstein, S., Perry, D., Bendell, D., Schanberg, S., Simmerman, E. & Kuhn, O. (1988). Infants of depressed mothers show "depressed behavior even with non-depressed adults. *Child Development*, 59, 1569–1579.

Field, T., Woodson, R., Greenberg, R. & Cohen, D. (1982). Discrimination and imitation of facial expressions by neonates. *Science*, 218, 179–181.

Freud, S. (1917). Mourning and melancholia. S.E., 14, 243–248.

Gazzaniga, M. & LeDoux, J. (1978). *The integrated mind*. New York: Plenum.

Goldberg, A. (1983). Self psychology and alternative perspectives on internalization. In J. Lichtenberg & S. Kaplan (Eds). *Reflections on self psychology* (pp. 297–312). Hillsdale, NJ: The Analytic Press.

Gottman, J. & Ringland, J. (1981). Analysis of dominance and bi-directionality in social development. *Child Development*, 52, 393–412.

Gianino, A. & Tronick, E. (1988). The mutual regulation model: The infant's self and interactive regulation and coping and defensive capacities. In T. Field, P. McCabe, & N. Schneiderman (Eds), *Stress and coping* (pp. 47–68). Hillsdale, NJ: Lawrence Erlbaum Associates.

Greco, C., Rovee-Collier, C., Hayne, H. Griesler, P. & Early, L. (1986). Ontogeny of early event memory: I. Forgetting and retrieval by 2- and 3-month olds. *Infant Behavior and Development*, 9, 441–460.

Hadley, J. (1983). The representational system: A bridging concept for psychoanalysis and neurophysiology. *International Review of Psycho-Analysis*, 10, 13–30.

Hadley, J. (1989). The neurobiology of motivational systems. In J. Lichtenberg (Ed), *Psychoanalysis and motivation* (pp. 227–372). Hillsdale, NJ: The Analytic Press.

Haith, M., Hazan, C. & Goodman, G. (1988). Expectation and anticipation of dynamic visual events by 3.5 month old babies. *Child Development*, 59, 467–479.

Hartmann, H. (1939). *Ego and the problem of adaptation*. New York: International Universities Press, 1958.

Hartmann, H. & Loewenstein, R. (1962). Notes on the superego. In H. Hartmann, E. Kirs & R. Loewenstein (Eds.), *Papers on psychoanalytic psychology. Psychological issues*. (Vol 4, No. 2, pp. 144–181). New York: International Universities Press.

Herzog, J. (1983). A neonatal intensive care syndrome: A pain complex involving neuro-plasticity and psychic trauma. In J. Call, E. Galenson & R. Tyson (Eds), *Frontiers of infant psychiatry* (pp. 291–299). New York: Basic.

Horner, T. (1985). The psychic life of the young infant: Review and critique of the psychoanalytic concepts of symbiosis and infantile omnipotence, *American Journal of Orthopsychiatry*, 55, 324–344.

Hirschfeld, N. & Beebe, B. (1987, April). *Maternal intensity and infant disengagement in face-to-face play*. Paper presented at the meeting of the Society for Research in Child Development, Baltimore, MD.

Hunt, J. McV. (1965). Intrinsic motivation and its role in psychological development. In D. Levine (Ed), *Nebraska Symposium on Motivation* (Vol 13, pp. 189–282). Lincoln: University of Nebraska Press.

Isabella, R. & Belsky, J. (1991). Interactional synchrony and the origins of infant-mother attachment: A replication study. *Child Development*, 62, 373–384.

Izard, C. E. (1979). *The maximally discriminative facial action coding system (MAX)*. Newark: University of Delaware, Instructional Resources Center.

Jacobson, E. (1964). *The self and the object world*. New York: International Universities Press.

Jaffe, J., Feldstein, S., Beebe, B., Crown, C. L., Jasnow, M., Fox, H., Anderson, S. W. & Gordon, S. (1991). [Final report for NIMH Grant No. MH41675]. Unpublished raw date.

Jasnow, M. & Feldstein, S. (1986). Adult-like temporal characteristics of mother-infant vocal interactions. *Child Development*, 57, 754–761.

Kegan, R. (1982). *The evolving self*. Cambridge, MA: Harvard University Press.

Klein, G. (1967). Peremptory ideation: Structure and force in motivated ideas. *Psychological Issues*, 5(2–3). Monograph 18/19. New York: International Universities Press.

Kohut, H. (1984). *How does analysis cure?* Chicago: University of Chicago Press.

Kronen, J. (1982). *Maternal facial mirroring at four months*. Unpublished doctoral dissertation. Yeshiva University, New York.

Lachmann, F. M. & Beebe, B. (1989). Oneness fantasies revisited. *Psychoanalytic Psychology*, 6, 137–149.

Lachmann, F. M. & Beebe, B. (1992). Reformulations of early development and transference: Implications for psychic structure. In D. Wolitzky, M. Eagle & J. Barron (Eds), *Psychoanalysis and psychology* (pp. 133–153). Washington, DC: American Psychological Association.

Lachmann, F. M. & Beebe, B. (1993). Interpretation in a developmental perspective. In A. Goldberg (Ed), *Progress in self psychology* (Vol 9. pp. 45–52). Hillsdale, NJ: The Analytic Press.

Lewis, M. & Lee-Painter, S. (1974). An international approach to the mother-infant dyad. In M. Lewis & L. Rosenblum (Eds). *The effect of the infant on its caregiver*. New York: Wiley.

Lewis, M. & Rosenblum, L. (Eds). (1974). *The effect of the infant on its caregiver*. New York: Wiley.

Lichtenberg, J. (1983). *Psychoanalysis and infant research*. Hillsdale, NJ: The Analytic Press.

Lichtenberg, J. (1989). *Psychoanalysis and motivation*. Hillsdale, NJ: The Analytic Press.

Loewald, H. (1960). On the therapeutic action of psychoanalysis. In H. Loewald (Ed), *Papers on psychoanalysis* (pp. 221–256). New Haven, CT: Yale University Press.

Loewald, H. (1962). Internalization, separation, mourning and the superego. In H. Loewald (Ed), *Papers on psychoanalysis* (pp. 257–276). New Haven, CT: Yale University Press.

Malatesta, C., Culver, C., Tesman, J. & Shepard, B. (1989). The development of emotion expression during the first two years of life. *Monographs of the Society for Research in Child Development*, 54 (1–2, Serial No. 219).

Malatesta, C. & Haviland, J. (1983). Learning display rules: The socialization of emotion in infancy. *Child Development*, 53, 991–1003.

Mandler, J. (1988). How to build a baby: On the development of an accessible representation system. *Cognitive Development*, 3, 113–136.

Meissner, W. (1981). *Internalization and psychoanalysis*. New York: International Universities Press.

Meltzoff, A. (1985). The roots of social and cognitive development: Models of man's original nature. In T. Field & N. Fox (Eds), *Social perception in infants* (pp. 1–30). Norwood, NJ: Ablex.

Mitchell, S. (1988). *Relational concepts in psychoanalysis*. Cambridge, MA: Harvard University Press.

Modell, A. (1984). *Psychoanalysis in a new context*. New York: International Universities Press.

Modell, A. (1993). *The private self in public space.* Cambridge, MA: Harvard University Press.

Ohr, P., Fleckenstein, L., Fagen, J., Klein, S. & Pioli, L. (1989). Crying-produced forgetting in infant: A contextual analysis. *Infant Behavior & Development*, 13, 305–320.

Oster, H. (1978). Facial expression and affect development. In M. Lewis & L. Rosenblum (Eds), *The development of affect* (pp. 43–75). Hillsdale, NJ: Lawrence Erlbaum Associates.

Oster, H. & Ekman, P. (1977). Facial behavior in child development. In A. Collins (Ed), *Minnesota Symposium on Child Development* (Vol 11, pp. 231–276). New York: Crowell.

Papousek, H. & Papousek, M. (1979). Early ontogeny of human social interaction. In M. Von Cranach, K. Koppa, W. Lepenies & P. Ploog (Eds), *Human ethology: Claims and limits of a new discipline* (pp. 63–85). Cambridge, England: Cambridge University Press.

Perris, E., Myers, N. & Clifton, R. (1990). Long-term memory for a single infancy experience. *Child Development*, 61, 1796–1807.

Piaget, J. (1954). *The construction of reality in the child* (M. Cook, Trans.). New York: Basic.

Pine, F. (1981). In the beginning: Contributions to a psychoanalytic developmental psychology. *International Review of Psycho-Analysis*, 8, 15–33.

Pine, F. (1986). The "symbiotic phase" in the light of current infancy research. *Bulletin of the Menninger Clinic*, 50, 564–569.

Reese, H. & Overton, W. (1970). Models of development and theories of development. In L. Goulet & P. Baltes (Eds), *Life-span developmental psychology* (pp. 115–145). New York: Academic Press.

Resch, R. (1988). The later creation of a transitional object. *Psychoanalytic Psychology*, 5, 369–387.

Ruff, H. (1980). The development of perception and recognition of objects. *Child Development*, 51, 981–992.

Sameroff, A. (1983). Developmental systems: Contexts and evolution. In W. Kessen (Ed.), *Mussen's handbook of child psychology* (Vol 1, pp. 237–294). New York: Wiley.

Sameroff, A. & Chandler, M. (1976). Reproductive risk and the continuum of caretaking casualty. In F.D. Horowitz (Ed). *Review of child development research* (Vol 4, pp. 187–244). Chicago: University of Chicago Press.

Sander, L. (1977). The regulation of exchange in the infant-caretaker system and some aspects of the context-content reslaitonship. In M. Lewis & L. Rosenblum (Eds), *Interaction, conversation and the development of language* (pp. 133–156). New York: Wiley.

Sander, L. (1983). Polarity paradox, and the organizing process in development. In J.D. Call, E. Galenson, & R. Tyson (Eds), *Frontiers of infant psychiatry* (pp. 315–327). New York: Basic Books.

Sander, L. (1985). Toward a logic of organization in psycho-biological development. In H. Klar & L. Siever (Eds)., *Biologic response styles: Clinical implications* (pp. 20–36). Washington, DC: American Psychiatric Press.

Sandler, J. & Sandler, A. (1978). On the development of object relations and affects. *International Journal of Psycho-Analysis*, 59, 285–296.

Schafer, R. (1968). *Aspects of internalization*. New York: International Universities Press.

Sherman, T. (1985). Categorization skills in infants. *Child Development*, 56, 1561–1573.

Shields, P. & Rovee-Collier, C. (1992). Longterm memory for context-specific category information at six months. *Child Development*, 63, 245–259.

Singer, J. & Fagen, J. (1992). Negative affect, emotional expression and forgetting in young infants. *Developmental Psychology*, 28(1), 48–57.

Socarides, D. & Stolorow, R. (1984/1985). Affects and self objects. In C. Kligerman (Ed), *The annual of psychoanalysis*, 12/13, 105–120.

Spinelli, D.N. & Jensen, F.E. (1979). Plasticity: The mirror of experience. *Science*, 203: 75–79.

Spitz, R. (1983). The evolution of dialogue. In R. Emde (Ed), *Rene A. Spitz: Dialogues from infancy. Selected papers* (pp. 179–195). New York: International Universities Press.

Sroufe, L.A. (1979). The ontogenesis of emotion. In J. Osofsky (Ed.), *Handbook of infant development* (pp. 462–516). New York: Wiley.

Sroufe, L.A. & Fleeson, J. (1986). Attachment and the construction of relationships. In W. Hartup & Z. Rubin (Eds), *Relationships and development* (pp. 51–71). New York: Cambridge University Press.

Stechler, G. & Kaplan, S. (1980). The development of the self. *Psychoanalytic Study of the Child*, 35, 85–105.

Stern, D. (1971). A microanalysis of the mother-infant interaction. *Journal of the American Academy of Child Psychiatry*, 10, 501–507.

Stern, D. (1977). *The first relationship*. Cambridge, MA: Harvard University Press.

Stern, D. (1982). Some interactive functions of rhythm changes between mother and infant. In M. David (Ed). *Interaction rhythms* (pp. 101–118). New York: Human Sciences Press.

Stern, D. (1983). The early development of schemas of self, other, and "self with other." In J. Lichtenberg & S. Kaplan (Eds), *Reflections on self psychology* (pp. 49–84). Hillsdale, NJ: The Analytic Press.

Stern, D. (1985a). Affect attunement. In J.D. Call, E. Galenson & R. Tyson (Eds), *Frontiers of infant psychiatry* (Vol 2, pp. 3–14). New York: Basic Books.

Stern, D. (1985b). *The interpersonal world of the infant*. New York: Basic Books.

Stern, D. (1988a). Affect in the context of the infant's lived experience: Some considerations. *International Journal of Psycho-Analysis*, 69, 223–238.

Stern, D. (1988b). The dialectic between the "interpersonal" and the "intrapsychic" with particular emphasis on the role of memory and representation. *Psychoanalytic Inquiry*, 8, 505–512.

Stern, D. (1989). The representation of relational patterns: Developmental consideration. In A. Sameroff & R. Emde (Eds), *Relationship disturbances in early childhood* (pp. 52–69). New York: Basic.

Stern, D., Jaffe, J., Beebe, B. & Bennett, S. (1975). Vocalizing in unison and alternation: Two modes of communication within the mother-infant dyad. *Annals of the New York Academy of Science*, 263, 89–100.

Stolorow, R., Brandchaft, B. & Atwood, G. (1987). *Psychoanalytic treatment: An intersubjective approach.* Hillsdale, NJ: The Analytic Press.

Strauss, M. (1979). Abstractions of proto-typical information by adults and 10 month old infants. *Journal of Experimental Psychology: Human Learning and Memory,* 5, 618–632.

Thomas, E.A.C. & Martin, J. (1976). Analyses of parent-infant interaction. *Psychological Review,* 83(2), 141–155.

Tobach, E. (1970). Some guidelines to the study of the evolution and development of emotion. In L. Aronson, E. Tobnach, D. Lehrman & J. Rosenblatt (Eds), *Development and evolution of behavior* (pp. 238–253). San Francisco: Freeman.

Tolpin, M. (1971). On the beginning of a cohesive self. In R. Eissler, A. Freud, M. Kris, S. Lustman & A. Solnit (Eds), *Psychoanalytic study of the child* (Vol 26, pp. 316–354). New York: International Universities Press.

Tomkins, S. (1980). Affect as amplification: Some modifications in theory. In R. Plutchik & H. Kellerman (Eds.), *Emotions: Theory, research and experience* (pp. 141–164). New York: Academic.

Tronick, E. (1980). The primacy of social skills in infancy. In D. Sawin, R. Hawkins, L. Walker & J. Penticuff (Eds), *Exceptional infant* (Vol 4, pp. 144–158). New York: Brunner/Mazel.

Tronick, E. (1982). Affectivity and sharing. In E. Tronick (Ed), *Social interchange in infancy* (pp. 1–8). Baltimore: University Park Press.

Tronick, E. (1989). Emotions and emotional communication in infants. *American Psychologist,* 44(2), 112–119.

Tronick, E., Als, H., Adamson, L., Wise, S. & Brazelton, T.B. (1978). The infant's response to entrapment between contradictory messages in face-to-face interaction. *American Academy of Child Psychiatry,* 17, 1–13.

Tronick, E. & Cohn, J. (1989). Infant-mother face-to-face interaction: Age and gender differences in coordination and miscoordination. *Child Development,* 59, 85–92.

Tronick, E. & Gianino, A. (1986). Interactive mismatch and repair: Challenges to the coping infant. *Zero to Three: Bulletin of the National Center Clinical Infant Programs,* 5, 1–6.

Watson, J. (1985). Contingency perception in early social development. In T. Field & N. Fox (Eds), *Social perception in infants* (pp. 157–176). Norwood, NJ: Ablex.

Weinberg, K. (1991). *Sex differences in 6 month infants' behavior: Impact on maternal caregiving.* Unpublished doctoral dissertation, University of Massachusetts, Amherst.

Werner, H. (1948). *The comparative psychology of mental development.* New York: International Universities Press.

Werner, H. & Kaplan, S. (1963). *Symbol formation.* New York: Wiley.

Wilson, A. & Malatesta, C. (1989). Affect and compulsion to repeat: Freud's repetition compulsion revisited. *Psychoanalysis and Contemporary Thought,* 12, 243–290.

Younger, B. & Cohen, L., (1985). How infants form categories. In G. Bower (Ed.), *The psychology of learning and motivation: Advances in research and theory* (pp. 211–247). New York Academic Press.

Younger, B. & Gotlieb, S. (1988). Development of categorization skills: Changes in the nature or structure of form categories? *Developmental Psychology*, 24, 611–619.

Zeanah, C., Anders, T., Seifer, R. & Stern, D. (1989). Implications of research on infant development for psychodynamic theory and practice. *Journal of the American Academy of Child Psychiatry*, 28(5), 657–668.

Zelner, S. (1982). *The organization of vocalization and gaze in early mother-infant interactive regulation*. Unpublished doctoral dissertation, Yeshiva University, New York.

Zelnick, L., & Bucholz, E. (1990). The concept of mental representations in light of recent infant research. *Psychoanalytic Psychology*, 7, 29–58.

Afterword*

The empirical microanalysis of mother–infant interaction has broadened our understanding of the analyst–patient interaction. A central contribution of infant research is its description of interaction as a continuous, reciprocally influenced process, co-constructed moment-to-moment by both partners, through both self- and interactive regulation. By studying the regulation of the dyad as well as the individual, infant research brings to psychoanalysis the perspective of the system. This perspective explicates the individual subjective experience of both patient and analyst within the dyad and the dyad's impact on the subjective experience of both.

The three organizing principles that we have postulated provide metaphors and analogies for adult treatment. They describe patterns of analyst–patient interactions and can further specify modes of therapeutic action in adult treatment. In a subsequent publication (Lachmann and Beebe, 1996) we used one case to illustrate how attention to the interactive process through the three principles can be integrated with dynamic interpretations.

The model of development derived from infant research cannot, of course, be directly translated into the adult psychoanalytic situation. In adults, the capacity for symbolization and the subjective elaboration of experience in the form of fantasies, wishes, and defenses further modify the organization and representation of interactive

---

* Portions of this afterword were originally published in Lachmann, F. & Beebe, B. (1996), Three principles of salience in the organization of the patient–analyst interaction. *Psychoanalytic Psychology*, 13:1–22.

patterns. However, what makes this model appealing for adult treatment is that it makes no assumptions about the dynamic content of adult experience. For example, the three principles do not address content issues such as oneness and separation or motivational issues such as needs, wishes, or defenses. Rather, this model focuses entirely on the process and patterning of interactions.

Furthermore, the three principles provide an overarching conceptual framework within which various psychoanalytic theories can be compared. Numerous well-established psychoanalytic concepts can be integrated within the three principles. Psychoanalysts have always paid attention to the issues covered by our three principles under other names. Ongoing regulations have been subsumed within discussions of patterns of transference and countertransference, the "holding environment" (Winnicott, 1965), and the "background of safety" (Sandler, 1960). Disruptions and their repair have been proposed as a basis for structure formation (Stechler and Kaplan, 1980; Kohut, 1984; Horner, 1985) and implicated in the analysis of resistance and the use of confrontation (Buie and Adler, 1973; Lachmann, 1990). Heightened affective moments (Strachey, 1934; Fenichel, 1938–1939; Pine, 1981, 1986) have been recognized as essential in making analysis emotionally meaningful.

The principle of ongoing regulations captures the characteristic, expectable pattern of repeated interactions in the treatment situation. Both partners actively contribute to the regulation of the exchange, moment-by-moment. The analyst has the greater range of flexibility in this process. The actions of both partners are intimately linked in time, space, affect, and arousal. Expectations are organized that each partner either can, or cannot, affect and be affected by the other in specific ways. These expectations determine the nature of interactive efficacy. Both partners come to expect and represent these ongoing characteristic regulations and their unique interactive efficacy with this partner.

In the treatment situation, ongoing regulations range from subtle nonverbal behaviors—postural and facial interchanges, intonations, and tone of voice and greeting and parting rituals—to verbal exchanges. Ongoing regulations include interactions where the patient narrates and discloses while the analyst attends, reflects, describes, and questions. The effects of such interactions are present throughout the treatment process. They can be most clearly illustrated, however, in the phase of understanding (Kohut, 1984), the process of listening (Schwaber, 1981), exploring and clarifying (Greenson, 1967). These patient–analyst interactions have generally been viewed as a preparatory phase. They have not been recognized as contributing directly to the formation of representations and internalization.

In these various kinds of interactions repetitive themes of the patient, for example, expectations of nonresponse, indifference, or rejection, are engaged, potentially disconfirmed, and woven into the patient–analyst relationship. Through this process these themes are altered; that is, they are provided, as a matter of course, with a new context (Loewald, 1980; Modell, 1984). We propose, then, that ongoing regulations can promote new expectations and constitute a mode of therapeutic action. Whereas the engagement and disconfirmation of expectations has been described as the interpretive work of analysis (Weiss and Sampson, 1986), it is also characteristic of ongoing regulations. That is, ongoing interactions that are never verbally explored or addressed can nevertheless potentially alter the patient's expectations.

The detailed study of ongoing regulations can further illuminate the processes of therapeutic action. The structure of the dialogue itself, irrespective of its verbal content, is the subject of study. Patient and analyst construct characteristic ways of asking each other questions, of wondering aloud together, of taking turns in the dialogue, and of knowing when to pause and for how long. In this process, both are constructing expectations and confirming or disconfirming fears of being ignored, steamrollered, intruded upon, misunderstood, or criticized. These interactively organized expectations and disconfirmations are represented and internalized, whether or not they are ever verbalized. This process constitutes the therapeutic action of ongoing regulations.

The disruption and repair of interactions is a specific extension of the principle of ongoing regulations. Rather than emphasizing what is expectable in the interaction, however, disruption and repair organizes violations of expectancies and ensuing efforts to resolve these breaches (Stechler and Kaplan, 1980; Horner, 1985; Tronick and Cohn, 1989; Beebe and Lachmann, 1994). Our review of infant research noted the wide range of disturbances encompassed by the term disruption. The continuum extends from mild disjunctions, rapidly rerighted, which are typical of successful interactions, to severe ruptures. Although these mild disjunctions can be considered normative, more severe and frequent disruptions may prejudice development (Tronick, 1989).

Interactions of disruption and repair are most clearly noted during phases of explanation (Kohut, 1984) and during the processes of confrontation, working through, and interpretation (Greenson, 1967). Depending on how, when, and where they occur, disruptions are variously understood. They may be seen as necessary for development, as emanating from the patient's resistance, or as due to the patient's inability to tolerate frustration. Others have ascribed disruptions to poor timing by the analyst, misunderstandings, specific transference–countertransference configurations, or the differently organized subjectivities of analyst and patient. Different notions of "repair" are associated with each of these views of "rupture" (Kohut, 1984; Blatt and Behrends, 1987; Stolorow, Brandchaft, and Atwood, 1987).

The disruption and repair model lies at the heart of formulations of structure formation and therapeutic action in psychoanalysis. Structuralization has been variously assumed to result from the internalization of the lost object, frustration of drive derivatives, or optimal frustration whereby functions of the relationship that were disrupted are constructed within the psyche of the analysand (Freud, 1917; Tolpin, 1971; Klein, 1976; Loewald, 1980; Kohut, 1984; Blatt and Behrends, 1987).

We consider disruption and repair to be only one avenue of structuralization and therapeutic action and as operating during all phases of the treatment. Furthermore, it is an activity of the patient–analyst interaction. Disruptions are neither solely a consequence of the analyst's countertransference nor a consequence of the patient's "resistance." Repairs are also jointly constructed. The therapeutic action of disruption and repair lies in the organization of a greater flexibility in negotiating a range of coordination and miscoordination in the process of interactive and self-regulation (Beebe and Lachmann, 1994).

Whereas affect is a component of the first two principles, we consider intense affect to be a sufficiently unique dimension to justify its inclusion as a third principle of organization (Singer and Fagen, 1992; Beebe and Lachmann, 1994). The term heightened affective moments was originally defined by Pine (1981); in our elaboration this principle refers to interactions that are organized when a person experiences a powerful state transformation, either positive or negative (Beebe and Lachmann, 1994; Lachmann and Beebe, 1993). "State" is used broadly to refer to arousal and activity level, facial and vocal affect, and cognition.

Heightened affective moments can, in the context of the patient–analyst interaction, provide opportunities for new experiences, refinding old loves, or, potentially, retraumatization (Lachmann and Beebe, 1992, 1993; Beebe and Lachmann, 1994). In the treatment of adults, we define affect broadly to include cognition and symbolic elaborations. For adults, the heightened moment may or may not include obvious nonverbal features and will include a symbolic context. Our integration is not designed to supplant these dynamic formulations. Instead, it can provide the analyst a view of the regulation of interactions and the organization of experience that goes beyond interpretation.

The application of this concept of interaction to adult treatment enriches our view of therapeutic action. At every moment there is the potential to organize expectations of mutuality, intimacy, trust, repair of disruptions, and hope, as well as to disconfirm rigid archaic expectations. At every moment both analyst and patient contribute significantly to this organization. Everything the analyst does, interpretive and noninterpretive, verbal and nonverbal, exploratory and descriptive, potentially contributes to the organization of the patient's experience.

Thus, despite the many differences between mother–infant and patient–analyst interaction, we propose similarities with respect to how these three principles function to organize interactions. The three principles operate together and can be considered different angles of the camera, in a foreground–background relationship. All three principles alter the context of rigid themes and promote the development of new interactive expectations, thus new internalizations and therapeutic change.

References

Beebe, B. & Lachmann, F. (1994), Representation and internalization in infancy: Three principles of salience. *Psychoanal. Psychol.*, 11:127–165.

Blatt, S. & Behrends, R. (1987), Internalization, separation-individuation, and the nature of therapeutic action. *International J. Psycho-Anal.*, 68:279–297.

Buie, D. & Adler, G. (1973), The uses of confrontation in psychotherapy of borderline cases. In: *Confrontation in Psychotherapy*, ed. G. Adler & P. Myerson. New York: Science House, pp. 123–146.

Fenichel, O. (1938–1939), *Problems of Psychoanalytic Technique*, trans. D. Brunswick. New York: Psychoanalytic Quarterly Press, 1969.

Freud, S. (1917), Mourning and melancholia. *Standard Edition*, 14:243–248. London: Hogarth Press, 1957.

Greenson, R. (1967), *The Technique and Practice of Psychoanalysis, Vol. 1.* New York: International Universities Press.

Horner, T. (1985), The psychic life of the young infant: Review and critique of the psychoanalytic concepts of symbiosis and infantile omnipotence. *Amer. J. Orthopsychiat.*, 55:324–344.

Klein, G. (1976), *Psychoanalytic Theory: An Exploration of Essentials.* New York: International Universities Press.

Kohut, H. (1984), *How Does Analysis Cure?* ed. A. Goldberg & P. Stepansky. Chicago: University of Chicago Press.

Lachmann, F. (1990), On some challenges to clinical theory in the treatment of character pathology. In: *The Realities of Transference: Progress in Self Psychology, Vol. 6*, ed. A. Goldberg. Hillsdale, NJ: The Analytic Press, pp. 59–67.

—— & Beebe, B. (1992), Representational and self-object transferences: A developmental perspective. In: *New Therapeutic Visions: Progress in Self Psychology, Vol. 8*, ed. A. Goldberg. Hillsdale, NJ: The Analytic Press, pp. 3–15.

—— & —— (1993), Interpretation in a developmental perspective. In: *The Widening Scope of Self Psychology: Progress in Self Psychology, Vol. 9*, ed. A. Goldberg. Hillsdale, NJ: The Analytic Press, pp. 45–52.

—— & —— (1996), Three principles of salience in the organization of the patient-analyst interaction. *Psychoanal. Psychol.*, 13:1–22.

Loewald, H. (1980), On the therapeutic action of psychoanalysis. In: *Papers in Psychoanalysis*, ed. H. Loewald. New Haven, CT: Yale University Press, pp. 221–256.

Modell, A. (1984), *Psychoanalysis in a New Context*. New York: Independent University Press.

Pine, F. (1981), In the beginning: Contributions to a psychoanalytic developmental psychology. *Internat. Rev. Psycho-Anal.*, 8:15–33.

Pine, F. (1986), The "symbiotic phase" in the light of current infancy research. *Bull. Menninger Clin.*, 50:564–569.

Sandler, J. (1960), Background of safety. *Internat. J. Psychoanal.*, 41:352–356.

Schwaber, E. (1981), Empathy: A mode of analytic listening. *Psychoanal. Inq.*, 1:357–392.

Singer, J. & Fagen, J. (1992), Negative affect, emotional expression, and forgetting in young infants. *Develop. Psychol.*, 28:48–57.

Stechler, G. & Kaplan, S. (1980), The development of the self. *The Psychoanalytic Study of the Child*, 35:85–105. New Haven, CT: Yale University Press.

Stolorow, R., Brandchaft, B. & Atwood, G. (1987), *Psychoanalytic Treatment: An Intersubjective Approach*. Hillsdale, NJ: The Analytic Press.

Strachey, I. (1934), The nature of the therapeutic action of psycho-analysis. *Internat. J. Psycho-Anal.*, 15:127–159.

Tolpin, M. (1971), On the beginning of a cohesive self. *The Psychoanalytic Study of the Child*, 26:316–354. New Haven, CT: Yale University Press.

Tronick, E. (1989), Emotions and emotional communication in infants. *Amer. Psycholog.*, 44:112–119.

—— & Cohn, J. (1989), Infant–mother face-to-face interaction: Age and gender differences in coordination and the occurrance of miscoordination. *Child Develop.*, 60:85–92.

Weiss, J. & Sampson, H. (1986), *The Psychoanalytic Process*. New York: Guilford Press.

Winnicott, D. W. (1965), *The Maturational Processes and the Facilitating Environment*. New York: International Universities Press.

Mentalization and the Changing Aims of Child Psychoanalysis

(1998)

Peter Fonagy
Mary Target

▼　▼　▼　▼　▼

Editors' Introduction

Peter Fonagy's work, with his frequent coauthor Mary Target and most recently with George Gergely and Elliot Jurist, is set at an interesting intersection of psychoanalysis, developmental psychopathology, and philosophy of mind. His earliest papers with Mary Target outlined a way of thinking about particular kinds of borderline phenomena, as the outcomes of interactive processes.

There are a number of important insights from Fonagy and Target's early work, which are now central to clinical understanding: the emergence of violence and aggression as an outcome of certain processes of interaction, vicissitudes of early interaction; the powerful impact of neglect on psychic functioning; the impact of neglect as brutal in its way as actual battering; and the ebb and flow of primary and secondary process, fantasy, and reality in interpersonal interactions and consequently in the developing child mind.

What has become a central to this emerging theoretical program is that the evolution of a capacity to think, or, more properly, to think and feel, is built out of the experience of being a focus of interest and respectful attention by another person. Mentalization is the term Fonagy and Target use to great effect to describe developmental outcomes in a wide variety of situations where a person's capacity to think reflectively, to represent experience and knowledge, and support feeling was contingent on the mentalizing capacity of another. Bind this process into the burgeoning reintegration of attachment theory (a reappraisal of Bowlby and his successors Ainsworth and Main and her colleagues), and Fonagy has located what seems a decidedly relational procedure at the heart of endogenous mind and strong ego functioning. Intrapsychic and interpersonal go hand in hand; they are mutually interdependent, as Fonagy and Target have illustrated in a brilliant series of clinical and theoretical papers.

Their work has opened the field to increasingly sophisticated perspectives on well-known problems of borderline functioning and management of aggression as well as on less well-theorized problems of affect and affect regulation. One might say that, from the relational matrices that Fonagy and Target embed individual functioning, a key aspect to attend to is affect regulation. How feelings are managed within and across dyads, individuals, and systems is now center stage in Fonagy's work.

Fonagy and Target are particularly interesting figures for us to include in this volume. While they are not self-described as relational analysts, relationality is at the core of their insights and their creative theorizing. We hope not to colonize or distort our colleagues' work. Their work remains very well rooted in the British object relations tradition in the work of Bio, in particular and at the same time is comfortably at home in various hybrid paradigms. Their recent book co-authored with George Gergely and Elliot Jurist, *Affect Regulation, Mentalization and the Development of the Self*, draws on empirical research on affect regulation, advances in neuroscience, clinical outcome studies, and attachment theory. Yet the kinds of interpersonal, or transpersonal or relational, processes Fonagy and Target describe seem highly compatible with the relational perspective originally in Mitchell's early formulations, which themselves did not have a strongly developmental focus. Fonagy and Target's work is thus placed in an interesting point of conversation with relational thinkers for whom issues of development may initially have taken a back seat.

Mentalization and the Changing Aims of Child Psychoanalysis*

▼   ▼   ▼   ▼   ▼

There has been general agreement on the indications for child psycho-analysis. Anxious, inhibited, neurotic children are thought clinically to be particularly suitable. Glenn (1978); Sandler, Kennedy, and Tyson (1980); Hoffman (1993); Kernberg (1995); and others have identified further criteria:

1) Superior intelligence, particularly verbal skills, and psychological mindedness.
2) A supportive and stable environment, including parents who can form an alliance with the analyst, respect the boundaries of the treatment, and support their child's participation in it.
3) Internal conflict, judged to be the primary cause of the child's symptoms.
4) An absence of major ego deviations—that is, developmental "deficits" that are not the result of unconscious conflict and thus cannot be "resolved" by insight.
5) Motivation to engage in a lengthy and sometimes difficult therapy, stemming from anxiety, guilt, or shame.
6) A capacity to form relationships and trust that help can be found in relationships with others.

A glance at such daunting criteria makes apparent that the number of children qualifying as adequate candidates for child analysis must be small indeed. Furthermore, such criteria beg the question of whether children, so endowed with inner resources and environmental supports do in fact require a very time-consuming and costly process. The "luxury" of child analysis appears more dissonant when mental health professionals face extraordinary pressures to cut costs—pressures intersecting with a rising clamor to do something to address the problems of violent, drug-using, impulsive youngsters and their overwhelmed parents, a population for whom child analysis can seem to have relatively little to offer.

* Originally published in *Psychoanalytic Dialogues*, 8:87–114. © 1998 The Analytic Press, Inc.

Child analysis' claims to legitimacy rest heavily on case reports that, however moving or dramatic, tend to resist objective assessment and controlled scrutiny. As the old quip goes, psychoanalytically oriented therapists can fail to realize that *data* is not the plural of *anecdote*.

An effort to remedy this state of affairs is the chart review and detailed examination of over 750 case records of children and adolescents in psychoanalysis and psychodynamic treatment at the Anna Freud Centre (Target, 1993; Target and Fonagy, 1994a, b; Fonagy and Target, 1994, 1996b). Our study confirmed that psychodynamic treatment was particularly effective for groups of children whose diagnosis included an emotional disorder. Over 80% of children with a single diagnosis of an emotional disorder and relatively high levels of adaptation—that is, those closest to what the child analytic literature considers optimal candidates for child analysis—showed reliable improvement. Surprisingly, however, they appeared as likely to benefit from nonintensive therapy—one to two sessions per week—as from intensive treatment—four to five sessions per week. Even more surprising was the finding that intensive treatment was remarkably effective for some children with relatively severe, long-standing, and complex psychosocial problems, including conduct disorder, given the presence of at least one emotional disorder diagnosis (anxiety disorder, dysthymia, etc.). This heterogeneous group of children with complex psychopathology was less likely to gain clinically significant change from nonintensive psychotherapy. Even more disturbing was our observation that nearly 60% showed negative outcomes following once- or twice-weekly treatment.

Inspired by our first reports of these findings in 1994, the Child and Adolescent Ambulatory Psychiatric Clinic in Heidelberg undertook a similar retrospective study, with many findings matching ours. They identified a similar difference between the effectiveness of intensive and non-intensive treatments, as well as the beneficial impact of length of treatment. They also found the same pattern of declining responsiveness to intensive treatment with age. Interestingly, they found an interaction between gender and treatment intensity (wherein girls were more likely to benefit from intensive treatment, having controlled for the age effect); we did not find this.

Ongoing detailed analysis of our therapeutic records is revealing further suggestive findings. The most helpful interventions for the cases with more complex disorders seem to differ from those previously described as central to child psychoanalytic technique. In particular, interpretations of unconscious conflict aimed at promoting insight long held as the centerpiece of analytic technique appear to be of limited value to these youngsters. Less severely disturbed youngsters with emotional disorders do seem to benefit from an interpretive approach.

We are in the process of replicating these findings with young adults, 18- to 25-year-old young people with more than two Axis I and at least one Axis II diagnoses, assigned to treatment either once per week or five times per week. Although the results of the project, led by Mrs. Anne-Marie Sandler, are only in the process of being analyzed, it is clear that once-weekly treatment frequently fails to prevent a deterioration of these young people's condition, whereas treatment five times per week has moderate to good therapeutic effects.

The current plans of the Centre, under its new director, Julia Fabricius, include a prospective study of treatment outcome, in collaboration with the local National Health Service Trust. The present director's vision, building on the earlier work of George Moran and Anne-Marie Sandler, is to make the outcome of child psychoanalysis a priority for the Centre's research work. We are now at a fairly advanced stage of planning a randomized controlled trial of child psychoanalysis, in comparison with once-weekly psychodynamic psychotherapy, cognitive behavior therapy, and treatment as usual. The theoretical framework we describe represents the conceptual underpinnings for this trial.

A Widening Scope for Psychoanalysis?

The children with "complex psychopathology" that appeared to benefit from intensive psychodynamic therapy in our chart review constituted a rather heterogeneous lot, not easily captured by DSM IV's diagnostic categories. These children's clinical and developmental characteristics suggested to us that many could be grouped by clusters of disturbance, with the common element of at least one emotional disorder (such as depression, dysthymia, generalized anxiety disorder, separation anxiety disorder, or social phobia).

These children generally present a severe disturbance of social and emotional development, including marked impairment of peer relationships, affect regulation, frustration tolerance, and self-image. Reading these records, together with discussions with Dr. Efrain Bleiberg, President of the Menninger Clinic, revealed two clusters (Bleiberg, Fonagy, and Target, 1997). Some of them, which we designate as Cluster A, show a more fragile reality contact and thought organization. Idiosyncratic or magical thinking pervades their lives, but it is more intense in emotionally charged contexts. They tend to retreat into an isolated world of bizarre fantasies, suspiciousness, and social anxiety. Their abilities to make sense of human exchanges and empathize with others are strikingly limited. They are often equally impoverished in their capacity to communicate, hampered by odd speech and inappropriate affect. Descriptively, they generally resemble a range of *DSM-IV* (American Psychiatric Association, 1994) diagnoses that include schizotypal and schizoid personality disorders and milder forms of pervasive developmental disorder. They also resemble the children described by Towbin et al. (1993) and Cohen et al. (1994) as showing "multiple complex developmental disorder."

By contrast, a second cluster of children, which we designate as Cluster B, show intense, even dramatic, affect and hunger for social response. Clinginess, hyperactivity, and temper tantrums are common features of their early development. By school age, they may meet diagnostic criteria for attention deficit hyperactivity disorder, conduct disorder, separation anxiety disorder, or mood disorder. Many appear anxious, moody, irritable, and perhaps explosive. This affective lability mirrors the kaleidoscopic quality of these children's sense of self and others. One moment they feel elated, in harmony with an idealized partner. But at the next moment, they plunge into bitter rage, self-loathing, or despair.

By the time they reach adolescence, drugs, food, or promiscuous sex may be used to block feelings of being out of control, fragmented, and lonely. Self-mutilation and suicidal gestures are common among girls, whereas aggression, coupled with hidden fears of rejection, is more typical of boys. We have some evidence to suggest that if analysts are successful in maintaining Cluster B children in treatment, their outcome is comparable to that of children with neurotic disorders. Children in Cluster A generally have a poorer outcome, although less likely to terminate prematurely (Fonagy and Target, 1996b).

Undoubtedly, no single pathogenic factor can explain this heterogeneous subgroup of the children we classified as showing severe emotional disorder. Constitutional vulnerabilities interact in various combinations with developmental factors, such as chronic illness or disability in the child, early parental loss, parental psychiatric disturbance, abuse and neglect, or restriction of autonomy. In spite of the heterogeneity, these youngsters seem to share a characteristic that we think is crucial and that we focus on: Some pervasively (Cluster A) and others intermittently (Cluster B) seem to lack the capacity to make use of an awareness of their own and other people's thoughts and feelings. This capacity is referred to as "mentalization" or "reflection function" by both cognitive developmentalists (Morton and Frith, 1995) and psychoanalysts (Fonagy, 1991; Fonagy and Target, 1995) and is maintained by neural structures that Baron-Cohen and others have termed "Theory of Mind

Mechanisms" and localized with functional Positron Emission Tomography scans to the frontal lobe (Baron-Cohen, 1995).

Mentalization:
A Protective Factor and a Focus of Psychotherapy

Mentalization or reflective function is the developmental acquisition that permits children to respond not only to another person's behavior, but to the child's conception of others' attitudes, intentions, or plans. Mentalization enables children to "read" other people's minds. By attributing mental states to others, children make people's behavior meaningful and predictable. As children learn to understand other people's behavior, they can flexibly activate, from the multiple sets of self-object representations they have organized on the basis of prior experience, the one(s) best suited to respond adaptively to particular relationships.

Exploring the meaning of others' actions, in turn, is crucially linked with the child's ability to label and find meaningful his[1] own psychic experiences, an ability that we suggest underlies affect regulation, impulse control, self-monitoring, and the experience of self-agency.

To appreciate the nature of this developmental process we have to delineate two levels of mental functioning not often distinguished in psychoanalysis. All mind is representation, but representations are themselves represented in the mind. In cognitive science, this is referred to as the distinction between cognition and metacognition. Some analytic authors, who contrast symbolic with concrete representations, touch on a similar dimension, although the concepts have become overburdened.

The deficit or dysfunction we address here is a difficulty in generating metarepresentations, a disorder of a mental process, in terms we have elaborated before (Fonagy, Edgcumbe et al., 1993). Patients with certain personality disorders in childhood or adulthood cannot reliably access an accurate picture of their own mental experience, their representational world. Children with limited mentalization or reflective abilities are unable to take a step back and respond flexibly and adaptively to the symbolic, meaningful qualities of other people's behavior. Instead, these children find themselves caught in fixed patterns of attribution; rigid stereotypes of response; nonsymbolic, instrumental uses of affect—mental patterns that are not amenable to either reflection or modulation.

---

[1] For clarity, we have sometimes referred to the child as he and to the caregiver or therapist as she. This makes it easier to follow and corresponds to the actual gender in the large majority of instances.

Most modern psychoanalytic theories of self-development (e.g., Fairbairn, 1952; Winnicott, 1960; Kohut, 1977; Target and Fonagy, 1996; Fonagy and Target, in press) assume that the psychological self (the part of the self-representation where the self is represented not as a physical entity but as an intentional being with goals based on thoughts, beliefs, and desires) develops through perception of oneself, in another person's mind, as feeling and thinking (Davidson, 1983). It is assumed that the parent who cannot think about the child's particular experience of himself deprives him of a core of self-structure that he needs to build a viable sense of himself. We suggest that developmental personality disturbances arise first from the child's failure to find the image of his mind, his experience of himself as a thinker of thoughts, believer of ideas, feeler of emotions, in the mind of the caregiver (see Fairbairn, 1952).

We assume that for the infant, internalization of this image performs the function of the "containment of mental states" (Bion, 1962), which Winnicott (1967) described as "giving back to the baby the baby's own self" (p. 33). Through the internalization of these perceptions the infant begins to learn that his mind is not a direct replica of the real world but a version of it (though this process is not complete until around four years of age; Target and Fonagy, 1996). The experience of containment involves the presence of another being who not only reflects the infant's internal state, but represents it as a manageable image, as something that is bearable and can be understood. The perception of self in the mind of the other becomes the representation of the child's experience, the representation of the representational world.

To give an example, like all emotion, anxiety for the infant is a confusing mixture of physiological changes, ideas, and behaviors. When the mother reflects, or mirrors, the child's anxiety, this perception organizes the child's experience, and he now "knows" what he is feeling. The mother's representation of the infant's affect is internalized and becomes the higher order representation of the child's experience. If the mirroring is too accurate, the perception itself can become a source of fear, and it loses its symbolic potential. If it is frequently absent, reluctant, or contaminated with the mother's own preoccupation, the process of self-development is profoundly compromised. We may presume that individuals for whom the symptoms of anxiety signify catastrophes (e.g., heart attack, imminent death, etc.) have metarepresentations of their primary emotional responses, which are ineffective in containing their intensity through symbolization, perhaps because the original mirroring by the primary caregiver exaggerated the infant's emotions.

Admittedly this is a speculative model, but it is also empirically testable and might help answer the thorny question of why individuals with panic disorders consistently attribute immense significance to physiologically relatively mild levels of disequilibrium. In collaboration with the eminent Hungarian developmentalist currently at the Anna Freud Centre, Dr. György Gergely, we are in the process of designing a series of studies of the infant's emotional understanding that will more directly test these ideas. In recent studies we have confirmed that mothers who soothe their distressed eight-month-old babies most effectively following an injection rapidly reflect the child's emotion, but this mirroring is "contaminated" by displays of affect that are incompatible with the child's current feeling (humor, skepticism, irony, and the like), which reflect coping, metabolization, or containment. In displaying such complex affect, they ensure that the infant recognizes their emotion as analogous, but not equivalent, to their experience, and thus the process of symbol formation can begin.

We believe that the security of attachment between infant and caregiver is the critical mediator. A secure bond is one where the infant's signals are accurately interpreted by the caregiver, thus giving them meaning in terms of the caregiver's response. Normal affect regulation develops from the expectation of re-equilibration following arousal, through physical proximity to the object. The infant's signal of distress and the caregiver's coping-mirroring are combined into a single representation that comes to signify distress and becomes a critical part of the child's capacity to autoregulate emotion.

But what of the child whose caregiver cannot be depended on in this way? Missing the normal experience of reflection of his own mental states the child is most likely to take as the core of his representation of himself the caregiver's distorted and often barren picture of the child. The child who fails to develop a representation of an intentional self is therefore likely to incorporate in his image of himself the representation of the other, sometimes mental, sometimes physical. The picture of the self will then be distorted, and the child's experience of himself is overly influenced by his early perceptions of what others think and feel, and strangely out of touch with what he himself or others are currently experiencing. We believe, along with Edith Jacobson, that prior to the establishment of firm boundaries between representations of self and other, the infant's perception of the other comes to be internalized as part of that representational domain that will eventually become the reflective part of the self.

Many of these children show apparent failures of object permanence, leading to primitive separation anxiety or feelings of merger or fusion with the object. In reality, they continue to existentially depend on the physical presence of the other both for self-sustaining auxiliary metacognitive function (to continue to seek and find their intentionality in the mind of the other) and, more subtly, as a vehicle for the externalization of parts of the self-representation that are experienced as alien and incongruent with the self. This is why it is essential, as Winnicott (1967) pointed out, that the other acts in harmony with the infant's self to the detriment of and, at times, the temporary abolition of her own self as an entity. If the other is consistently incongruent with the state of self, the other's presentation is still internalized as part of the self structure, but without the appropriate links and associations that would enable a coherent functioning of the infant's self-representation.

The ultimate consequences of this process can be clearly discerned, we suggest, in later borderline personality structure. In order for the self to be coherent, the alien and unassimilable parts require externalization; they need to be seen as part of the other where they can be hated, denigrated, and even destroyed. The physical other who performs this function must remain present for this complex process to operate. The borderline child or adult cannot feel that he is a self unless he has the other present (often the analyst) to frighten and intimidate, to seduce and excite, to humiliate and reduce to helplessness. The other's departure signals the return of these "exterojects" and the destruction of the coherence the child achieves by such projection. This we believe is the root of that type of projective identification where the patient feels an overriding need to control the other, as his self is only actualized when the other's behavior can be forced to be consistent with this projective process. One of Cynthia Carlson's cases treated at the Anna Freud Centre used to take such control to extremes. This nine-year-old boy's mother permitted him to treat her as an extension of himself both physically and psychologically. In the analysis, he had to resort to far cruder devices, revealing the same underlying need. He frequently tied the therapist up as well as constantly ordering her to do things for him. In our view, with cases as severely impaired as this child was, understanding such behavior as an extension of the eroticized transference is unlikely to be sufficient. In this case, what turned out to be important was the child's need to make Cynthia's thoughts and feelings (of rage, hatred, disgust, helplessness) predictably present and to eliminate other ideas or feelings that Cynthia presented to him, which he found unpredictable and therefore terrifying.

At the root of disturbance such as this boy's is, we suggest, a failure to achieve mentalization, which we see as the integration of two more primitive forms of representing psychic reality (Fonagy and Target, 1996a; Target and Fonagy, 1996). In early childhood, reflective function is characterized by two modes of relating internal experiences to the external situation.

In a serious frame of mind, the child expects the internal world in himself and others to correspond to external reality, and subjective experience will often be distorted to match information coming from outside (psychic equivalence mode), (e.g., Perner, Leekman, and Wimmer, 1987; Gopnik and Astington, 1988). While involved in play, the child knows that internal experience may not reflect external reality (e.g., Bartsch and Wellman, 1989; Dias and Harris, 1990), but then the internal state is thought to have no relationship to the outside world and to have no implications for it (pretend mode).

In normal development the child integrates these two modes to arrive at the stage of mentalization, or reflective mode, in which mental states can be experienced as representations. Inner and outer reality can then be seen as linked, yet they are accepted as differing in important ways and no longer have to be either equated or dissociated from each other (Gopnik, 1993; Baron-Cohen, 1995).

We have hypothesized that mentalization normally comes about through the child's experience of his mental states being reflected on, prototypically through experience of secure play with a parent or older child, which facilitates integration of the pretend and psychic equivalence modes through an interpersonal process that is perhaps an elaboration of the complex mirroring of the infant by the caregiver. In playfulness, the caregiver gives the child's ideas and feelings (when he is "only pretending") a link with reality by indicating the existence of an alternative perspective, which exists outside the child's mind. The parent or older child also shows that reality may be distorted by acting upon it in playful ways, and through this playfulness a pretend but real mental experience may be introduced.

In traumatized children, intense emotion and associated conflict can be thought of as having led to a partial failure of this integration, so that aspects of the pretend mode of functioning become part of a psychic equivalence manner of experiencing reality. This may be because where maltreatment or trauma has occurred within the family, the atmosphere tends to be incompatible with the caregiver playing with the most pressing aspects of the child's thoughts; these are often disturbing and unacceptable to the adult, just as they are to the child. The rigid and controlling behavior of the preschool child with a history of disorganized attachment, as with Cynthia's patient, thus is seen as arising out of a partial failure on the part of the child to move beyond the mode of psychic equivalence in relation to specific ideas or feelings, so that he experiences them with the intensity that might be expected had they been current, external events.

We believe, the almost impossible challenge patients present is rooted in this aspect of the transference. For the relationship to serve a function and to be tolerable, the analyst must do something fresh and creative, "an act of freedom" (Symington, 1983), which has as one component the real impact of the real patient on the analyst, yet through its novelty reassures the patient that his attempt at control and tyranny has not completely succeeded. Through identification with the externalized part of the patient's self, the analyst has validated the patient's psychic reality, yet by bringing a new perspective, the patient is forced to see his own action with another dimension and thus overcome the one-to-one correspondence between thought and reality in his mind. Without such a creative spark the analysis is doomed to become an impasse, a rigid stereotypic repetition of pathological exchanges.

The challenge is the preservation of the "as if" nature of the therapeutic exercise, and sometimes playfulness is the only ally. A man with a violent disposition was greatly distressed by a rather clumsy interpretation made to him. Aiming to be empathetic, the analyst referred to the pain he felt about a canceled session. The patient promptly got up, shoved his fist under the analyst's nose, and said, "I'll show you what pain is, you little shit!" Without thinking, the analyst said "You know, as I get older I can't see things so clearly when they are too close to my eyes," and with that gently moved the clenched fist away from his face. To the analyst's relief and surprise, the patient immediately calmed down and smiled. On reflection, the analyst realized what was critical to this exchange: forcing this patient to experience the world through the analyst's somewhat long-sighted perspective and thus to see him as a real person, allowing the patient to enter his mental world.

Self, Action, and the Body

Over 10 years ago, Stern (1985) summarized findings and offered theories tracing self-development back to the actions of the four-month-old. A sense of authorship of one's own actions, whether derived from the experience of forming plans, proprioceptive feedback, or the consequences of physical action, contributes to the continuity of the sense of self. Where actions are significantly curtailed, self-agency and continuity are threatened. Bolton and Hill (1996), in their outstanding book *Mind, Meaning and Mental Disorder*, make a strong case for the "close connection between thoughts and action, and of the experience of effective agency as crucial to the sense of self" (p. 368). This crucial link of intentionality between thought and action cannot be totally sustained by actions of the child, as these usually continue to be limited because of his immature physical and cognitive capacities, in certain respects until adolescence. Playful interpersonal interaction that permits (a) the registration of perceptions, thoughts, and emotions as causes and consequences of action and (b) the contemplation of these mental states without fear provides the basis of self-agency.

Coercive, rigid, frightening, and, at an extreme, abusive parenting can undermine not just the understanding of mental states, but also the establishment of a firm connection between the self and action, as this connection crucially depends on the perceived bidirectional link between mental state and action. Disorders of conduct may be understood as the consequence of the child having failed to link his sense of self with his actions. In the case of abuse, the meaning of intentional states is also commonly compromised by the parent's denial of the child's internal reality. Abuse, particularly within the family, prevents the child testing representations of mental states for their applicability, truth, and possible modification. The representations thus become rigid and unhelpful and are partially and sometimes almost fully abandoned.

The experience of helplessness and defensive decoupling of painful bodily experiences associated with maltreatment may cause the individual to blame his body for the abuse. The body is less likely to be experienced as a potent agent of action, and actions on it are less integrated with the self. It is nonetheless perceived as the cause of difficulties, and thus action directed against it relieves both frustration and anger.

Another possible outcome is that the representation of the body may be used as if it was part of the psychic apparatus. In these cases the child's own body is used in representing and expressing feelings, ideas, and wishes. The child's or another's body may be attacked in an effort to grapple with feelings and ideas in others (most commonly in boys) and in the self (mostly in girls). Young women with apparently uncontrollable insulin-dependent diabetes often fall into this group (Moran, 1984; Fonagy and Moran, 1993). In other young children, the search for the psychological self in the other may lead to the physical image of the object being internalized as part of the child's identity, and gender identity disorder, for example, may be the consequence (Coates, Friedman, and Wolfe, 1991).

The decoupling of self-representation and action because of the disruption of the child's intentional stance is as relevant for violence against the other as for violence against the self. In conduct-disordered children, the broken link between action and psychological self is painfully clear, as those of you who have treated kicking and biting children would probably testify. A critical obstacle to interpersonal aggression, the innate responsiveness to another person's suffering through identifying with his or her state of mind, is lost. This is not, as is often claimed, to be attributed to the absence of empathy, although to be sure there is little evidence of this. Rather, violence reflects the absence of a critical precursor of empathy, the capacity to link action and mental state, which normally begets the psychological self.

Another consequence of the weak link between thinking or feeling and action is that violence or aggression may be resorted to as the only acts that succeed in linking intentional state to external events. Both violent and self-harming individuals feel real when attacking someone physically. We believe (Fonagy, Moran, and Target, 1993; Fonagy and Target, 1995) that violent acts combine two powerful motivations for such people: The aggression and damage can lend a sense of coherence to the self (self-actualization) and at the same time it expresses the need to attack externalized, alien aspects of the self, felt to be either in one's own body or represented by somebody else.

Empirical Support

There is a certain amount of empirical data, from experimental studies of the development of social cognition in normal and abnormal children and from studies of parent-child attachment, that is consistent with this model.

As we mentioned, developmentalists for the most part refer to mentalizing as maintained by a theory of mind mechanism (ToMM). There is substantial accumulating evidence that ToMMs are dysfunctional in children with autism (Baron-Cohen, 1995), some of whose symptoms children with developmental disturbances share to a milder degree. Dennett (1978) convincingly argued that the understanding of mental states, such as belief, could only be unequivocally demonstrated by the individual showing an understanding that someone else could have a false belief. The capacity to mentalize is thus operationalized as the child being able to pass a false belief task, to show understanding that someone else would act or desire something based on a mental state the child knows to be mistaken. The child is shown a tube that normally contains chocolate, but this time it has a pencil inside it. When asked what his friend will say when shown the tube, most three year olds reply, "A pencil." Four year olds, having acquired the capacity to represent false belief, will say, "Chocolate!" Various versions of this task exist. Our interest is principally in belief-desire reasoning, which tests the child's capacity to attribute appropriate emotion based on false belief.

We believe that lesser degrees of ToMM deficit, with a large psychosocial component, are prevalent in the group of children with developmental disturbances we considered previously. This suggestion fits the expectations of developmental psychologists working on the development of ToMM in normal children, who have explored the likely consequences of a child not "discovering the mind" in the normal way: impairment of family and peer relationships, the capacity to learn, and emotional control (see, e.g., Astington, 1994, pp. 146–147). A number of distinct lines of evidence converge to underline the plausibility of the model we are proposing.

1) In a program of work over the last 10 years several laboratories, including the London Parent-Child Project initiated by Miriam Steele, have been able to demonstrate the importance of the caregiver's capacity to think about their own past relationships in terms of their own and others' mental states to ensure the child's security of attachment. We have developed a reliable coding scheme (Fonagy, Steele, et al., 1997) that assesses reflective capacity from the autobiographical narratives obtained from Adult Attachment Interviews (George, Kaplan, and Main, 1985):
   (i) In the London Parent-Child Project of 100 first-time parents, the large majority of both mothers and fathers, who were rated above the median in reflective function before the birth of their first child were observed to have secure relationships with these children 12 to 18 months later (Fonagy, Steele, et al., 1991).
   (ii) The presence of social deprivation in the mother's background greatly increases the importance of reflective capacity; all the children of reflective mothers with a history of deprivation had infants who were securely attached to them, but only 1 of 17 low reflective mothers with similar histories did so (Fonagy et al., 1994). Thus the capacity to mentalize permits the individual to cope with disadvantage. The parent's efforts to make sense of the infant's behavior convey to him that mental states underlie behavior and that finding this meaning is the most effective strategy to relate and cope with the social environment. The child's sense of himself as an intentional being evolves to the extent that he can clearly perceive those intentions in the mind of the parent.
2) Harris (1994) and Dunn (1996), in their recent review of emotional development, identified many of the social determinants of the capacity to understand mental states, particularly emotional states. For example, recent evidence has demonstrated that mother-child and sibling-child relationships influence the rate of development of ToMM as assessed by both young children's spontaneous conversation about feelings (Brown and Dunn, 1991) and the false-belief task (Perner, Ruffman, and Leekman, 1994).

3) Studies of parent-child attachment have demonstrated that mentalization is a biologically prepared capacity triggered by an attachment figure who treats the child as an intentional being. A secure attachment relationship creates the emotional environment within which the child's opportunity to discover his intentional state, mentalizing capacity, or theory of mind is maximized:

   (i) Insecure attachment at five years has been shown to be negatively correlated with performance on ToMM tasks (Fonagy, Redfern, and Charman, 1997).

   (ii) Insecure attachment to the mother at one year predicts poor performance on ToMM tasks at five years (Fonagy et al., submitted) and limited metacognitive capacities in an autobiographical task at 10 years (Main, 1991).

   (iii) Insecure attachment at 1 year predicts poor social adaptation at 10 years (Sroufe, 1988) and identity problems and low ego resilience once in adolescence (Grossmann et al., 1993).

4) The capacity to mentalize not only permits the individual to cope with disadvantage, but ensures the transgenerational transmission of this protective capacity:

   (i) Parents' mentalizing ability (or reflective function), assessed before the birth of the child, predicts the child's mentalization capacity (performance on ToMM measures) at five years (Steele et al., 1995).

   (ii) This process is mediated by the quality of the child's attachment to the primary caregiver at 12 to 18 months and is independent of verbal skill in either caregiver or child (Fonagy et al., submitted).

5) In a number of clinical papers (Fonagy, 1991; Fonagy and Target, 1995), we reported that individuals with features of borderline personality disorder appear to have specific difficulties in understanding mental states both in themselves and in others and that this dysfunction may be seen as an adaptation to intolerable experiences of maltreatment and abuse in childhood. Rather than contemplate the intolerable idea of what may be going on in the mind of their abuser, these children opt to inhibit their capacity to think about minds altogether; decouple the link between self-representation and action, and turn away from the world of thoughts, feelings, beliefs, and desires, at least in the context of intense attachment relationships:

   (i) Studies of maltreated children show that they have both disrupted attachment (Cicchetti and Barnett, 1991) and a specific difficulty in acquiring mental state words (Beeghley and Cicchetti, 1994).

(ii) A study of adult nonpsychotic psychiatric in-patients show that those who have documented histories of severe maltreatment with current significant impairments in understanding mental states almost invariably meet *DSM-IV* diagnostic criteria for borderline personality disorder (Fonagy, Leigh, et al., 1996).

(iii) Our recent studies of young incarcerated adults have shown even more dramatic reductions in the reflective capacity amongst criminals contrasted to a group matched for psychiatric diagnosis, with the lowest levels amongst those individuals convicted for violent offenses (Levinson and Fonagy, submitted).

We are currently involved in prospective work at the Menninger Clinic to demonstrate that the difficulties of children with developmental disorders may be understood in terms of insecure attachment in infancy and the sequelae of this which seem to include impairment in the full development of mentalizing. This, in turn, leaves them vulnerable to subsequent psychosocial stress (or may contribute to the generation of such stress) to which they respond by the sometimes dramatic inhibition of mentalizing function. It is our view that a metacognitive deficit brought about by psychosocial experiences, which undermine the healthy development of the ToMM, may account for self-regulation deficits such as problems of affect regulation, frustration tolerance, impulsiveness, and self-esteem problems, as well as social deficits, such as poor peer relationships, poor communication skills, and aggressive or violent behavior (Bleiberg et al., 1997).

It is our premise that a crucial therapeutic aspect of psychoanalysis, for both children and adults, lies in its capacity to activate people's ability to find meaning in their own and other people's behavior. Child psychoanalysis has always aimed at strengthening children's capacity to recognize mental states. We believe that a therapeutic program that engages in a systematic effort to enhance mentalization holds the promise of increasing the effectiveness of psychoanalysis for the children with more severe and complicated difficulties by more specifically tailoring therapeutic intervention to their particular configuration of clinical and developmental problems.

So what does a child analytic approach focused on enhancing mentalization look like? Work at the Anna Freud Centre for over three decades has evolved a set of techniques for helping children with primarily developmental disturbances, or more borderline pathology, and our formulations began with studying this work in the records of completed cases. In collaboration with Rose Edgcumbe and Jill Miller, as well as George Moran and Hansi Kennedy, together with vital input from other clinical staff at the Centre, we have tried to provide an integrated view of both traditional technique and what has come to be known as developmental help (Fonagy et al., in press). For now we only consider three aspects, which are covered at greater length in a recent article by Efrain Bleiberg and the two of us (Bleiberg, Fonagy, and Target, 1997).

Enhancing Reflective Processes

How does one go about enhancing mentalizing capabilities? First of all, such patients need to learn to observe their own emotions and understand and label their emotional states, including their physiological and affective cues. They need help to understand the both the conscious and the unconscious relationships between their behavior and internal states, for instance of frustration or anxiety.

As part of that process, the analyst focuses children's attention on the circumstances that lead them, for example, to be aggressive in particular situations in which they feel misunderstood or made anxious by those around. The analyst introduces a mentalizing perspective that focuses on children's minds as well as the mental states of people who are important to them.

The focus is kept, at least initially, on simple mental states. These children are unable to accept complex mental states of conflict or ambivalence but may understand simple states of belief and desire. They will typically fail to grasp how mental states may change over time. Thus, working with current, moment-to-moment changes in children's mental states within the therapy is crucial. Likewise, analysts generally refrain, early in the process, from linking children's feelings with dynamically unconscious thoughts. An individual who fails to recognize his subjective experience can hardly relate to an even more inaccessible realm. Of course, by definition, the analyst is always addressing a nonconscious realm—feelings and ideas that the patient has limited capacity to become aware of.

Clinical experience has shown that some patients find it helpful to focus interventions around their perceptions of the analyst's mental states, as a precursor to self-reflection (Steiner, 1994). They can get to know the way they are seen by others, which can then become the core of their own self-perceptions. Analysts, of course, do not necessarily reveal to the children what they actually experience; rather, they speculate about how the child might be experiencing their state of mind at that moment. Some analysts have used guessing games along these lines (Moran, 1984), "What do you think I am thinking about you today?"

Play Helps Children to Strengthen Impulse Control and Enhance Self-Regulation

Children with mentalizing problems tend to require considerable help in curbing impulsivity. Rosenfeld and Sprince (1965) described a six-year-old child, Pedro, who frequently urinated over the analyst and her possessions. Other features of the material led the analyst to understand this as a crude attempt to coerce her into mutual activity, or simply to maintain a sense of connection. Neither interpretation nor physical restraint reduced the behavior. The analyst then devised a way of meeting what she had felt to be his need by saying that she would continue with the interrupted joint activity while he went to the lavatory, and she would give him a running commentary on what she was doing while he was there. He then stopped urinating in the treatment room and was still able to feel in contact through her voice. Pedro's analyst identified the gap in mentalization that triggered impulsivity and compensated for it.

Cluster B children often seem more impaired in their impulse control and self-regulation as their attachment to the analyst becomes more intense. The temporary impairment of mentalization appears linked to the activation of traumatic responses triggered by closeness to or separation from attachment figures (van der Kolk, 1989, 1994; Terr, 1994; van der Kolk and Fisler, 1994). For example, Joe, a 13-year-old boy, had been subjected to brutal physical and sexual abuse by an alcoholic father, while his mother pursued her theatrical career. Almost in spite of himself, he began to feel more comfortable with the analyst, even to look forward to the sessions. Yet desires for closeness were almost unbearable for him; thus, he began to carefully look for "mistakes" (e.g., the analyst interrupting him or "invading" his space while walking). These would trigger hateful barrages. He let the analyst know of his plans to run away and find out the analyst's address ("I have good sources, you know") so he could set the analyst's house on fire after raping his wife and murdering his children with slow, intravenous injections of cocaine. He would spare the analyst's life, but only to ensure that he would suffer the devastation of the loss of everything he held dear.

Sensing his desire to maintain a relationship, while overtly disowning it, the analyst commented on the meanness and cruelty of his imagery. Where did that come from? Joe looked at him with a mix of contempt and amusement and proceeded to describe, in a wildly exaggerated fashion, the toughness of his neighborhood and its brutal gang wars. He was sure that the analyst's wimpy, nerdy self had been shielded from such roughness. The analyst entered the role and created play. He replied with an even more fantastic account of his own heroic battles as a gang kingpin—a secret identity hidden behind his deceptively mild appearance. The banter continued over several sessions, but gradually the analyst was able to return Joe's attention to the rage he had experienced and the abuse he inflicted on the analyst.

This vignette illustrates how these youngsters often require a transitional area of relatedness akin to Winnicott's (1953) transitional experience. In this transitional, as-if area (often jointly created by patient and analyst) standing between fantasy and reality, patients can both own and disown their rejection feelings and experiences and test out the analyst's attunement, respect, and responsiveness to the vulnerable aspects of the self. The essence of the interaction appears to be the provision of a safe context in which to play with ideas and come to experience them as ideas.

The patient's threat, even if it is verbal rather than physical, is experienced by him as action; its modulation by the analyst into an idea allows it to be played with, mentalized, thus creating the potential for understanding. For the abused child, the adult's mental world is too real a threat to permit play and is thus shunned and avoided. The analyst's attitude and verbalization permit the opening of a window on the mental world of self and other, but the child has to find the courage to use this, to look through it and find in his own feelings and ideas something that has never before felt safe. In other words, the therapeutic intent is to facilitate the establishment of a beachhead, an area of self-other relatedness. Prematurely confronting the patient's defenses before this beachhead is established only exacerbates the need for distance, control, or devaluation of the analyst and the therapy.

The capacity to take a playful stance may be a critical step in the development of mentalization as it requires holding simultaneously in mind two realities: the pretend and the actual, in synchrony with a moment-by-moment reading of the other person's state of mind. Analysts often need to create a context in which an attitude of pretense is possible. For example, they may exaggerate their intonations to mark for children the pretend nature of interactions or may choose objects that are clearly incapable of adopting any intentional stance (e.g., crude toys).

Gradually, children are nudged to introduce small modifications in their play to better encompass the complexities, limitations, conflicts, and frustrations of reality. The transitional space of play and fantasy offers borderline children the magic of anonymity in which to attempt to bring together split-off representations of the self and others.

Working in the Transference

Finally, the emphasis is on working in the transference, not "transference" in the classic sense of expecting children to "transfer" their thoughts and feelings about their parents onto the analyst. The relationship with the analyst, however, remains central because the clarification of children's feelings about themselves and about the analyst is the most effective route toward acquiring mentalizing capacity.

The analyst uses her relationship with the child as a vehicle for all the processes described earlier, helping him to find, through involvement in a therapeutic relationship, a way of thinking, understanding, and coping with feelings; of recognizing the connections and differences between oneself and somebody else; and of being with another person. Accepting and recognizing the mental chaos of the patient and abandoning the traditional stance of recovering forgotten memories is the first step of the process. The past makes no sense as a cause of the present, as it is the present that cannot be thought or felt about. The analyst has to teach the patient about minds, principally by opening his mind to the patient's explorations. "Deep interpretations" will be experienced as persecutory taunts, intrusions, distractions, or seductions. The appropriate focus of work is the exploration of triggers for feelings, small changes in mental states, highlighting differences in perceptions of the same event, bringing awareness to what would be almost conscious for most people. Work takes place strictly in the analyst-patient relationship and focuses on the mental states of patient and analyst. Interpretations are not global summaries, but rather attempts at placing affect into a causal chain of concurrent mental experiences. The patient's actions on the analyst are not intended as communications (and interpreting them as such is therefore not appropriate). They are desperate attempts at coping with the intolerable closeness that analysis brings.

The analyst adopts a nonpragmatic, elaborative, mentalistic stance that places a demand on the patient to focus on the thoughts and feelings of a benevolent other. This stance, in and of itself, enhances, frees, or disinhibits the patient's inborn propensity for reflection and self-reflection. Perhaps more important, he is able to find himself in the mind of the analyst as a thinking and feeling being, the representation that never fully developed in early childhood and was probably further undermined by subsequent painful interpersonal experience. In this way, the patient's core self-structure is strengthened, and sufficient control is acquired over mental representations of internal states so that psychotherapeutic work proper can begin. Even if work were to stop here, much would have been achieved in terms of making behavior understandable, meaningful, and predictable. The internalization of the analyst's concern with mental states enhances the patient's capacity for similar concern toward his own experience.

Conclusion

Psychoanalysis is under savage attack in most countries where it is practiced. Yet intensive psychosocial treatments for severe psychological disorders are increasingly seen as essential by behaviorists, cognitive therapists, and those practicing systemic work with families. We recommend a shift in analytic technique for certain particularly disturbed or traumatized children, from the conflict- and insight-oriented approach to a focused, mentalization-oriented therapy, which we believe is already widely used by those treating severe psychological disturbance. Psychoanalytic training, supervision, and personal treatment remain crucial in enabling clinicians to use their emotional reactions to better understand their patient's subjective world, rather than be entrapped in the quicksand of rigid, unthinking patterns of relatedness. The techniques suggested here and the theoretical ideas on which they are based may also be put to good effect in prevention, informing parenting training, home visitation programs, nursery education, and crime prevention initiatives.

The change of aims and priorities we are suggesting is not radically new or exclusive of other approaches, which of course includes more classical technique with the "good, neurotic case." At its strongest, our claim is that severe disorders of character require modifications of technique in the direction of prioritizing a mentalizing approach. At its weakest, we are introducing new jargon into an area already bursting with terminological confusion. However, even here, there may be value added by harmonizing our language with that of developmental cognitive science.

Of course, as analytic readers, you will see through this false modesty. Deep down we do believe that we are doing analysis with these patients, in that we are trying to understand the roots of psychological problems in early emotional development, encompassing the whole range of conscious and unconscious motivations within the intense relationship with the analyst. Thus, we believe that we may contribute to the advancement of Freud's vision of development, psychopathology and therapeutic action. But then we would think that, wouldn't we?

References

American Psychiatric Association (1994), *Diagnostic and Statistical Manual of Mental Disorders* (4th ed.). Washington, DC: American Psychiatric Association.

Astington, J. W. (1994), *The Child's Discovery of the Mind*. London: Fontana Press.

Baron-Cohen, S. (1995), *Mindblindness: An Essay on Autism and Theory of Mind*. Cambridge, MA: MIT Press.

Bartsch, K. & Wellman, H. M. (1989), Young children's attribution of action to beliefs and desires. *Child Devel.*, 60:946–964.

Beeghly, M. & Cicchetti, D. (1994), Child maltreatment, attachment, and the self system: Emergence of an internal state lexicon in toddlers at high social risk. *Dev. Psychopath.*, 6:5–30.

Bion, W. R. (1962), *Learning from Experience*. London: Heinemann.

Bleiberg, E., Fonagy, P. & Target, M. (1997), Child psychoanalysis: Critical overview and a proposed reconsideration. *Psych. Clins. N. America*, 6:1–38.

Bolton, D. & Hill, J. (1996), *Mind, Meaning and Mental Disorder*. Oxford: Oxford University Press.

Brown, J. R. & Dunn, J. (1991), "You can cry, mum": The social and developmental implications of talk about internal states. *Brit. J. Dev. Psychol.*, 9:237–257.

Cicchetti, D. & Barnett, D. (1991), Attachment organisation in preschool aged maltreated children. *Dev. Psychopath.*, 3:397–411.

Coates, S., Friedman, R. C. & Wolfe, S. (1991), The etiology of boyhood gender identity disorder: A model for integrating temperament, development and psychodynamics. *Psychoanal. Dial.*, 1:481–523.

Cohen, D. J., Towbin, K. E., Mayes, L. & Volkmar, F. (1994), Developmental psychopathology of multiplex developmental disorder. In: *Developmental Follow-Up: Concepts, Domains and Methods*, ed. S. L. Friedman & H. C. Haywood. New York: Academic Press, pp. 155–182.

Davidson, D. (1983), *Inquiries into Truth and Interpretation*. Oxford: Oxford University Press.

Dennett, D. C. (1978), Beliefs about beliefs. *Beh. Brain Sc.*, 4:568–570.

Dias, M. G. & Harris, P. L. (1990), The influence of the imagination on reasoning by young children. *Brit. J. Dev. Psychol.*, 8:305–318.

Dunn, J. (1996), The Emanuel Miller Memorial Lecture 1995. Children's relationships: Bridging the divide between cognitive and social development. *J. Child Psychol. Psychiat.*, 37:507–518.

Fairbairn, W. R. D. (1952), *An Object-Relations Theory of the Personality*. New York: Basic Books.

Fonagy, P. (1991), Thinking about thinking: Some clinical and theoretical considerations in the treatment of a borderline patient. *Internat. J. Psycho-Anal.*, 72:639–656.

—— Edgcumbe, R., Moran, G. S., Kennedy, H. & Target, M. (1993), The roles of mental representations and mental processes in therapeutic action. *The Psychoanalytic Study of the Child*, 48:9–48. New Haven, CT: Yale University Press.

—— Kurtz, A., Bolton, A. M. & Brook, C. (1991), A controlled study of the psychoanalytic treatment of brittle diabetes. *J. Amer. Acad. Child Psychiat.*, 30:241–257.

————— Leigh, T., Steele, M., Steele, H., Kennedy, R., Mattoon, G. & Target, M. (1996), The relationship of attachment status, psychiatric classification, and response to psychotherapy. *J. Consult. Clin. Psychol.*, 64:22–31.

————— & Moran, G. S. (1993), Childhood diabetes. In: *Textbook of Psychiatry*, ed. A. J. Solnit. Philadelphia: Lippincott.

————— Redfern, S. & Charman, T. (1997), The relationship between belief-desire reasoning and a projective measure of attachment security (SAT). *Brit. J. Dev. Psychol.*, 15:51–61.

————— Steele, H., Steele, M. & Holder, J. (submitted), Quality of attachment to mother at 1 year predicts belief-desire reasoning at 5 years. *Child Dev.*

————— ————— Moran, G., Steele, M. & Higgitt, A. (1991), The capacity for understanding mental states: the reflective self in parent and child and its significance for security of attachment. *Inf. Ment. Health J.*, 13:200–217.

————— Steele, M., Steele, H., Higgitt, A. & Target, M. (1994), Theory and practice of resilience. *J. Child Psychol. Psychiat.*, 35:231–257.

————— ————— ————— & Target, M. (1997), Reflective-functioning manual, version 4.1, for application to Adult Attachment Interviews. Unpublished manuscript, University College, London.

————— & Target, M. (1993), Aggression and the psychological self. *Internat. J. Psycho-Anal.*, 74:471–485.

————— & ————— (1994), The efficacy of psychoanalysis for children with disruptive disorders. *J. Am. Acad. Child Adolesc. Psychiat.*, 33:45–55.

————— & ————— (1995), Towards understanding violence: The use of the body and the role of the father. *Internat. J. Psycho-Anal.*, 76:487–502.

————— & ————— (1996a), Playing with reality: I. Theory of mind and the normal development of psychic reality. *Internat. J. Psycho-Anal.*, 77:217–234.

————— & ————— (1996b), Predictors of outcome in child psychoanalysis: A retrospective study of 763 cases at the Anna Freud Centre. *J. Amer. Psychoanal. Assn.*, 44:27–77.

————— & ————— (in press), Attachment and reflective function: Their role in self-organisation. *Dev. Psychopath.*

————— ————— Miller, J. & Moran, G. S. (in press), *Contemporary Psychodynamic Child Therapy. Theory and Technique*. New York: Guilford.

Freud, A. (1962), Assessment of childhood disturbances. *The Psychoanalytic Study of the Child*, 17:149–158. New York: International Universities Press.

————— (1965), *Normality and Pathology in Childhood*. Harmondsworth, England: Penguin Books.

George, C., Kaplan, N. & Main, M. (1985), The Adult Attachment Interview. Unpublished manuscript, Department of Psychology, University of California, Berkeley.

Glenn, J. (1978), *Child Analysis and Therapy*. New York: Aronson.

Gopnik, A. (1993), How we know our minds: The illusion of first-person knowledge of intentionality. *Beh. Brain Sci.*, 16:1–14, 29–113.

————— & Astington, J. W. (1988), Children's understanding of representational change and its relation to the understanding of false belief and the appearance-reality distinction. *Child Devel.*, 59:26–37.

Grossmann, K. E., Loher, I., Grossmann, K., Scheuerer-Englisch, H., Schildbach, B., Spangler, G., Wensauer, M. & Wimmermann, P. (1993), The development of inner working models of attachment and adaptation. Presented at symposium of the Society for Research on Child Development, New Orleans.

Harris, P. L. (1994), The child's understanding of emotion: Developmental change and the family environment. *J. Child Psychol. Psychiat.*, 35:3–28.

Hoffman, L. (1993), An introduction to child psychoanalysis. *J. Clin. Psychoanal.*, 2:5–26.

Kernberg, P. F. (1995), Child psychiatry: individual psychotherapy. In *Comprehensive Textbook of Psychiatry*, ed. H. I. Kaplan & B. J. Sadock. Baltimore, MD: Williams & Wilkins, pp. 2399–2412.

Kohut, H. (1977), *The Restoration of the Self*. New York: International Universities Press.

Levinson, A. & Fonagy, P. (submitted), Attachment classification in prisoners and psychiatric patients. *Brit. J. Psychiat.*

Main, M. (1991), Metacognitive knowledge, metacognitive monitoring, and singular (coherent) vs. multiple (incoherent) models of attachment: Findings and directions for future research. In: *Attachment Across the Life Cycle*, ed. C. M. Parkes, J. Stevenson-Hinde & P. Marris. London: Tavistock/Routledge, pp. 127–159.

Moran, G. S. (1984), Psychoanalytic treatment of diabetic children. *Psychoanalytic Study of the Child*, 38:265–293. New Haven, CT: Yale University Press.

Morton, J. & Frith, U. (1995), Causal modelling: A structural approach to developmental psychology. In: *DevelopmentalPsychopathology, Vol. 1: Theory and Methods*, ed. D. Cicchetti & D. J. Cohen. New York: Wiley, pp. 357–390.

Perner, J., Leekman, S. & Wimmer, H. (1987), Three-year-olds' difficulty in understanding false belief: Cognitive limitation, lack of knowledge, or pragmatic misunderstanding? *Brit. J. Dev. Psychol.*, 5:125–137.

———— Ruffman, T. & Leekman, S. R. (1994), Theory of mind is contagious: You catch it from your sibs. *Child Devel.*, 65:1228–1238.

Rosenfeld, S. & Sprince, M. (1965), Some thoughts on the technical handling of borderline children. *The Psychoanalytic Study of the Child*, 20:505–512. New York: International Universities Press.

Sandler, J. (1962), The Hampstead Index as an instrument of psychoanalytic research. *Internat. J. Psycho-Anal.*, 43:287–291.

———— Kennedy, H. & Tyson, R. (1980), *The Technique of Child Analysis: Discussions with Anna Freud*. London: Hogarth Press.

Sroufe, L. A. (1988), The role of infant-caregiver attachment in development. In: *Clinical Implications of Attachment. Child Psychology*, ed. J. Belsky & T. Nezworski. Hillsdale, NJ: Lawrence Erlbaum Associates, pp. 18–38.

Steele, M., Fonagy, P., Yabsley, S., Woolgar, M. & Croft, C. (1995), Maternal representations of attachment during pregnancy predict quality of childrens' doll play at 5 years of age. Presented to Society for Research in Child Development, Indianapolis.

Steiner, J. (1994), Patient-centered and analyst-centered interpretations: Some implications of containment and countertransference. *Psychoanal. Inq.*, 14:406–422.

Stern, D. N. (1985), *The Interpersonal World of the Infant: A View from Psychoanalysis and Developmental Psychology*. New York: Basic Books.

Symington, N. (1983), The analyst's act of freedom as agent of therapeutic change. *Internat. Rev. Psycho-Anal.*, 10:783–792.

Target, M. (1993), The outcome of child psychoanalysis: A retrospective investigation. Unpublished doctoral dissertation, University of London.

——— & Fonagy, P. (1994a), The efficacy of psychoanalysis for children: Developmental considerations. *J. Amer. Acad. of Child Adolesc. Psychiat.*, 33:1134–1144.

——— ——— (1994b), The efficacy of psychoanalysis for children with emotional disorders. *J. Amer. Acad. Child Adolesc. Psychiat.*, 33:361–371.

——— ——— (1996), Playing with reality. II: The development of psychic reality from a theoretical perspective. *Internat. J. Psycho-Anal.*, 77:459–479.

Terr, L. (1994), *Unchained Memories: True Stories of Traumatic Memories, Lost and Found*. New York: Basic Books.

Towbin, K. E., Dykens, E. M., Pearson, G. S. & Cohen, D. J. (1993), Conceptualising "borderline syndrome of childhood" and "childhood schizophrenia" as a developmental disorder. *J. Amer. Acad. Child Adolesc. Psychiat.*, 32:775–782.

van der Kolk, B. (1989), The compulsion to repeat the trauma: re-enactment, revictimization, and masochism. *Psych. Clins. N. America*, 12:389–411.

——— (1994), The body keeps the score: Memory and the evolving psychobiology of post-traumatic stress. *Harvard Rev. Psychiat.*, 1:253–265.

——— & Fisler, R. (1994), Childhood abuse and neglect and loss of self-regulation. *Bull. Menn. Clin.*, 58:145–168.

Winnicott, D. W. (1953), Transitional objects and transitional phenomena. *Internat. J. Psycho-Anal.*, 34:1–9.

——— (1960), Ego distortion in terms of true and false self. In: *The Maturational Processes and the Facilitating Environment*. New York: International Universities Press, 1965, pp. 140–152.

——— (1967), Mirror-role of mother and family in child development. In: *The Predicament of the Family*, ed. P. Lomas. London: Hogarth, pp. 26–33.

Having a Mind of One's Own and Holding the Other in Mind: Commentary on Paper by Peter Fonagy and Mary Target*

(1998)

Susan W. Coates

▼   ▼   ▼   ▼   ▼

Editors' Introduction

In this essay, Coates, exploring new models for psychoanalytic developmental theory and developmental lines, draws on theories of mind, intersubjective processes of mentalization, and a keen eye for the complex transmissions, sometimes owned, sometimes disowned, that can jump from mind to mind, body to body. This essay marks a shift in her work from gender development to a wider ranging interest in intergenerational transmission of trauma.

Coates's work on matters of development from a psychoanalytic and psychodynamic perspective began with her clinically sophisticated and theoretically innovative work on gender dysphoria in young children, initially and primarily in boys. Perhaps because gender is one of those interpersonal, interfamilial, and intrapsychic matters where implicit and explicit communication are often strangely at odds, this clinical population gave Coates a complex puzzle to unravel. With both a scientist's eye and a clinician's heart, she is able to hold the complexity of confusing ruptures in identity expectation for parents and for children. Her model holds in tension constitutional patterning, critical stages, the dangers of parental depression and distorted or ruptured mentalization, and a child's brilliant solution to use gender to maintain the structural integrity and capacities of the interacting adult, usually the mother.

Coates is reacting to and deepening a new and important perspective on child analysis developed by Fonagy and his colleagues, particular Mary Target, his coauthor of the essay Coates is commenting on. Her critique clarifies the heart of Fonagy and Target's analysis: namely, that disturbances in children of a wide and serious variety can be linked to disturbances in the mentalizing containers in which they are interpersonally and emotionally embedded. To think, to reflect—a core capacity with which children negotiate the internal and interpersonal world—emerges from being thought about, held in mind. This deceptively simple idea brings together a variety of child syndromes and disturbances, a variety of disruptions in family systems, and a set of techniques for remediation.

Coates elaborates on this conceptual work but goes beyond it. She ties these ideas to the work of Winnicott and Stern. She links this material to the work of Bion in particular and underscores the relational and transgenerational process of these difficulties in children. Coates connects this work to the older tradition of Fraiberg and, most important to the old and new literature on attachment. Far from encompassing simple ego deficits, this idea that thinking requires being kept in mind and that reflective functioning is at the heart of affect regulation, and psychic health is powerfully linked to our understanding of the abiding transgenerational experience of attachment security (or insecurity).

In this model Coates shows that a relational perspective neglects neither the individual intrapsychic dimension nor the interpersonal. She adds wonderful detail and theory to Fonagy's example of his handling of a menacing encounter with a patient. The charged, intense moment is built on Fonagy's both knowing and showing his internal state, here fear. Thus the patient has the experience of an agentic impact on another who nonetheless neither retaliates nor collapses but talks and interprets. Countertransference is the awareness and careful titration of knowledge and emotion from analyst to analysand about minds and impact of self and other. For Coates it is crucial that mentalization is always thinking and feeling, a point she makes very strongly in relation to Fonagy's and Target's theoretical stance.

One final note in introducing Coates's essay. She focuses on an element of Fonagy and Target's analysis that has to do with outcome assessment and the question of change in types of treatment. Coates sounds the moral dimension—the ethic inherent in asking for both accountability about our work and its effectiveness—and an extension of our ideas to matters of social policy. Coates is thus in a long tradition of child practitioners whose interests are both in the intricacy of a case and in the larger social settings in which children may thrive or suffer.

Having a Mind of One's Own and Holding the Other in Mind: Commentary on Paper by Peter Fonagy and Mary Target*

Peter Fonagy and Mary Target's contribution, "Mentalization and the Changing Aims of Child Psychoanalysis," is a remarkable and important article. Fonagy and Target are continuing to report on an important body of programmatic research that they and their collaborators, notably George Moran and Miriam and Howard Steele, have been producing for more than a decade (Fonagy, 1991; Kennedy and Moran, 1991; Fonagy, Steele et al., 1993; Fonagy et al., 1995; Fonagy and Target, 1995; Fonagy and Target, 1996). Their work is a part of a broad effort within psychoanalysis to integrate modern developmental research and thought into the psychoanalytic theory of development (Stern, 1985; Lyons-Ruth, 1991; Silverman, 1991; Slade and Aber, 1992; Diamond and Blatt, 1994; Main, 1995; Osofsky, 1995; Mayes and Cohen, 1996; Beebe, Lachmann, and Jaffe, 1997). Fonagy and Target provide us with an integrative article of the highest caliber: It pulls together a number of seemingly disparate ideas and findings and unites them in an overall conception of intensive treatment; its mode of operation; and, important to identify in an age of restrictive access to mental health care, the kind of

* Originally published in *Psychoanalytic Dialogues*, 8:115–148. © 1998 The Analytic Press, Inc.

patients most likely to benefit from such treatment. The synthesis presented in this article is novel and refreshing, and it opens up new ways of thinking about the complex clinical challenges that we all face daily. It is a vision of the future of intensive psychoanalytically oriented work with children that challenges our traditional ways of thinking.

In what follows I first attempt to address the originality of Fonagy and Target's vision by singling out for discussion those parts of their presentation that may be unfamiliar to most clinical readers. To be sure, I do not attempt to be exhaustive; instead, I emphasize what I think are the most interesting points and leave it to others to explore those facets of the presentation that I have left unexamined. Second, at the same time, I try to articulate my fundamental agreement with both the aims of Fonagy and Target's paper and their constituent arguments based on my own clinical and research experience, as well as that of others in the field. Despite the novelty of this article, it is also organically related to recent developments within the field of intensive psychoanalytically oriented intervention with children that hold great therapeutic promise. From a theoretical perspective it widens the lens of the applicability of psychoanalytic intervention, creating a space, both conceptually and technically, for working with children who historically have been considered not well suited to psychoanalytic intervention. Finally, I argue that a deeper appreciation of their work also has the potential to facilitate more constructive engagements with family systems in clinical work while preserving the integrity of the individual encounter with the child.

Therapeutic Efficacy

I start with what may potentially be most unsettling about Fonagy and Target's presentation to traditional child psychoanalysts. They report on treatment outcome in a systematic, empirically sound way. Many child analysts are unaccustomed to being held to scientific accountability in this manner. Rather, the field has chiefly relied on individual case reports, which are essentially anecdotes no matter how convincing they may be. But psychoanalysis is not just an investigatory tool for the study of the development of meaning-making; it is most importantly a healing art. Cooper (1993, p. 381) justly remarked that, as psychoanalysts and psychoanalytic psychotherapists, we do more than simply investigate; we charge fees and make implied promises that the investigation will be of some benefit to the child. This stance takes us into a realm of accountability that, as Cooper further noted, demands scientific documentation of our claims.

I am not arguing against the value of the individual case report. Case reports are enormously important for studying the intricacies of meaning-making in the individual child, but in and of themselves, they neither provide sufficient information for the field to understand the processes of development broadly conceived nor do they allow us to specify what in the treatment is truly efficacious. As Fonagy and Target note with an appealing wry sense of humor, *data* is not the plural of *anecdote*. In today's contracting economic environment, not to mention the context of renewed public debates about psychoanalysis in general, we will be left behind unless we have outcome data demonstrating the efficacy of intensive psychoanalytic treatment. Moreover, as thoughtful clinicians have begun to recognize, such systematically obtained outcome data represent the best avenue for bringing into clearer relief what we do that is most helpful to troubled children and their parents and why. It is worth noting that Fonagy and Target's research in many ways confirms aspects of the methodological vision of Anna Freud. For it was her foresight in insisting on detailed records at the Hampstead Clinic that made possible the subsequent research by Fonagy and Target that underlies the present communication.

What the data show is that intensive treatment, (i.e., child analysis conducted three and four times a week) did prove of benefit for children with single emotional disorders. However, it makes clear the fact that less intensive treatment conducted once or twice a week is equally beneficial to such children. Moreover, although the mechanism of therapeutic action that is perhaps most cherished by many analytically oriented clinicians—insight—did in fact seem to be of benefit to these children, it turns out that the children could also derive this benefit from the less intensive forms of treatment. Thus, there was no differential advantage for child analysis, at least not for those children with single emotional disorders.

However, of equal or perhaps even greater import for child psychoanalysis is the further finding that the more intensive form of treatment was found to be of benefit for the more seriously troubled children, (i.e., children with pervasive ego deficits and multiple emotional and interpersonal difficulties). Why this should be the case and its implications for our continuing efforts to refine child analytic techniques I address shortly. Let us first note a further, quite unexpected finding that emerged from the research: The less intensive forms of treatment were actually disadvantageous to the more seriously disturbed children. Sixty percent of the time, such treatment actually made more than half of the children worse. This is a disturbing finding of course, but it is critical that we all know about it. Also to be noted, and for the experienced child analyst this may not be a totally unexpected finding, is that these more seriously disturbed children, even though they did well in analysis, did *not* seem to profit from insight.

Considered just as a report on outcome, though it is clearly much more than that, Fonagy and Target's article is consonant in a number of ways with what has already been argued by others with regard to adult treatment. I am referring to the repeated findings that psychoanalysis per se has not been shown to be differentially more effective than other forms of psychotherapy in general. But it is beginning to emerge that psychoanalysis with adults may be differentially more effective with *more* seriously disturbed patients, such as severely depressed patients or borderline patients, over the long haul. Here an historical note may be in order. It is to the credit of psychoanalysts, and not other clinicians, that they first identified the type of patients now characterized as borderline. They did so because they observed that there was a group of patients, seemingly presenting as hysterics, for whom analysis, at least as it was then conducted, was *not* suitable. Now it turns out, after several conceptual revolutions within psychoanalysis—in understanding disorders of the self, the common developmental antecedents of such disorders, and the special techniques they require in treatment—that it may be just these patients once thought to be unanalyzable" who may be most helped by psychoanalysis, as compared to briefer and less intensive forms of treatment. Thus, one way of viewing Fonagy and Target's research is that they have extended this way of thinking about the differential effectiveness of analysis for adults to analysis for children.

Reflective-Functioning

To be truly useful to individual practitioners, the outcome findings need some interpretation. Here is where Fonagy and Target's analysis is both highly original and generative of new ways of thinking about child psychopathology and child intervention. They argue for a particular understanding of the kind of deficits shown by the more seriously troubled children—the very ones who will benefit most from intensive treatment and who may well get worse with less intensive treatment—and on the basis of that understanding they then proceed to a particular view of the mutative factors in analytic intervention. Specifically, Fonagy and Target draw our attention to an affective-cognitive processing function, which they identify as reflective-function, that is absent or deficient in these children. Further, they argue that the development of this capacity in intensive treatment is central to therapeutic transformation.

Reflective-functioning as Fonagy and Target define it entails the ability to understand mental states as essentially propositional and intentional, (i.e. as entailing beliefs and wishes). These two aspects of mental functioning are derived from well-established philosophical analyses. Let me explain them briefly by taking an instance from toddlerhood. There is a difference between being utterly repelled by a particular food such as spinach and recognizing that I as an individual am having a particular reaction to this food. Being utterly repelled is essentially a matter of perception that does not know itself as such. One feels menaced by the spinach; its repugnant qualities are apprehended as immanent truths of the universe. Having a personal dislike of spinach is different. One recognizes one's own state of mind as such; one is aware of one's own beliefs and intentional preferences. Implied in this recognition is the possibility that others may feel quite differently about spinach.

There is thus a kind of stepping back from or reflecting on direct experience that is involved in coming to appreciate one's own mind as possessing beliefs and wishes—or in the language of philosophy as entailing a propositional or intentional stance (Dennett, 1978). An important corollary of developing this appreciation is that one also comes to grasp that mental states may be variable from one time to the next and from one context to the next. Further, mental states may also be fallible, and they may differ from one person to the next.

Very young children necessarily lack this ability to understand mental states as propositional and intentional. The clinical consequences of this lack can be far-reaching if circumstances are not favorable. Consider, for example, that this lack will have major consequences for a young child's understanding of a parent's negative affect and negative attributions. A two year old ordinarily cannot think of a parent's angry behavior as a consequence of the parent's bad mood. The child is even less likely to think that the parent's angry behavior stems from something that happened in his or her own past. The child cannot readily suppose that the parent is simply wrong. That is to say, the child cannot think, "My Mom is in one of those bad moods that she sometimes gets into and I am not really as bad a kid as she is saying I am." The child cannot say, "My Mom is wrong." He or she is simply stuck with the reality of a mother saying he or she is a bad kid; the child's inability to take a perspective on the attribution means that it is experienced as simply true.

The development of reflective-functioning is a gradual process. From a research standpoint, the child's growing capacity to understand his or her own and others' mental states can be assessed through standard procedures. Wimmer and Perner (1983) used the following task. They told a child a variation of this story: Max is in the kitchen helping his mother put some chocolate in a cupboard. When he leaves the room she takes all the chocolate out of the cupboard and puts it in a large bowl to make a chocolate cake. The child is asked, "Where will Max look for the chocolate when he returns to the kitchen?" A child who can grasp that Max will think wrongly, that the chocolate is still in the cupboard, is providing evidence of reflective-functioning. That is to say, he or she can construct and hold in mind the experience of the other, in this case Max. He or she understands that Max will have a different state of mind or perspective based on a different set of experiences than he or she has had hearing the story. The child will also grasp the emotional consequence that Max will likely be very surprised and disappointed indeed when he opens the cupboard and sees that the chocolate is gone.

The ability to understand another's state of mind as a state of mind, or the capacity to have a theory of mind as it has been referred to by philosophers and developmental psychologists, ordinarily only develops in the late preschool years. Its precursor may begin in the affective resonance of the first months of life (Stern, 1985), but its true origins begin once an infant can communicate intentionality, and, for this to be possible, a framework of meaning must be established spanning the interface between mother and child. This occurs roughly by the end of the first year of life (Bretherton, McNew, and Beeghly-Smith, 1981). It can be seen in an infant's capacity to share a focus of attention with another, as when the infant can follow the trajectory of a mother's pointing finger to discover what she is pointing at and, by implication, what she has in mind. Or the infant can point to something and try to get the mother—"Look Mommy"—to see what he or she has in mind. Further evidence of a child's dawning capacity to understand the state of the mind of the other can be seen in the second year as the infant begins to move from parallel play to cooperative play. The capacity to attribute a belief to another person that one does not hold oneself develops in the third or fourth year. In tests where a child is presented with a situation where another child has been excluded from having a critical piece of information, most children under the age of three are not able to take account of the other person's lack of information and they operate as if everybody has the same knowledge (Mossler, Marvin, and Greenberg, 1976; Wimmer and Perner, 1983). By age four most become able to keep in mind the fact that the other person is missing a critical piece of information, and that will inform their decision making. Veridical conceptual perspective taking, the capacity to understand another's state of mind with regard to the mind of a third person (e.g., being able to think about another person's thought about a third person's thoughts) does not mature until the sixth year (Mossler et al., 1976). Clearly, what is important clinically is not whether a child possesses the interrelated abilities to understand the states of mind of self and other in the abstract, but whether the child can utilize them to negotiate the world of emotions and interpersonal relatedness. A child may have the capacity to hold the experience of the other in mind in a relatively neutral situation but may not be able to hold onto the same cognitive ability when the stimuli are emotionally laden or involve conflict.

How do these capacities develop? Developmental research from a variety of domains has converged on an understanding of these abilities as maturational possibilities that become activated in the context of parent–child and parent–sibling interactions. If, as Trevarthen (1987) put it, young brains are designed to learn from older brains, it is becoming clear that young *minds* first learn about minds—both their own and others'—by being exposed to the reaction of other minds to themselves. Winnicott (1967) put the matter elegantly: What does the baby see when he or she looks at the mother's face? I am suggesting that, ordinarily, what the baby sees is himself or herself. In other words, the mother is looking at the baby and what she looks like is related to what she sees (p. 112).

But Winnicott's famous metaphor of the mother as "mirror" deserves further elucidation. For the mother is more than a mirror in the sense of simply reflecting the infant's behavior; she is rather something like a magical mirror, for she intuitively sees in the infant something that is only still potential, that she both recognizes and shapes, thereby creating a space for the infant to experience his or her mind as his or her own. Thus the mother's ability to see the potential in the infant is what allows the infant to find it for himself or herself, in the face of the mother. (Just as the child's understanding of his or her self is characteristically shaped by what the parents can and cannot find in their child, so, too, the child's capacity to regulate affect is characteristically shaped by parental attunement and parental capacity to recognize and contain affect.)[1]

Just what the child observes in the mother's face is, of course, widely variable, depending on, among other things, the mother's own past experience and consequent capacity to understand and more or less accurately reflect and expand on the child's experience. Optimally, the mother reflects something in the child that is easily and pleasurably integrated into the child's experience. Consider the following example wherein a child discovers something new about his mind through his mother. A young toddler, barely two, is playing in the backyard; he excitedly pulls at and sniffs some flowers while making excited but unintelligible utterances. His mother can see his pleasure, a pleasure that differs from her own, and smiles in recognition saying, "You really love those colors,

---

[1] Perner, Ruffman, and Leekam (1994) demonstrated that siblings as well as parents influence the child's developing understanding of other minds.

don't you? You are a guy who loves flowers." Now, in addition to the flowers and the child's excitement, there is a third space (Ogden, 1994) where the boy moves from a spontaneous sensory experience to a discovery of the experience (of his enjoying colors and the flowers) in the intersubjective space as it is held in the mind of his mother. The child looks at the mother, sees himself, and smiles; there is a recognition and a discovery of a part of the self held by the other. By virtue of being sensitively met, the child comes to experience loving colors and flowers as a part of his notion of himself, and this notion has emerged in the transitional space created by the mother's attuned response. He has been met by his mother in an unobtrusive way such that her needs have not been imposed upon him; thus he has the experience of his own creativity.

What happens when, due to her own anxieties, the mother responds to her child in a way that is out of synch with the child's experience? A typical example from early childhood is the reaction of an anxious mother whose toddler, after falling, is briefly startled but not frightened. The mother, in response to her own anxieties, panics and runs to the child with far more intense affect than the child originally experienced, picks him up, holds him, rocks him, and asks him where it hurts while lecturing to him about the need to be careful. This mother has partly responded to the child's experience of being startled when he fell, but she has intensified it almost beyond recognition, up-regulating the child's affect rather than helping him to contain it. The child in this intersubjective space is forced to incorporate into the experience of falling the additional experience of his mother's anxiety and hypervigilant defenses. The original reaction, although it may not be completely obliterated, gets both intensified and overshadowed by the mother's reactions, making it difficult for the child to differentiate his own experience from that of the mother.

For an extreme example, consider the experience of another child who discovers a litter of kittens and, excitedly picking one of them up, accidentally drops it. The mother in this case races toward him in horror and outrage, telling him that he is going to grow up to be a "killer." The mother has not met the child's sense of wonder and discovery but has imposed her own fears on the child's experience such that she obliterates the child's original impulse. In its place the mother's fears, anxieties, and preoccupations have been substituted—only in treatment does the mother trace these back to traumatic physical abuse suffered from men in adolescence—with no way for the child to sort things out. Such repeated experiences can leave a child not only with a sense of inauthenticity, but also with impaired development of reflective-functioning and with little or no sense of having a mind of his or her own. The child is likely to take on these negative attributions—himself as "killer," his mother as enraged victim—as alien introjects or presences that have not been worked over and metabolized. The self attributes are not made into his own as occurs in identification (Sandler, 1987), but they are enduring nonetheless. Such profound failures of mirroring when they occur over and over again lead to severe distortions in the sense of self and can lead to self-fulfilling prophecies.

The child who does not find his or her mind in the mind of the mother is left without an awareness of his or her own mind and without a personalized, authentic, and vitalized sense of self. At the heart of these disorders is a relative void where an experience of self should be found but where instead reside parental preoccupations that are experienced as alien unmetabolized introjects, leaving the child without a sense of him- or herself as a person in his or her own right. These children often appear devitalized, seem to have no blood in their veins, or act like automatons without an internally authorized sense of agency. Yet in other instances, children with very similar or even identical internal worlds present with an inauthentic overly bright pseudovitality. Not infrequently, this pseudovitality reflects the child's taking on of the mother's defensive attempt to compensate for her own depression (Stern, 1995).

But the polar examples of devitalized or overly bright children scarcely exhaust the possibilities. In fact, the clinical consequences can be enormously varied—as varied as the manifold developmental tasks the child faces and as idiosyncratic as a parent's specific traumatic heritage. A child whose reflective-functioning has remained underdeveloped and compromised by the parent's preoccupations and defenses will be prone not only to breakdowns in functioning around important general domains involving issues like separation, autonomy, and self-regulation, or the management of aggression, but also to breakdowns around those particular affect-event experiences where the parent's capacity to hold the baby in mind is profoundly compromised. The consequence in either case is likely to be the development of significant symptoms that are not simply symbolic expressions of conflict but rather repetitive enactments with primary caretakers who are experienced as unmetabolizable introjects or alien presences (Britton, 1992) (i.e., others who do not mirror the child's self). One way of grouping the manifold serious disturbances that can arise is suggested by Fonagy and Target's ad hoc differentiation of two types of disturbances among the group of seriously disturbed children in their sample. In one group, we find those children manifesting tenuous reality contact; magical thinking; and marginal ability to understand, anticipate, or empathize with others. In the second group, we find those children who show object hunger but who are anxious, moody, irritable, and explosive to the point that they compel responses from the environment. The cluster of symptoms in both groups rightly deserve to be understood, as Fonagy and Target argue, in terms of the basic failure to develop a mind of one's own. A child, or for that matter an adult, who lacks the ability to understand the mental states of self and other is obviously going to live in a quite different experiential world. This world may be characterized by such things as schizoid detachment and quite magical means for maintaining self-regulation of a quite rudimentary kind. It also may be characterized by unmetabolizable emotions that can readily be experienced with traumatic intensity and impinging or impenetrably remote others who are of use only insofar as they can be pressed into service for purposes of self-management via enactments.

The converse possibility also deserves our attention. Consider the child who has a well-developed reflective-function in Fonagy and Target's terms and can readily make use of it in situations that are emotionally charged, highly stressful, or both. It is still conceivable that such a child might become symptomatic if the nature of the stress exceeded his or her capacity to cope. Nonetheless, one would expect, first, that the resulting symptomatology would be of the nature of a circumscribed disorder and not entail serious ego distortions, and second, that the child would readily be able to use treatment, even circumscribed treatment, aimed at helping him or her relieve that distress and find more effective means of coping. We would expect these children to behave more or less like the group described by Fonagy and Target as suffering from single emotional disorders and as being likely to benefit from child analysis but also from less intensive treatment.

Given what has just been said in regard to both prevention and treatment responsiveness, we might well consider the development of reflective-function from what might be called a public health perspective. That is to say, we would want to encourage those child rearing practices that fostered this capacity in the child, and discourage those that interfered with its development, provided we knew what these were. We could not eliminate all child psychopathology this way, but we could significantly reduce its risk and could significantly raise the proportion of children who would benefit from less intensive forms of treatment when and if they became symptomatic. In fact, we are beginning, though only just beginning, to acquire just this kind of knowledge. As I outline later, what we are learning has implications not only from a public health perspective, but also for how we conceptualize analytic intervention in relation to the ordinary processes of parenting.

Fostering Reflective-Functioning

Thus far, I have been presenting Fonagy and Target's conception of reflective-functioning as essentially consonant with similar and related conceptions of how the self develops and acquires a degree of autonomy and resiliency, which have been advanced by Winnicott, Stern, and others. This concept is indeed consonant with much of contemporary psychoanalytic theorizing. Fonagy and Target's theory builds on this previous work while offering us a more highly specific understanding of how structures are built and how our technique should be shaped to meet the individual child patient. If we can appreciate that, in the moment, the child does not "know" what he or she feels but only feels it, then we can begin to understand how the therapeutic task is neither simply to facilitate self-expression nor to offer interpretation aimed at promoting insight into internal conflicts. Rather, the therapeutic task is to provide the child with an experience of being understood—and even here we have to qualify further that being understood is not the same thing as being responded to. Rather, being understood entails having the therapist reflect back to the child an understanding of what the child feels in a way that simultaneously reflects comprehension of the feeling and demonstrates a capacity to contain the feeling; in other words, the therapist must not only demonstrate that he or she appreciates what the child is experiencing but must also communicate this understanding in a way that implies that the child can potentially have a similar experience of mastery of the state.

A further note of clarification may be helpful here in regard to what it means for the child (or adult) to understand that the therapist understands his or her feelings. It is not enough that the therapist gets what the child intends (or would be intending if the behavior could be reflected on as intentional). The therapist must get what the child feels. And this kind of "getting" has to be immediate and direct. It must come about through a kind of affect contagion. It must accord with the real quality and intensity of the patient's affect. One might more accurately say that, rather than get the patient's feeling, what the therapist must do is let the patient's feeling *get* to him or her (i.e., take him or her over in a way that is recognizable to the patient). Speaking of work with seriously disturbed children, Fonagy and Target write, "Therapists' ingenuity and creativity are called upon to connect with these children at an emotional level. Words often fail without the analyst conveying, in the emotional coloring of their expression, both their appreciation of the child's affect and a capacity to cope with it." One cannot foster the development of a patient's capacity for reflective-functioning simply by standing outside the patient's emotional world and observing and commenting on his or her mind. In another context, Fonagy (personal communication) described the process that needs to unfold in the relation between patient and therapist as follows:

> One must permit and even in some circumstances encourage the patient to colonize one's mind and then recover to be able to offer the patient a fresh perspective upon their own mental functioning.

Let me use Fonagy's own example of a borderline man who threatens him with a clenched fist some few inches from Fonagy's face after he has made an interpretation referring "to the pain he was experiencing in relation to a canceled session." The patient lurched from his seat and shoved his fist under Fonagy's nose saying, "I'll show you what pain is, you little shit!" Fortunately I have heard him lecture on the same case and can add to the description of the written report what I learned from his imitation of both himself and the man; Fonagy's response was to grab the man's fist and very firmly, yet slowly, almost gently push it away from him while saying, "You know, as I get older I can't see things so clearly when they are too close to my eyes." At first, the example sounds like limit-setting accompanied by whimsy, and indeed, both are involved. But what was also present in the communication—by physical means and by the intonation of Fonagy's voice and the expression on his face— was that he was genuinely threatened in that moment. The experience of his own fear in turn helped Fonagy to get what the patient was feeling and how intensely his patient felt. Through affect contagion from Fonagy, the patient recognized that Fonagy got it. Fonagy met the man's sense of vulnerability with an intense sense of vulnerability of his own while stepping outside of the confrontation and creatively containing it. This interchange with Fonagy allowed the man to get hold of his own experience by seeing it in Fonagy's face and mind and by witnessing another way of handling it. In the moment of this recognition, the patient presumably felt known, respected, and envisioned as a person who could find a mind of his own.

On one level, one could say about this kind of interaction that there is finally a meeting of minds. But one could say with even more precision that a true meeting of minds requires a small mismeeting of the minds if the patient is to be recognized and authentically met. It is this slight mis-meeting that allows a symbolic stance to occur and provides the "creative spark" allowing the man to begin to understand his own mind. In effect, by responding in a way that suggests a degree of freedom in relation to the affect, the therapist is providing an intentional stance of his or her own that invites the patient to do the same. Stern (1985) provided an essentially consonant vision of this kind of mismeeting of minds in his description of how affect attunement also entails a degree of misattunement in a well-functioning mother-child dyad.

To return to the arena of treatment, the conception offered by Fonagy, Target, and their various collaborators offers a detailed and sophisticated way of trying to appreciate—at the very border between intelligible and opaque interactions—what it is we do with patients, both children and adults, that leads to therapeutic improvement. Space does not permit a more detailed discussion here, but one would want to extend this same kind of reasoning more fully into a discussion of various play interactions with children as well as to other kinds of interventions. To some extent, Fonagy and Target have already started down this road in their article. To be sure, what they have to say about encouraging reflective processes in the child in relation to affects and the circumstances that provoke them will not by itself be novel to most child clinicians. Less familiar perhaps is their suggestion of the usefulness of inviting the child to consider the therapist's mind. But both of these processes, as they emphasize, must be continually adapted to the moment-by-moment unfolding of the child's experience and to the nuances of the relation to the therapist. As for the multitude of ways in which play can help strengthen impulse control and enhance self-regulation, one only wishes their article were longer. In regard to the interaction of play in the therapeutic setting and the developmental vulnerabilities of a child's symbolic capacities, Fonagy and Target provided a more detailed and quite fascinating discussion elsewhere. A feature of that discussion, which has particular relevance for the clinician, is their technical recommendations for working with young children who do not understand the concept of pretend, and who thus are likely to misconstrue the meaning of symbolic play (see Fonagy and Target, 1996). One also wishes that the authors had extended their discussion in other directions. For example, the variations in the development of reflective-function that they observe invite us to consider the various uses of fantasy more deeply, particularly as concerns the child who is moving from dyadic to triadic fantasies and is beginning to engage the conflicts seen in oedipal configurations.

Forgoing these and other discussions for lack of space, I instead focus on another aspect of their article that I believe to be important because it helps offer us a vision not only of how child analysis works, but also of how to situate it conceptually with regard to some of the processes mediating the origins of severe psychopathology in children. The latter feature, in turn, offers a new perspective for beginning to reconceptualize how best to work with families in conjunction with treating the child.

Transmission of Attachment Security and Its Relation to Reflective-Functioning

The idea of reflective-functioning did not emerge on an ad hoc basis from the data set to which it is currently being applied in Fonagy and Target's article. It comes out of a synthesis of psychoanalytic theory of object relations (Bion, 1962; Sandler and Rosenblatt, 1962; Winnicott, 1965, 1971; Bretherton, 1985) and attachment research (Bowlby, 1973, 1980; Ainsworth et al., 1978; Main, 1995). Within attachment research, moreover, it comes out of a series of studies of the mechanisms in the transmission of security from one generation to the next (Main and Hesse, 1990) that Fonagy and his colleagues have adapted in such a way as to make it highly clinically relevant. One of Fonagy's specific contributions has been to take a look at the microprocesses involved in the intergenerational transfer of secure and insecure attachment from one generation to the next. What he has found to be particularly relevant from a clinical standpoint is a component of parental sensitivity—sensitive parenting has previously been linked to secure parent-child attachment (Ainsworth et al., 1978; Haft and Slade, 1989)—which goes beyond affection, concern, and affect attunement and involves the capacity to hold in mind the mental state of the other (Fonagy et al., 1991). This capacity in the parent is potentially critically involved in the transmission of security from one generation to the next, whereas its absence is associated with the development of serious psychopathology. This is a most important strength of their work.

To appreciate the ways in which the concept of reflective-functioning intersects with attachment research requires some background in the latter. Here I review this area of research quite briefly. The study of internal working models of attachment—begun by Bowlby, operationalized by Ainsworth at a behavioral level, and more recently investigated at the level of representation by Main—has opened up the possibility of understanding how object relations are constructed in early development and has provided the first powerful empirical window on how intersubjective experience becomes transformed into intrapsychic structures. Current research finds that children can be reliably classified as securely or insecurely attached to specific caregivers as early as one year of age and that these differential relations reflect not only the child's previous experience with the particular caregiver in question but the strategies that have been successful in maintaining proximity to that caregiver (van IJzendoorn, 1995). It has become clear that the quality of the attachment bond, whether secure or insecure, is likely to endure across the first years of development and to be very highly correlated with a host of personality variables, with children who have secure attachment relationships with their caregivers having the most favorable outcomes.[2] These strategies for maintaining proximity to the caregiver can now be reliably related to psychological processes in the caregiver which can be independently assessed thanks to the pioneering work of George, Kaplan and Main (1985) in developing the Adult Attachment Interview (AAI).

The foregoing may be familiar to most readers, but the full implications of this work may not be. Of importance, is that insecure attachment in the child is not the same thing as psychopathology, and secure attachment, either in the child or in the adult, is not the same thing as mental health. To appreciate the significance of a particular working model of attachment, one must put attachment in relation to psychopathology. Perhaps the simplest way of relating the two domains is to say that an insecure attachment style plus severe stress is very likely to result in psychopathology. Insecure attachment is not the same as psychopathology, but it does raise the risk of it. Conversely we could say that, in general, secure attachment status is a protective factor against the development of psychopathology so that, for secure child, the stress has to be much greater to produce psychopathology.

Main and others (Main, Kaplan, and Cassidy, 1985; Kobak and Sceery, 1988; Kobak et al., 1993; Cassidy, 1994; Diamond and Blatt, 1994; Slade, 2003) view both secure and insecure styles of attachment as a means of regulating a variety of behaviors including affect. The regulatory styles are useful in highlighting differential outcomes of secure and insecure patterns of attachment. Securely attached children are thought to regulate affect in an open, direct, and flexible way. The avoidant strategy, which develops in the relational context of consistent parental rejection of a child's attachment behaviors, appears to reflect the child's efforts to tamp down the attachment system by minimizing emotional expression of distress (Cassidy, 1994). Such a child typically neither protests a parent's departure nor is reassured by the parent's return in an experimental situation, the so-called Strange Situation, that is tailor-made to elicit these behaviors. The ambivalent/resistant strategy,

---

[2] When there is great change in the family situation or context, one would not expect the quality of attachment to endure.

which develops in the context of inconsistent parental response to the child's attachment behaviors (i.e., response that is governed more by the parent's needs than by the child's), appears to represent the child's attempt to activate the attachment system by maximizing emotional expression of distress, but without achieving a satisfactory resolution (Cassidy and Berlin, 1994). Such a child is visibly upset by the parent's departure in the Strange Situation, but fails to calm down after the parent's return. The third category of insecure attachment, the disorganized-disoriented style, is behaviorally different from the two previously described categories. Disorganized—disoriented attachment, the relational context for which I examine in greater detail next, represents a breakdown in a consistent strategy for managing attachment motivation so that the child does not fit the secure, avoidant, or ambivalent/resistant styles, but instead exhibits contradictory behaviors simultaneously or in rapid succession. Disorganized attachment represents a truly grave risk for the development of psychopathology. Even in the absence of frank symptoms, a child who has been disorganized with respect to attachment will inevitably attempt to forge a resolution of this critical state through the adoption of more or less severe distortions of the self, distortions that will allow the attachment system to reorganize in some more coherent form.

Thus far, I have been concerned with the different styles of attachment (secure, avoidant, ambivalent/resistant and disorganized-disoriented), which can be measured in the infant and toddler and which gradually consolidate over time into intrapsychic regulatory structures as the child develops toward adolescence and adulthood. But, one can also turn matters around and work from the other direction. That is to say, one can begin with the parents' attitudes toward their own attachment experiences and the ways the parents integrate these in their conceptions of self and seek to predict how their children will behave in the Strange Situation as one year olds. In other words, if the child's attachment strategy represents his or her cumulative experience of the real characteristics of the parent, one should be able to predict the former from the latter and, in so doing, see how the parents' attitudes toward attachment are transmitted to their children. In fact, this is how Main's AAI (George et al., 1985) was first constructed (i.e., with a view to predicting the transmission of attachment security from one generation to the next).

The AAI is a semistructured interview that takes about one hour and includes 18 questions that deal directly with memories of early attachment experiences. Subjects' responses are primarily categorized according to the degree to which semantic memory of the adults' own experience with significant caretakers is integrated successfully with episodic memories of the same figures to form coherent discourse. In scoring the AAI, persons are categorized as being either autonomous or insecure (a category that is further subdivided into three styles: dismissive, preoccupied/enmeshed, and unresolved with respect to loss or trauma). It is the quality of the adult's narrative and his or her ability to integrate disparate memories while staying in meaningful relation to the interviewer that determine the categorization of secure and insecure, not the specifics of the memories themselves. Thus it is possible for a person to have had a highly distressed or traumatic childhood and at the same time be judged autonomous as an adult and thus be likely to have children who are themselves securely attached.

Autonomous adults are easily able to recall early relationships; they speak about attachment in a way that suggests prior reflection and integration and do not unrealistically overidealize their parents or past experiences. They are able to provide convincing event or episodic memories supporting their semantic generalizations about their relationship with their own parents. They demonstrate "autobiographical competence" (Holmes, 1995). They are unencumbered by pervasive defensive processes such as blanket denial or manic reversal of affect, and their style of regulating affect is flexible. Their past experiences can be remembered and reflected on flexibly and openly, sometimes resulting in a change of opinion or judgment during the course of the interview. This capacity to consider and reflect Main (1991) termed "metacognitive monitoring." One way of thinking about metacognitive monitoring, as suggested by Main and Hesse, is that it entails the ability to move back and forth between maintaining a coherent dialogue with the interviewer and accessing one's own memories, memories that may in some cases be painful and upsetting.

A parent with a dismissive style is predicted to foster an avoidant attachment relationship with his or her child. Such parents in the interview minimize the importance of their early experiences in shaping their current behavior and often tend to describe their childhood relationships in globally positive and idealized terms (e.g., "It was great"). In general, however, they dismiss attachment relationships as being of little concern, value, or influence, and they often have great difficulty remembering specific early relationship experiences or describing them with any feeling or insight. It is thought that a dismissive style is likely to consolidate in a context of parental rejection with the further implication being that this style obscures the reality of that rejection and thus softens or obviates the memory of disappointment and hurt. When negative memories do surface during the interview, the common strategy for regulating affect is to minimize and discount such memories as unimportant. These adults seem detached from the feelings that are activated by these memories.

From the point of view of narrative coherence, the representation of early memories offered by dismissive subjects is judged to be unpersuasive because the negative aspects of them are not integrated into the narrative. Either semantic generalization (e.g., "My childhood was just great") is discrepant with the apparent reality of the relationships being described or else episodic memories are simply not available to support the semantic generalizations. This strategy of minimizing the impact of attachment experiences preserves the individual's sense of autonomy but compromises his or her capacity for intimacy. The children of such parents will exhibit much the same strategy in their behavioral reaction to the Strange Situation (i.e., they will act hyperindependent and will not seek comfort when the parent returns after an absence). Yet, the appearance is deceiving; when studied closely, their cortisol levels reveal that such avoidant children are in fact highly stressed (Spangler and Grossmann, 1993).

Individuals with a preoccupied/enmeshed style as categorized by the AAI are still preoccupied with their parents and memories of their relationship with their parents and are still actively struggling to please them, still angrily struggling against them, or both. Narrative incoherence in describing early experiences is highest in this group and affect is maximized in their narratives. Such a parent is often flooded with memories of early affect-laden experiences but lacks the capacity to place these in any perspective. It is thought that in general, a preoccupied/enmeshed style is constructed in the context of often intense but highly inconsistent parental attunement. Emotional availability is determined primarily by the parents' needs and not by the needs of the child.

Unlike parents judged to be dismissive, parents judged to be preoccupied/enmeshed are able to access their emotional memories. What they have difficulty doing is accessing their memories and simultaneously organizing them in such a way as to allow them to maintain a relatedness with the interviewer in the sense of getting closure and returning the conversational turn. They seem at times to be drowning in their feelings, and often the interviewer feels the same way. Put another way, these parents seem to be ambivalently attached to their own emotional histories, just as one would expect their children to be ambivalently but intensely preoccupied with them in the Strange Situation.

Parents who are unresolved with respect to trauma or abuse are considered by Main to differ from both autonomous parents and those with dismissive or preoccupied attachment styles in that they are unable to prevent breakdowns in their attempt to maintain a coherent strategy vis-à-vis their attachment experiences. The AAI has specific questions with regard to trauma, loss, and abuse, and some individuals who would otherwise be classified as secure (or insecure) will show momentary lapses in responding to these questions that seem to reflect the intrusion of typically sealed-off memories or else an unusual absorption in these memories. Talking about a dead parent as if he or she were still alive is an example; lapsing into eulogistic speech is another. The lapse in metacognitive monitoring is suggestive of a momentary state change triggered by the memory; it is as if the person is suddenly somewhere else. There is growing evidence that affect in these individuals is partly regulated by dissociation (Main and Hesse, 1992; Liotti, 1995; Schuengel et al., 1997). However, in the interview situation the person quickly regains his or her composure, and the conversation resumes. More recent evidence suggests that in individuals with histories of abuse during childhood, the lapses appear to be more pervasive and also show a more global lack of organization in comparison with individuals burdened with unresolved loss (Hesse, 1996).

Attachment researchers have found that unresolved loss of significant attachment figures through death and also unresolved experiences of physical and sexual abuse in the parent's history are linked to disorganized/disoriented behavior in children. Main and Hesse (1990) have put forth the hypothesis that "the traumatized adult's continuing state of fear together with its interaction/behavioral concomitant (frightened or frightening behavior or both) is the mechanism linking unresolved trauma to the infant's display of disorganized/disoriented behavior" (p. 163).

Very recent studies from Leiden University (Schuengel et al., 1997) carry this work even further by directly testing Main and Hesse's transmission hypothesis. The Leiden researchers studied a group of mothers known to have had important losses and made direct observations of their frightening, frightened, and dissociated behaviors while interacting with their children. These observations were correlated with the mothers' AAI status. The results showed first, as expected, that among insecurely attached mothers the presence of unresolved loss led to a *greater* incidence of frightening maternal behaviors and a correspondingly greater incidence of infant disorganization. But the second finding, far less intuitively obvious, is that securely attached (autonomous) mothers with unresolved loss actually showed less frightened and frightening behaviors than did securely attached mothers without this history of unresolved loss. This fascinating finding demonstrates the important protective role of a secure attachment and suggests that unresolved but otherwise secure mothers must call on some mechanism, some strategy, to protect their children from the impact of their disorganized and dissociated states. It seems likely that securely attached mothers with unresolved loss must be more vigilant than their counterparts with no unresolved loss in preventing their own affective experience from contaminating their child's experience. It also seems likely that the mothers must be able to regulate intense negative affect even when the child may be the direct stimulus to activating their affect. Fonagy's theoretical proposals provide a powerful explanation for how this might come about. Fonagy would argue that securely attached mothers despite their unresolved traumas are able to hold their child's experience and needs in mind in such a way that prevents them from discharging or dumping their own unresolved fears and anxiety onto the child. The study of the micromechanisms involved in these processes will be an important avenue for future research.

The remarkable achievement of attachment researchers is that they have been able to demonstrate beyond all doubt—and do this cross-culturally—that security of attachment is an intergenerational phenomenon. That is to say, the security of attachment in the child is directly correlated with the parent's state of mind in relation to attachment in a way that suggests that working models of attachment are often handed from one generation to the next. Statistically, the clearest concordance is between autonomous adults and their securely attached children on one hand and between insecure adults, taken in aggregate, and their insecurely attached children, also taken in aggregate, on the other hand. (It is important to remember, however, that though the child of an autonomous parent is likely to be securely attached to *that parent*, he or she will not necessarily display the same pattern in relation to the other parent or other attachment figures.) The degree of concordance between parent and child within the various insecure subcategories is somewhat less impressive—a matter still under investigation. Nonetheless, it does appear that, as predicted, parents classified as dismissive in general tend to have children exhibiting an avoidant style and, also as predicted, that parents classified as unresolved tend to have children exhibiting a disorganized-disoriented attachment style. But in addition, a sizable minority of parents classified as unresolved who would otherwise have been classified as secure except for a few momentary lapses on the AAI do in fact have securely attached children.

The findings in relation to the disorganized-disoriented attachment style are of the greatest importance in working with seriously disturbed children from an object relations perspective. A characteristic style in attachment relationship reflects an amalgam of the child's history with the parents. Thus, encapsulated within a particular style is not only whether a parent has been able to function as a secure base for the child, but how he or she has managed the inevitable disruptions in the attachment relationship, no matter whether these have been brought on by actual separations, negative affective reactions in the child, or factors within the parent. That is to say, we have within each style characteristic strategies for managing negative affect and characteristic patterns for negotiating situations of disruption and repair. To put it another way, in the child's reactions to the parent in the Strange Situation we have, in a single episode, the cumulative history of the child's experience of the disruption and repair (Beebe et al., 1997) of his or her relationship with that particular caregiver, a history moreover that is now evidenced in the child's intrapsychic organization. Where the child exhibits an insecure form of attachment, it is an indication that the history is one of systematic failures to meet the child empathically. Even more important, where the child exhibits a disorganized-disoriented attachment style, it is a signal that that history has been so fraught with contradiction that the child has been unable to find any stable means for working out a strategy for regulating his or her attachment needs in the context of that relationship.[3] Moreover, the greater likelihood is that at least one parent of this child is insecurely attached and unresolved for loss or abuse; rather than reacting to the child, he or she is likely, in matters large and small and over a greater or lesser extent of time, not responding to the child at all, but is responding instead, whether consciously or unconsciously, to the reactivated memories of his or her own past.[4]

Clinicians, however, have been slow to appreciate the importance of this research into the intergenerational transmission of attachment security. It is here where the programmatic research of Fonagy, Target, and their colleagues is, in my view, particularly valuable. To begin with, following the suggestion of Miriam Steele, they have been able to accurately predict the attachment status of first born infants at 12 months in

---

[3] Space does not permit a fuller discussion here, but the reader should be alerted to the fact that attachment researchers ordinarily assign a secondary classification (i.e., secure/autonomous, avoidant/dismissive, ambivalent/enmeshed), on a best fit basis both to children classified as disorganized/disoriented or adults who are classified unresolved. Though undoubtedly important, the clinical implications of the various different types of combinations of primary and secondary classifications remained to be explored.

[4] The theory that has generated—and often confirmed—these powerful hypotheses is still, however, relatively young, and our understanding of the complexities of adults' state of mind in relation to attachment is as yet unrefined. Among many of the interesting areas currently being researched is the question of multiple working models of attachment in children and adults and the related issue of how and under what circumstances these are integrated.

75% of cases by assessing the mother's security of attachment during pregnancy. This is a remarkable accomplishment in its own right, not only in the history of psychoanalytic research but also in developmental research in general. We have an incontestable demonstration that the child's sense of security is, in fact, a function of measurable psychological characteristics in the parents. For the clinician who proceeds on an object relational basis, this demonstration has been long overdue.

Second, Fonagy and colleagues have been able to show that in the child the development of reflective self-functioning is, in fact, a demonstrable correlate of secure attachment. That is to say, children who are securely attached to at least one parent develop a theory of mind earlier, and they are better able to use it in situations that are emotionally charged. Conversely, children who are insecurely attached to their parents develop this dimension more slowly, and it is more subject to disruption in situations that are laden with emotional conflict. Thus, Fonagy and Target's suggestion that the more severely disturbed children suffer from a lack in reflective-function whereas the less severely disturbed children possess it to a greater or lesser degree falls in line with what has otherwise been learned about the relation of attachment security and insecurity to the presence or absence of psychopathology.

Third, and most important, Fonagy and colleagues have been able to demonstrate that the presence of reflective-functioning in the parents is highly protective for the next generation. That is to say, parents who themselves have suffered significant loss or abuse in childhood but who are high in reflective-functioning tend to have children who are securely attached. Such parents coming from a disadvantageous past, when they lack this capacity, are at significant risk to pass on patterns of abuse or the sequelae of unresolved loss to their children.

In a separate study relating to adult psychopathology, Fonagy and his colleagues (1995) showed that where there is a preexisting history of abuse and this is coupled with low reflective-functioning, the overwhelming likelihood is that the adult will meet the criteria for a diagnosis of borderline personality disorder. By demonstrating that this epidemiological finding explicates the phenomenology of typical borderline transference constellations in significant ways, Fonagy and colleagues have made a major contribution to our understanding of borderline psychopathology.

Taken together, the findings in regard to attachment suggest that reflective-functioning is not just a philosophical or developmental concept but rather an essential, if heretofore unrecognized, aspect in the transmission of attachment security from one generation to the next. Moreover, it is of particular relevance in those situations where the existence of loss or abuse in the parents' histories might otherwise work to derail the normal functioning of the attachment bond. Conversely, its absence is of particular relevance in those situations that lead to severe psychopathology in the child. Thus, not only have Fonagy, Target, and their colleagues advanced attachment research generally, but they have done so in a way that is directly relevant for clinicians.

In this context, one can offer a reconceptualization of Fonagy and Target's recommendations pertaining to technical interventions in child psychoanalytic psychotherapy by comparing these interventions with processes ordinarily found in the secure attachment bond. Fonagy and Target are suggesting that the therapist provide experiences that will strengthen the development of reflective-functioning in the child and thereby repair defects that have accrued from the child's attachment history. In this way, the therapist enables the child to catch up with other children who presumably have had these experiences provided for them by their parents. Since Winnicott, we are familiar with the analogies between the analyst and the "good enough" mother. The transformative feature of therapeutic process that Fonagy and Target theorize can be seen as a more refined estimate of "good enough" specifically tailored for the therapeutic encounter. Experiences that promote reflective-functioning, one could argue, are that facet ordinarily found in secure attachment relationships that can in fact be provided in intensive therapy. I believe that it is a measure of the validity of this overall vision of how therapeutic activity might relate to ordinary "good enough" parenting that Fonagy and Target are able to delineate their understanding in terms of specific technical recommendations.

The Widening Scope of Child Psychoanalysis

The foregoing brings us to another way of appreciating what Fonagy and Target and their colleagues are bringing to the psychoanalytic table. They are inviting us to understand the more severely impaired child in terms of what is known about attachment processes in general and what can be inferred about his or her personal attachment histories in particular. To be sure, in their article Fonagy and Target do not discuss the two types of severely disturbed children who show profound deficits in reflective-functioning explicitly in terms of their attachment histories. The possibility of adopting such a vantage point is only implied, though it has been addressed more directly in their other publications. Yet, the implications are there to be drawn, and I think it is important to begin to draw them out.

If what distinguishes the more severely disturbed children from those who have single emotional disorders is, in fact, a deficit in reflective-functioning, and further, if the development of reflective-functioning is ordinarily contingent on the ongoing functioning of the attachment relationships and the continuing negotiation of situations of disruption and repair in that relationship, then what we encounter in the more seriously disturbed child—the very child for whom analytic intervention may be differentially helpful—are distortions in his or her sense of self that have arisen in the context of a severely impaired or derailed attachment relationship. If this is true—and the data increasingly converge around this understanding—then there are profound implications not only for how we work with these children individually but also for how we work with their families.

In this respect, Fonagy, Target, and their colleagues have revived Fraiberg, Adelson, and Shapiro's (1975) classic and brilliant understanding of "ghosts in the nursery" while extending it in a way that potentially offers a much more detailed understanding of the micro-processes involved. What Fraiberg et al. observed clinically was the phenomenon of intergenerational transfer of trauma. That is to say, experiences in the lives of parents were being replayed in the next generation, leaving the child highly traumatized. For Fraiberg, the critcal aspect of this transfer of trauma from one generation to the next was the mother's inability to recall her own affect from when she was a child. This incapacity rendered the mother unable, as Fraiberg poignantly put it, to hear her child crying.

To Fraiberg's conceptualization, Fonagy, Target and their colleagues have now added a second variable involved in the transfer of trauma—the mother's deficits in reflective-functioning. Besides the mother's inability to appreciate, let alone contain, the child's affective experience, they have identified the mother's further inability to keep her child's mind in mind. Combined, these deficits lead to repeated failures to grasp the child's own incipient effort to establish himself or herself as an intentional being in his or her own right. But these deficits can arise in more than one way and in more than one context. Here the conceptualizations that have been operationalized in attachment research offer a scaffolding that can enable the psychoanalytic clinician to frame increasingly detailed and subtle hypotheses as to what is going on, and has gone on, in a particular family.

To take a pertinent example, in the classic article by Fraiberg and her colleagues (1975), one can see what is clearly a dismissive and perhaps a dissociated style in the parent. The mother does not hear her child crying because she does not recall her own feelings. Having been herself traumatized but lacking the prophylactic ability to see her child's mind apart from her own, the dismissal of her own emotional memories, which is characteristic of a dismissive style, leaves her unable to grasp what her child is going through. But there can be other parents who do the opposite, who lose themselves in ongoing rumination about their parents and in an absorption in their emotional memories and yet who do not really hear their child cry either. Moreover, there can be parents who simply are unable to maintain a coherent style consistently. A mother who otherwise adopts a dismissive style may lapse into quite different mental states when memories of trauma and abuse are triggered. In these moments, she is after a fashion no longer in her "right mind." More important, in these moments, she no longer provides her child with a mirror in which he can see himself or herself as an incipiently intentional and propositional being, as someone potentially with a mind of his or her own. Thus, what registers as an unresolved classification on the AAI becomes in the nursery the basis for a disorganized-disoriented attachment style in the child and the beginnings of severe distortions in the child's self, distortions that not only will require intensive psychotherapeutic intervention at a later date, but will be perpetuated in the ongoing relationship between parent and child.

In general, I argue that the new research not only allows us to frame more refined hypotheses, as to the etiology of the child's difficulties, but also suggests new avenues for framing collateral work with parents. To begin with, it now becomes possible to try to understand parents in terms of their general orientation toward attachment and to see how their attachment styles have informed and fostered particular defensive strategies in the child, especially in the realm of affect regulation. Moreover, in some subgroups of otherwise well-functioning parents the failures in mirroring and affect containment can be observed to be specifically triggered by certain behaviors in the child (often a particular child) and in at least some instances can be most efficaciously addressed in that context. Consider for example the mother I mentioned earlier who screams at her child that he is a "killer." The roots of this mother's panic—a severe assault in early adolescence—can of course be addressed in her own treatment. More than likely, however, her treatment will take time, perhaps a great deal of time, and as Fraiberg et al. (1980) pointed out, it cannot be done fast enough for the rapidly developing child. From a child analytic perspective we need to help this mother to see that her panic is triggered whenever her boy does something that is assertive or aggressive and to help her work in a focal way on the unresolved trauma that his behavior is reactivating in her. From my own experience in working with traumatized children and their parents, this focal work can create surprisingly rapid changes in both the mother (and/or father) and the child. Moreover, insofar as this work is successful, it enables the mother (and/or father) to become an ally of treatment in a new way—by recognizing whatever it is that is triggering the inability to mirror the child's intentions in a way that helps the parent to see the child's experience more accurately and, in turn, to help the child to have a mind of his or her own.

Widening the scope of treatment along these lines is essentially consonant with recent innovations in psychoanalytically informed approaches to parent–child intervention. The past few years have seen a proliferation of exciting new approaches to working with parents (Cramer and Stern, 1988; Hopkins, 1992; Lieberman, 1992; Seligman, 1994; Stern, 1995; Slade, in press) that are based on the recognition that having the child in treatment can permit one to access the parents' difficulties more directly and often much more efficaciously than simply seeing the parents in their own treatment. This does not take away from the value of direct intensive psychoanalytic treatment of the child—far from it. The whole point of Fonagy and Target's articles, with which I am entirely in agreement, is to underline how vitally important intensive analytic intervention is with these children. But in future work, we need to begin to determine how the child's treatment can be supplemented and perhaps greatly enhanced by work with the parents. I am suggesting that as we begin to grasp the extent to which the child's difficulties are the sequellae of a derailed attachment system, we can become more sensitively attuned to the specific places where work with parents can be most profitable.

Fonagy and Target close their presentation by noting that what they are arguing for is not radically new. Indeed, it is not. Their suggestion that severe disorders in children require modifications of technique in the direction of prioritizing the enhancement of reflective-functioning, specifically through the relationship with the therapist but also through other means, is in line with much current thinking. Ultimately, Fonagy and Target's claim is a modest one: If their conceptualization and terminology enjoy a relative advantage over what has been advanced by others, this consists in the harmonization with the findings of contemporary developmental psychology. But I believe the authors are being too modest. From my point of view, the empirical link to attachment research allows this approach to become highly generative in a way that goes beyond our traditional conceptualizations. For by cross-correlating our clinical intuitions and observations with what is now known about parenting and early development, both in health and in illness, we can begin to frame far more detailed hypotheses about what is creating serious psychopathology in the children that we work with. Potentially we can also begin to generate technical interventions with parents that can be thought about more selectively and fruitfully than before. This is a major challenge to our field, but it is a challenge in the very best sense; it opens up the possibility for theoretical and technical creativity as we try to find out under what circumstances and with which cases and at what ages such interventions will prove most efficacious. This work will take many thoughtful clinicians to explore its many implications.

References

Ainsworth, M. D. S., Blehar, M. C., Waters, E. & Wall, S. (1978), *Patterns of Attachment: A Psychological Study of the Strange Situation*. Hillsdale, NJ: Lawrence Erlbaum Associates.

Beebe, B., Lachmann, F. & Jaffe, J. (1997), Mother–infant interactive structures and presymbolic self-object representation. *Psychoanal. Dial.*, 7:133–182.

Bion, W. R. (1962), *Learning from Experience*. London: Heinemann.

Bowlby, J. (1973), *Attachment and Loss: Volume II Separation*. New York: Basic Books.
——— (1980), *Attachment and Loss: Volume III Loss*. New York: Basic Books.

Bretherton, I. (1985), Attachment theory: Retrospect and prospect. In: *Growing Points of Attachment Theory and Research. Monographs for the Society for Research in Child Development*, ed. I. Bretherton & E. Waters. Serial No. 209, Vol. 50, Nos. 1–2, pp. 3–35.

——— McNew, S. & Beeghly-Smith, M. (1981), Early person knowledge as expressed in gestural and verbal communication: When do infants acquire a "theory of mind"? In: *Infant Social Cognition*, ed. M. E. Lamb & L. R. Sherrod. Hillsdale, NJ: Lawrence Erlbaum Associates, pp. 333–373.

Britton, R. (1992), In: *Clinical Lectures on Klein and Bion*, ed. R. Anderson. London: Tavistock/Routledge.

Cassidy, J. (1994), Emotion regulation: Influences of attachment relationships. In: *Biological and Behavioral Foundations of Emotion Regulation. Monographs of the Society for Research in Child Development*, ed. N. Fox. Serial No. 240, Vol. 69, pp. 228–250.

——— & Berlin, L. J. (1994), The insecure/ambivalent pattern of attachment: Theory and research. *Child Devel.*, 65:971–991.

Cooper, A. (1993), On empirical research. *J. Amer. Psychoanal. Assn.*, 41 (Suppl.): 381–391.

Cramer, B. & Stern, D. N. (1988), Evaluation of changes in mother–infant brief psychotherapy: A single case study. *Infant Mental Health J.*, 9:20–45.

Dennett, D. C. (1978), *Brainstorms*. Cambridge, MA: MIT Press.

Diamond, D. & Blatt, S. (1994), Internal working models and the representational world in attachment and psychoanalytic theories. In: *Attachment in Adults: Clinical and Developmental Perspectives*, ed. M. Sperling & W. Berman. New York: Guilford, pp. 72–98.

Fonagy, P. (1991), Thinking about thinking: Some clinical and theoretical considerations in the treatment of a borderline patient. *Internat. J. Psycho-Anal.*, 72: 639–656.

———— Steele, M., Moran, G., Steele, H. & Higgitt, A. (1993), Measuring the ghost in the nursery: An empirical study of the relation between parents' mental representations of childhood experiences and their infants' security of attachment. *J. Amer. Psychoanal. Assn.*, 41:929–989.

———— ———— Steele, H., Leigh, T., Kennedy, R., Mattoon, G. & Target, M. (1995), Attachment, the reflective self, and borderline states: The predictive specificity of the Adult Attachment Interview and pathological emotional development. In: *Attachment Theory: Social, Developmental and Clinical Perspectives*. ed. S. Goldberg, R. Muir & J. Kerr. Hillsdale, NJ: The Analytic Press, pp. 233–278.

———— ———— ———— Moran, G. & Higgitt, A. (1991), The capacity for understanding mental states: The reflective self in parent and child and its significance for security of attachment. *Infant Mental Health J.*, 12:201–217.

———— ———— (1996), Playing with reality. I. *Internat. J. Psycho-Anal.*, 77:217–234.

———— & Target, M. (1995), Towards an understanding of violence: The use of the body and the role of the father. *Internat. J. Psycho-Anal.*, 76:487–501.

Fraiberg, S., Adelson, E. & Shapiro, V. (1975), Ghosts in the nursery: A psychoanalytic approach to the problems of impaired infant-mother relationships. *J. Amer. Acad. Child Psychiat.*, 14:387–421.

———— Shapiro, V. & Cherniss, D. S. (1980), Treatment modalities. In: *Clinical Studies in Infant Mental Health: The First Year of Life*, ed. S. Fraiberg. New York: Basic Books, pp. 49–77.

George, C., Kaplan, N. & Main, M. (1985), The Berkeley Adult Attachment Interview. Unpublished manuscript, Department of Psychology, University of California, Berkeley.

Haft, W. & Slade, A. (1989), Affect attunement and maternal attachment: A pilot study. *Infant Mental Health J.*, 10:157–172.

Hesse, E. (1996), Discourse, memory, and the adult attachment interview: A note with emphasis on the emerging cannot classify category. *Infant Mental Health J.*, 17:4–11.

Holmes, J. (1995), Something there is that doesn't love a wall: John Bowlby, attachment theory and psychoanalysis. In: *Attachment Theory: Social, Developmental, and Clinical Perspectives*, ed. S. Goldberg, R. Muir & J. Kerr. Hillsdale, NJ: The Analytic Press, pp. 19–45.

Hopkins, J. (1992), Parent-infant psychotherapy. *J. Child Psychother.*, 18:5–17.

Kennedy, H. & Moran, G. (1991), Reflections on the aim of child analysis. *The Psychoanalytic Study of the Child*, 46:181–198. New Haven, CT: Yale University Press.

Kobak, R. R. & Sceery, A. (1988), Attachment in late adolescence: Working models, affect regulation, and representation of self and others. *Child Devel.*, 59:135–146.

———— Cole, H. E., Ferenz-Gillies, R. & Fleming, W. S. (1993), Attachment and emotion regulation during mother-teen problem solving: A control theory analysis. *Child Devel.*, 64:231–245.

Lieberman, A. F. (1992), Infant-parent psychotherapy with toddlers. *Devel. & Psychopath.*, 4: 559–574.

Liotti, G. (1995), Disorganized/disoriented attachment in the psychotherapy of the dissociative disorder. In: *Attachment Theory: Social, Developmental, and Clinical Perspectives*, ed. S. Goldberg, R. Muir & J. Kerr. Hillsdale, NJ: The Analytic Press, pp. 343–367.

Lyons-Ruth, K. (1991), Rapprochement or approchement: Mahler's theory reconsidered from the vantage point of recent research on early attachment relationships. *Psychoanal. Psychol.*, 8:1–23.

Main, M. (1991), Metacognitive knowledge, metacognitive monitoring and singular (coherent) vs. multiple (incoherent) model of attachment: Findings and directions for future research. In: *Attachment Across the Life Cycle*, ed. C. Parkes, J. Stevenson-Hinde & P. Marris. London: Routledge, pp. 127–160.

—— (1995), Discourse, prediction and studies in attachment: Implications for psychoanalysis. In: *Research in Psychoanalysis: Process, Development, Outcome*, ed. T. Shapiro & R. N. Emde. Madison, CT: International Universities Press, pp. 209–245.

—— & Hesse, E. (1990), Parents' unresolved traumatic experiences are related to infant disorganized attachment status: Is frightened and/or frightening parental behavior the linking mechanism? In: *Attachment in the Preschool Years: Theory, Research, and Intervention*, ed. M. T. Greenberg, D. Cicchetti & E. M. Cummings. Chicago: University of Chicago Press, pp. 161–182.

—— —— (1992), Disorganized/disoriented infant behavior in the Strange Situation, lapses in the monitoring of reasoning and discourse during the parent's Adult Attachment Interview, and dissociative states. In: *Attachment and Psychoanalysis*, ed. M. Ammaniti & D. Stern. Rome: Gius, Laterza & Figli, pp. 86–140.

—— Kaplan, N. & Cassidy, J. (1985), Security in infancy, childhood, and adulthood: A move to the level of representation. In: *Growing Points of Attachment Theory and Research. Monographs of the Society for Research in Child Development*, ed. I. Bretherton & E. Waters. Serial No. 209, Vol. 50, Nos. 1–2, pp. 66–104.

Mayes, L. & Cohen, D. J. (1996), Children's developing theory of mind. *J. Amer. Psychoanal. Assn.*, 44:117–142.

Mossler, D. G., Marvin, R. S. & Greenberg, M. T. (1976), Conceptual perspective taking in 2–6-year-old children. *Devel. Psychol.*, 12:85–86.

Ogden, T. H. (1994), *Subjects of Analysis*. Northvale, NJ: Aronson.

Osofsky, J. D. (1995), Perspective on attachment and psychoanalysis. *Psychoanal. Psychol.*, 12:347–363.

Perner, J., Ruffman, T. & Leekman, S. (1994), Theory of mind is contagious: You catch it from your sibs. *Child Devel.*, 65:1228–1238.

Sandler, J., ed. (1987), *Projection, Identification, Projective Identification*. Madison, CT: International Universities Press.

—— & Rosenblatt, B. (1962), The concept of the representational world. *The Psychoanalytic Study of the Child*, 18:128–148. New York: International Universities Press.

Schuengel, C., van IJzendoorn, M. H., Bakermans-Kranenburg, J. & Blom, H. (1997), Frightening, frightened, and dissociated behavior, unresolved loss and infant disorganization. Presented at biennial meeting of the Society for Research in Child Development, Washington, DC.

Seligman, S. (1994), Applying psychoanalysis in an unconventional context: Adapting infant-parent psychotherapy to a changing population. *The Psychoanalytic Study of the Child*, 49:481–510. New Haven, CT: Yale University Press.

Silverman, D. K. (1991), Attachment patterns and Freudian theory: An integrative proposal. *Psychoanal. Psychol.*, 8:169–194.

Slade, A. (2003), Representation, symbolization and affect regulation in the concomitant treatment of a mother and child: Attachment theory and child psychotherapy. *Psychoanal. Inq.*, 23:521–529.

———— & Aber, J. L. (1992), Attachments, drives, and development: Conflicts and convergences in theory. In: *Interface of Psychoanalysis and Psychology*, ed. J. W. Barron, M. N. Eagle & D. L. Wolitzky. Washington, DC: American Psychological Association, pp. 154–185.

Spangler, G. & Grossmann, K. E. (1993), Biobehavioral organization in securely and insecurely attached infants. *Child Devel.*, 64:1439–1450.

Stern, D. (1985), *The Interpersonal World of the Infant*. New York: Basic Books.

———— (1995), *The Motherhood Constellation: A Unified View of Parent-Infant Psychotherapy*. New York: Basic Books.

Trevarthen, C. (1987), Brain development. In: *The Oxford Companion to the Mind*, ed. R. L. Gregory. Oxford: Oxford University Press, pp. 101–110.

van IJzendoorn, M. H. (1995), Adult attachment representation, parental responsiveness, and infant attachment: A meta-analysis on the predictive validity of the Adult Attachment Interview. *Psychol. Bull.*, 117:387–403.

Wimmer, H. & Perner, J. (1983), Beliefs about beliefs: Representation and constraining function of wrong beliefs in young children's understanding of deception. *Cognition*, 13:103–128.

Winnicott, D. W. (1965), *The Maturational Processes and the Facilitating Environment*. New York: International Universities Press.

———— (1967), Mirror-role of mother and family in child development. In: *Playing and Reality*. New York: Basic Books, 1971, pp. 111–118.

———— (1971), *Playing and Reality*. New York: Basic Books.

The Two-Person Unconscious: Intersubjective Dialogue, Enactive Relational Representation, and the Emergence of New Forms of Relational Organization

(1999)

Karlen Lyons-Ruth

▼ ▼ ▼ ▼ ▼

Editors' Introduction

In this essay rigor is combined with creativity to outline a model for early "relational knowing." Psychoanalysts reading this essay are carefully inducted into a world of empirical work on early dyadic life, early forms of representation of relational dialogic patterns, and the status and function of affect development and its impact on meaning making. The core activity of psychoanalytic work—meaning making—is in this essay set out as a relational creation. Relational psychoanalysts can now appreciate the developmental grounding of social constructionist ideas of the cocreation of psychic reality and meaning. For Lyons-Ruth, the individual psychic experiences of agency, of intentionality, of meaning making arise in a dynamic dyadic form, laid down through processes of relational transaction.

Lyons-Ruth is interested here in working out a particular picture of development. She stresses fluidity and nonlinearity. When she describes the continuous and transformational interplay of the nonverbal and symbolic, always elaborated across persons as well as within minds, she is proposing a developmental model more consistent with dynamic systems theory than with linear stage models. While procedural, or relational, knowing and symbolic representation are both parallel and interdependent processes, Lyons-Ruth notes the transformative potential in procedural knowing as a mechanism for psychic transformation. She thus contributes to the growing debate on the power of attachment and relational processes over the power of interpretation as sites for mutative action in psychoanalysis. She makes this contribution with a clear appreciation for the subtle interplay of these forces of change while emphasizing the power in the procedural realm.

Since this essay was written, Lyons-Ruth has gone on to develop a very complex and sophisticated account of the particular intrapsychic and interpersonal outcome of one kind of attachment pattern: disorganized attachment. She has been developing a clinically relevant picture of the impact of a frightened and frightening caregiver on mental and relational processes in a young child. The impact of these kinds of distortions in attachment appear both in the long range and in the short range. Such early patterned experiences have effects on mentalization, on capacities to be self-regulating, and on capacities to be intimately connected to other beings.

The Two-Person Unconscious:
Intersubjective Dialogue, Enactive Relational Representation, and the Emergence of New Forms of Relational Organization*

❧   ❧   ❧   ❧   ❧

Recent psychoanalytic theory has moved increasingly toward a relational, intersubjective, and social–constructivist stance. In this view the psychoanalytic encounter is seen as mutually co-constructed between two active participants, with the subjectivities of both patient and analyst

* Originally published in *Psychoanalytic Inquiry*, 19:576–617. © 1999 The Analytic Press, Inc.

contributing to the form and content of the dialogue that emerges between them (McLaughlin, 1991; Hoffman, 1992; Ogden, 1994). The current emphasis in analytic writing on the importance of enactments in the treatment situation attempts to keep the lens focused squarely on the point of contact between the two analytic participants and on the form of the implicit transactions that emerge between them (e.g., Ogden, 1994). Clinical descriptions acknowledge the active contributions of both partners to the co-construction of the enactment, even though the primary clinical interest may be in those features of the enactment that echo problematic aspects of the patient's interactions with other important people (Jacobs, 1991; Hoffman, 1992). Enactments have been viewed as important opportunities to gain a window on unconscious motivation; and meanings held by the patient that have not been previously recognized or articulated (McLaughlin, 1991).

In this shift to a more fluid and mutual view of therapeutic process the need for a psychoanalytic model of development has increasingly been questioned (e.g., Mitchell, 1988). Converging pressures or psychoanalytic theories of mind and of development have come from the increasing sophistication of both behavioral and neuroscientific research. New findings regarding the development and organization of mind, brain, and behavior have outstripped the pace of change in psychoanalytic theory, further undermining the credibility of older developmental models. In contrast to these changes that have fostered scepticism about the role of developmental theory, longitudinal attachment research has provided recent consistent support for the view that important dimensions of relational behavior are grounded in relational history. This emerging developmental research base supports the continued relevance of developmental history to psychoanalytic process and the concomitant need to refashion a psychoanalytic metatheory that is consistent both with the new research base and with a more fluid, mutual, and constructivist view of relational change in adulthood.

The initial questions that led to the concerns in this paper were questions taken as a focus by the Process of Change Study Group of Boston, namely: what are the noninterpretive mechanisms of change that operate in the psychoanalytic situation, and how might the study of development illuminate these mechanisms of change? These questions are more directly addressed in related papers (Boston Process of Change Study Group, 1998; Stern et al., 1998). In struggling with these questions, however, it became apparent that to consider how noninterpretive mechanisms lead to change, one also has to grapple with the issue of what changes.

Psychoanalysis has always been concerned with understanding the organization of meaning, with affects viewed as the central guides and directors of meaning. New research is now pressing psychoanalytically oriented scholars to expand accounts of how meaning systems are organized to include implicit or procedural forms of knowing. Procedural knowing refers to knowing how to do something and how to behave adaptively, rather than knowing information or images that can be consciously recalled and recounted (Cohen and Squire, 1980). The organization of memory and meaning in the implicit or enactive domain only becomes manifest in the doing. In accord with the current psychoanalytic interest in enactments in psychoanalytic treatment, I will refer to "knowing how to do" as enactive representation (see also Bruner, Olver, and Greenfield, 1966).

The central postulates of this paper will be (1) that much of our relational experience is represented in an implicit procedural or enactive form that is unconscious, though not necessarily dynamically unconscious; (2) that in both development and psychoanalysis, the increasing integration and articulation of new enactive "procedures for being with" destabilize existing enactive organization and serve as a primary engine of change; and (3) that enactive procedures become more articulated and integrated through participation in more coherent and collaborative forms of intersubjective interaction. Put another way, at the level of unconscious enactive procedures, the medium is the message; that is, the organization of meaning is implicit in the organization of the enacted relational dialogue and does not require reflective thought or verbalization to be, in some sense, known. In accord with infant observers such as Beebe and Lachmann (1994), enactive representation is viewed here as the earliest medium through which the "shadow of the object" becomes part of the "unthought known" of the infant's early experience (Bollas, 1987).

This paper will attempt to make more explicit a model of the development and change of enactive relational procedures that is consistent both with recent psychoanalytic literature and with recent findings in attachment research, early parent–infant interaction, cognitive neuroscience, and nonlinear dynamic systems theory. Attachment research has concentrated on describing and validating a range of organized strategies of caregiver–infant interaction around attachment needs that are represented by the infant by the end of the first year. More recent work has extended these descriptions of the infant's enactive representations around attachment needs to include the parent's corresponding enactive strategies for ways of responding to an interview about his or her own early attachment-related experiences. Although the details of these patterns of enactive relational representation in the realm of attachment experiences are important in themselves, they have been well described in the literature and will not be reviewed here (see Bretherton, 1988; Main, 1993; Lyons-Ruth and Jacobvitz, 1999). Instead, the focus of this paper will be on the implications of such enduring attachment-oriented enactive relational procedures for a general developmental-psychoanalytic theory of relational process and enactive representation. Attachment research has provided the most extensive empirical basis for this synthesis, but work on early face-to-face interaction and work on context-sensitive models of brain development and cognitive development, as well as research on adult cognition, also contribute to the emergence of the model.

Because it seems premature to rigidify a set of terms for describing this new conceptual territory, I will refer interchangeably to enactive representations, relational procedures, or implicit relational control systems. I use the term *representation* in relation to enactive knowing because, in keeping with prior psychoanalytic insights, this form of representation preserves knowledge of the affective-perceptual and spatio-temporal contingencies in the environment. I will also use *implicit* and *unconscious* interchangeably here to refer to the nondynamic procedural unconscious.

A central contention of this paper is that enactive knowing develops and changes by processes that are intrinsic to this system of representation and that do not rely on translation of procedures into reflective (symbolized) knowledge. This is not to contend that translating enactive knowledge into words may not be an important therapeutic tool or developmental step; it is to contend that development does not proceed only or primarily by moving from procedural coding to symbolic coding (*or* from primary to secondary process *or* from preverbal to verbal forms of thought). Procedural forms of representation are not infantile but are intrinsic to human cognition at all ages and underlie many forms of skilled action, including intimate social interaction.

The elaboration of symbolic forms of thought, including both images and words, contains the potential to contribute to the reorganization of enactive knowing. However, I would contend that retranscription of implicit relational knowing into symbolic knowing is laborious, is not intrinsic to the affect-based relational system, is never completely accomplished, and is not how developmental change in implicit relational knowing is generally accomplished. Rather, I would argue that procedural systems of relational knowing develop in parallel with symbolic systems, as separate systems with separate governing principles. Procedural systems influence and are influenced by symbolic systems through multiple cross-system connections, but these influences are necessarily incomplete. Furthermore, enactive relational knowing is grounded in goal-directed action, along with the affective evaluations guiding that action, and so is likely to exert as much or more influence on how symbolic systems are elaborated as symbolic systems exert on how relational systems are elaborated (see Anderson, 1982; Schacter and Moscovitch, 1984; Damasio, 1994).

I sketch the outlines of a theory of psychoanalytic and developmental change based on unconscious or implicit enactive representation and patient–therapist transactions rather than on symbolized meaning and interpretation. This focus on the two-person process is intended to establish a theoretical framework through which long-standing clinical insights on the interplay of affect, conflict, defense, and resistance can be further extended into a two-person realm and given a scientifically credible developmental base. Although constructs of motivation and, to some extent, affect are not dealt with extensively here, they are intrinsic to any theory of enactive representation, and the current framework is intended to augment, not replace, the extensive literature on affect and motivation in analytic treatment. Similarly, many points of interface where the model described in this paper might converge with or complement self psychological or conflict models of intrapsychic organization are not made explicit here. Instead, the paper focuses on extending our conceptualization of the transactional space and its representational forms in development and in psychoanalytically oriented treatment.

The paper is divided into two parts. The first section focuses on the two-person dialogue in early development. Three central implications of current attachment research are highlighted. First, more flexible and inclusive enactive representations emerge from more collaborative forms of parent–child dialogue. Second, adult neuroscience converges with infant research to confirm the separate and dissociable status of conscious symbolized knowledge and nonsymbolized implicit or procedural knowing throughout the lifespan. Third, prior to the outset of symbol use, the infant's implicit relational procedures include indicators of conflict and defense that are tied to particular restrictions or distortions in the parent-infant affective dialogue.

The second section of the paper explores noninterpretive mechanisms of change in implicit relational control systems. The developmental models of Fischer (1980) and Case (1991) are reviewed which emphasize the context-dependent and fractionated nature of the development of skilled behavior, in both relational and nonrelational domains. Most importantly, Fischer and Case elaborate developmental models of how more complex control systems are elaborated from infancy to adulthood by coordinating enactive procedures with one another to form progressively more flexible and inclusive skills. A strength of these models is their emphasis on the analysis of task complexity, a complexity that is independent of whether the task requires verbalized knowing or more implicit procedural problem solving. The increasing articulation and coordination of task components in these models offers a view of how enactive procedures may become more coordinated, articulated, flexible, and inclusive as they are repeatedly applied, without verbal articulation of the procedure itself. Some unique features of enactive procedures for doing things with others are also considered, features that are central to psychoanalytic concerns but that have not been articulated in the literature on cognition.

Finally, nonlinear dynamic systems principles are evoked to account for how the slow transactional process of repeated relational encounters in the psychoanalytic situation can result in increased complexity and organization in the patient's (and analyst's) relational procedures. From a self-organizing systems perspective, this increased articulation destabilizes old forms of organization and eventually crystallizes a shift to an emergent new form of procedural organization that is more complex and coherent.

Part I: Developmental Origins of Enactive Relational Procedures

Collaborative Dialogue and Coherence in Enactive Representations

Both the analyst–patient relationship and the parent–infant relationship share a focus on facilitating developmental change—for our purposes here, change particularly in the area of constructing new possibilities for adaptive regulation of intersubjective experiences. In addition, the analyst has the much more demanding charge of facilitating the deconstruction of established but unsatisfying ways of "being with" while simultaneously moving toward the new.

This focus on understanding and deconstructing the old has captured much of the attention of psychoanalytic writers in the past. Psychoanalytic clinicians have inherited a well-articulated descriptive language of individual psychopathology. With this has come an indispensable understanding of how to read some of the intricate and creative defensive maneuvers available to adapt to painful and constricting environments. To some extent, however, psychoanalytic theorists have concentrated on exploring the internalized forms of pathological representations and their emergence in the transference with less attention to articulating the developmental requirements for the co-construction of more flexible, coherent, and adaptive ways of being with others.

Attachment research has demonstrated that the development of coherent "internal working models of attachment" or implicit relational procedures is tied to participation in coherent forms of parent–child dialogue (see van IJzendoorn, 1994, metaanalysis; Main and Goldwyn, 1994). *Dialogue* is being used here in its broadest sense to encompass all avenues of interpersonal communication, including the affective communications inherent in movement, timing of behavior, and speech contour, as well as in gestural and affective signals. *Coherence* is being used as defined in relation to adult attachment representations by Main and Goldwyn (1994), following the philosopher Grice (1975). According to Grice (1975), coherence in communication is achieved by adhering to maxims governing quantity, quality, relation, and manner, that is, being truthful, clear, relevant, and succinct, yet complete. These qualities serve to maximize the overriding communicative principle of cooperation between participants. Thus, coherent dialogue is truthful and collaborative. This definition might also serve as a first-level working model for capturing essential attributes of coherent clinical dialogue as defined in contemporary two-person models.

The attachment research literature offers a perspective on what might be termed some essential features of collaborative dialogue. Studying the early parent–child communication process provides one laboratory for observing how various organizations of dialogue play out over developmental time. Longitudinal attachment studies give some insight into the kinds of parent–child dialogue associated with the child's development of coherent and flexible enactive procedural models for negotiating in relationships. Collaborative and flexible parent–infant dialogues have been termed *open communication* in the developmental attachment literature but this term is subject to misinterpretation. Coherent, or "open," dialogue is characterized, not by parental "openness" in the sense of unmonitored parental self-disclosure, but by parental "openness" to the state of mind of the child, including the entire array of the child's communications, so that particular affective or motive states of the child (anger, passion, distress) are not foreclosed from intersubjective sharing and regulation.

Attachment studies typically assess parental "sensitivity" as the aspect of parental behavior associated with infant attachment security (van IJzendoorn, 1994). However, it became clear in our own work on early interaction that what is required from the parent to merit this description is a continuing attempt to apprehend the infant's current subjective reality (affect state, current desired goal, and level of understanding) and an attempt to devise a response that acknowledges and comments or elaborates on that state ("You want the glass? No, you can't have the glass; it might break. Take this cup." "Maybe this block could be a house. Do you want this to be a house? What kind of house shall we make?") (Lyons-Ruth, Bronfman, and Atwood, 1999; Lyons-Ruth, Bronfman, and Parsons, 1999). Collaborative dialogue, then, is about getting to know another's mind and taking it into account in constructing and regulating interactions. The process of creating adequate intersubjective recognition in development requires close attention to the child's initiatives in interaction because, through these initiatives, the child communicates his or her local and general goals (motives) and their associated meaning structures. Without recognition of one person's initiatives or communications by another, no intersubjectivity or dyadic regulation is possible.

Observation of videotapes of parents and infants during the first year further reveals that the parent actively scaffolds the infant's ability to articulate and communicate his mental states somewhat ahead of the infant's ability to do so himself. Thus, the parent inducts the infant into the role of communicative partner (building on the infant's preadapted ability to participate as a social partner) by responding carefully to infant nonlinguistic initiatives as communications and by taking the infant's turn in conversation until the infant can fill the turn himself, for example, to a 2-month-old: "Does that noise mean you're hungry? Maybe you're hungry. Let's see if you want this water? No? No water? How about juice? Ok, you like that!"

The goodness of fit of the parent's scaffolding activity depends on the parent's ability to develop a sense of the infant's current cognitive capacities, developed likes and dislikes, and store of past experiences. That this knowledge is difficult to attain, approximate at best, fraught with error, and subject to constant revision makes this a challenging process and one easily open to distortion and misattribution by the parent. Another's mind is a terrain that can never be fully known. The difficulty of knowing another's mind guarantees that communication will be fraught with error and require many procedures for disambiguating messages, detecting and correcting misunderstandings, and repairing serious communicative failures, "What's the matter? You don't want your bear? Do you want your blanket? No? Are your new teeth hurting? Maybe you're tired." Thus, empathy should not be viewed as a simple apprehension of one person's state by another but as a complex outcome of a number of skilled communicative procedures for querying and decoding another's subjective reality.

Developmental work, then, has given us systematic access for the first time to the details of collaborative and flexible or incoherent and inflexible verbal and nonverbal interactive processes between parent and child.

Developmental research on attachment relationships has also documented the features of developmental dialogue that are associated with flexibility and resilience in the child's later development. The convergence across studies and across different research traditions is unmistakable. Developmental communication systems that are open to the entire array of affective communications (e.g., Ainsworth et al., 1978); that include both participants' initiatives in a balanced, mutually regulated dialogue (Baldwin, Cole, and Baldwin, 1982); that are characterized by active negotiation and repairing of miscues, misunderstandings, and conflicts of interest (Tronick, 1989; Crockenberg, and Litman, 1990); and that are actively scaffolded by the developmentally more advantaged partner toward more flexible and inclusive forms (e.g., Wood, Bruner, and Ross, 1976) are associated with positive developmental outcomes for the child. These outcomes include affectively positive interpersonal relationships and enactive procedural models for conducting relationships that are coherent, integrated, flexible, and open to new information (see Bretherton, 1988, for a review of this literature).

Based on these emerging studies of communication processes in early development, "coherent communication" in a developmental relationship can be described as having the following features:

1. Active structuring of dialogue around eliciting the child's current and emerging wants, needs, views, likes: Both the importance and the difficulty of knowing another's mind are explicitly acknowledged.
2. Active pursuit of repairs when misunderstanding occurs: Need for mutual contribution to regulation and repair is explicit.
3. Active bridging of dialogue to new levels of awareness by developmentally advantaged partner: Paradox that relationship is mutually regulated in the face of developmental inequality.
4. Active engagement and struggle with the child through trans-formational periods when awareness of self and others is being reorganized, with attendant recalibration of the extent of the child's initiative and direction of the relationship: Paradox that relationship initiatives are balanced in the face of inequality of power.

Attachment research has further demonstrated that attachment-related encounters in intimate social relationships are regulated by "internal working models" or enactive procedural representations of how to do things with others (van IJzendoorn, 1995, for review). At the adult level, these models are revealed through the verbal discourse of the adult, as research on the Adult Attachment Interview has described (Main, 1993). Because these models are revealed in verbal dialogue, however, does not mean that the models themselves are symbolically represented by the subject, even though they may be symbolically represented by the observing researcher or psychoanalyst. This research has further established that such models can be observed in operation in caregiver–infant transactions, begin to be represented in implicit procedural form early in life, and are mentally reaccessed in new social encounters (see Bretherton, 1988, and Lyons-Ruth, 1991, for reviews). These models also tend to persist into adolescence and adulthood in the absence of major changes in close relationships (see Main, 1993). This work begins to make explicit the partial isomorphism of process and structure, of medium and message, of features of the relational dialogue, and features of the resulting enactive relational procedure.

Attachment research thereby provides general empirical support for the psychoanalytic construct of "internalized objects" while at the same time underscoring the early origins of these models in actual relational transactions. However, "internalization" is occurring at a presymbolic level, prior to the capacity to evoke images or verbal representations of "the object." Thus, the primary form of representation must be one, not of words or images, but one of enactive relational procedures governing "how to do," or what Stern et al. (1998) have called "implicit relational knowing" (see also Lyons-Ruth, 1998).

Enactive Representation and the Implicit Procedural Unconscious

If "objects" are "internalized" from the earliest months of life, not simply as a way of coping with malevolent objects, as Fairbairn (1952) proposed, but as a process of normal development, then a language and a set of constructs are needed to capture how these objects are represented and how such representations change with development. An adequate theory also needs to retain a view of the individually idiosyncratic nature of life experience and the unique elaborations of enactive strategies, internal fantasy, and symbolic meaning that mark the individual. Can cognitive developmental science converge with psychoanalytic thinking to fashion a general theory of the development of enactive relational representation from the earliest months of life?

Both psychoanalytic theory and cognitive science agree that meaning systems include both conscious (e.g., verbalizable or attended to) aspects of experience and unconscious, or implicitly processed, aspects of experience. Implicit processing in modern cognitive science is applied to mental activity that is repetitive and automatic, provides quick categorization and decision making, and operates outside the realm of focal attention and verbalized experience (e.g., Marcel, 1983; Rumelhart and McClelland, 1986; Kihlstrom, 1987). Although not discussed in the cognitive literature, implicit processing may be particularly relevant to the quick and automatic handling of nonverbal affective cues, which are recognized and represented early in infancy in complex social "proto-dialogues" (Trevarthen, 1980), and so have their origins prior to the availability of symbolic communication.

Cognitive–developmental researchers also view thought as involving both conscious and unconscious, or implicit, procedures (Fischer and Pipp, 1984). However, developmental researchers are less quick to equate implicit processing with more repetitive and superficial decision making. For example, Fischer and Pipp (1984) specifically argue against the equation of unconscious processing with the "developmentally primitive" unconscious of Freud, claiming instead that "unconscious thought does not remain static during childhood but demonstrates systematic developments that are structurally parallel to the developments in conscious thought" (p. 89).

The neuropsychology literature approaches the issue of different and parallel forms of mental processing from the study of brain-damaged adults and comes to a converging conclusion. As Schachter and Moscovitch (1984) point out, "The psychological and neurobiological reality of multiple memory systems is . . . consistent with a wide range of data from cognitive psychology, neuropsychology, physiological psychology, and we will argue, developmental psychology" (p. 175). They argue for the existence of "at least two distinct and dissociable forms of memory" (p. 174), variously termed procedural versus declarative memory (Cohen and Squire, 1980), "knowing how" versus "knowing that" (Cohen and Squire, 1980), perceptual versus autobiographical memory (Jacoby and Dallas, 1981), "memory in the wide sense" versus "memory in the narrow sense" (Piaget and Inhelder, 1973), or implicit versus explicit memory (Schacter and Buckner, 1998). The implicit form of memory described as "knowing how" refers to the acquisition of skills, maps, and rule-governed adaptive responses that are evident in behavior but remain unconscious, in that they are not represented in symbolic form and are rarely fully translated into language; the explicit form of memory described as "knowing that" involves symbolic or imagistic knowledge that allows facts or experiences to be called into conscious awareness in the absence of the things they stand for. Not surprising to psychoanalysts, the domain of knowledge that is available to conscious awareness through symbolic representation constitutes but a small part of the individual's acquired adaptive knowledge base.

While implicit procedural and explicit declarative forms of knowing interpenetrate one another in normal adult functioning, studies of amnesic adults with a variety of neurological conditions, as well as studies of normal infants, demonstrate the potential dissociability of the two forms of knowledge. For example, amnesics' performances in completing fragmented versions of words benefitted from prior exposure to the word list as much as did normal subjects' performances. However, amnesics' ability to say whether they had seen a specific word before or had even seen the word list before was severely impaired. Implicit procedural knowledge was accrued in the absence of any conscious recall (declarative knowledge) of the learning experience itself. Similar learning effects in the absence of conscious recall occurred on even more complex tasks such as assembling a jigsaw puzzle, learning to apply a complex mathematical rule (the Fibonacci rule), or learning to solve the Tower of Hanoi puzzle (see Schachter and Moscovitch, 1984). Examples cited by Schachter and Moscovitch (1984) that are closer to the concerns of psychoanalysts include a patient of Claparède (1911) who refused to shake Claparède's hand but did not know why she refused. She was not able to recall that the day before she had been pricked with a pin hidden in Claparède's extended hand. In another case, an amnesic was told unusual stories about a series of presented pictures. The next day the patient could not recall that any stories had been told to him. However, he consistently chose titles for the pictures that reflected the unusual themes of those stories.

Cognitive psychologists continue to struggle with numerous issues involved in the more precise specification of these dissociable memory systems (see Anderson, 1982; Schachter and Buckner, 1998). For the purposes of this paper, however, these data make clear that implicit learning, operating outside conscious awareness, is fundamental to complex adult functioning, as well as to infant functioning. In addition, complex new learning occurs in adulthood through implicit procedural mechanisms, new learning that is not mediated by translation of implicit knowing into symbolic or conscious form, even though words or images may be involved as part of the procedural memory. Particularly relevant to our concerns here, some processes that influence procedural knowing have little effect on declarative memory (such as modality of initial learning), and some processes influencing declarative memory have little effect on implicit learning (such as delay interval after initial learning and level of processing involved in initial learning). Based on all the above data,

Schacter and Moscovitch argue for the relative independence of the two memory systems. The implications for our discussion is that change in implicit procedural forms of relational knowing may come about through somewhat different mechanisms than change in conscious declarative forms of knowing.

In recent psychoanalytic writing, the increasing participation of the analyst has been predicated partly on an increasing sense that we gain much more access to these implicit enacted knowings, one's own as well as the patient's, in a more participatory frame. This emerging sense of the implicit procedural unconscious is consistent with modern cognitive research, but its implications for prior models of the unconscious have not yet been explicitly worked out. Such implicit enacted procedures for being with others are central to therapeutic work but are not well captured by previous divisions between primary and secondary process, between ego and id, between verbal and nonverbal, or even by the construct of the dynamic unconscious. Implicit relational procedures are often neither conscious and verbalizable nor repressed in a dynamic sense. They are not reducible to unacceptable drives or impulses and do not have their origins or essence in fantasy. However, implicit relational knowing is likely to be visible in the structure of fantasied interactions, as well as in the enactive structure of real interactions. Seligman (1995) notes that Freud's preconscious may have prefigured this aspect of the unconscious. Stolorow, quoted in Seligman (1995), has advanced the notion of the "pre-reflective unconscious," and Sandler and Sandler (1994) distinguish between the "past unconscious" and the "present unconscious." The Sandlers also offer a careful discussion of Freud's usages of the terms *unconscious* and *preconscious*. An excellent synthesis of the literature on procedural memory from a psychoanalytic viewpoint is also available in Clyman (1991).

Infant research, in particular, has shown us that, long before words are relevant, procedures for being with others are being acquired that vary widely along many dimensions, such as in the likelihood of engaging others in positive exchanges, in the affects that are exhibited or not exhibited to others, in the social and affective information that is elicited from others, or in the effectiveness of procedures for eliciting help or comfort from others. While these procedures develop in adaptation to particular caregiving partners, they are not necessarily equally effective in regulating internal physiological arousal (Spangler and Grossman, 1993; Hertsgaard et al., 1995; Gunnar et al., in press), in protecting exploration and mastery (Cassidy and Berlin, 1994), in adapting to the range of environments encountered in the peer group (Lyons-Ruth, Alpern, and Repacholi, 1993), or in relating to others in adolescence

(Kobak and Sceery, 1988). In psychoanalytic work, paying close attention to all transactions in the hour is in keeping with the need to understand the multiple implicit procedural maps of the patient and their breadth, flexibility, and range of application or their discontinuities and inflexibilities. However, if development is not primarily about translating primary process into symbolic form, but about developing implicit adaptive procedures for being with others in a wide range of emotionally charged situations, then making the unconscious conscious does not adequately describe developmental or psychoanalytic change.

Dialogue and Defense

As Ainsworth, Main, and others have further demonstrated, procedural models guiding the early parent–child affective dialogue exhibit various kinds of deletions and distortions or "incoherencies," distortions that analysts have long understood from a one-person, intrapsychic model as defensive (Ainsworth et al., 1978; see Bretherton, 1988, for review). This literature makes clear that implicit two-person processes are integral to the developmental origins of some defenses. This developmental work, tieing nonverbal affective discourse to defensive structure, mirrors the current analytic interest in closely following the process of the two-person dialogue within the hour as it instantiates the deletions and distortions of both participants' implicit relational models.

In the case of less coherent parent–child dialogues, attachment studies have demonstrated that a particular character stance or a particular defensive strategy may constitute one component of a much broader interpersonal arrangement that has endured over a significant period of the patient's life. Thus, some defensive strategies are not best viewed as resulting from a particular intrapsychic conflict or a particular interpersonal perturbation confined to a specific developmental epoch. For example, developmental research has revealed that a child's tendency to suppress vulnerable feelings of anger or distress and to displace attention away from relationships and onto the inanimate world should not be viewed as an obsessional style resulting from control struggles in toddlerhood. Instead, for a sizable number of children (van IJzendoorn, 1994), this stance is reliably evident in the child's behavior by 12 months of age and is related to particular forms of parent–child affective dialogue over the first year of life, including parental suppressed anger and discomfort with close physical contact (Main, Tomasini, and Tolan, 1979) and parental mock surprise expressions to infant anger (Malatesta et al., 1989). These restrictions in parent–child dialogue are further foreshadowed by the parent's style of discourse in attachment-related interviews prior to the child's birth (see van IJzendoorn, 1994, for meta-analytic review).

Even in cases where a traumatic event at a particular developmental period has played a crucial pathogenic role, the continued physiological and intrapsychic effects of traumatic events are related to the quality of parent–child dialogue in relation to the painful event available subsequent to the trauma. For example, recent data tie excessive and sustained reactivity of the stress-responsive hypothalamic-pituitary-adrenal system to impaired collaborativeness in the parent–infant dialogue (Spangler and Grossmann, 1993; Hertsgaard et al., 1995; see Lyons-Ruth and Jacobvitz, 1999, for review). The collaborativeness of the ongoing parent-child dialogue, then, emerges as one potent mediator of whether particular aspects of traumatic experience will be segregated outside the process of ongoing regulation in the parent–child dialogue.

This research literature indicates that implicit two-person processes must be integral to any theory of the development of defenses. However, most theorizing has remained intrapsychically oriented. Attachment theorists have discussed defensive processes as processes that result in the distortion, exclusion, or lack of integration of information or affective experience, with a particular emphasis on the formation and maintenance of multiple inconsistent models of relational experience. From an attachment perspective, Bretherton (1991) cites Stern (1985), Tulving (1972), Craik (1943), and others who point to the potential for multiple models inherent in the representational and memory systems that store human experience.

Other approaches to this issue from both psychoanalytic and attachment theorists stress the role of conflict and intense affect rather than the availability of different modes of mental representation in leading to multiple incompatible models. For example, Main and Hesse (1990), discussing disorganized/disoriented attachment behaviors, stress the role of fear and conflict, in that fear aroused by the attachment figure leads the infant to both activate and inhibit behavioral approaches to the attachment figure when stressed. The simultaneous activation and inhibition postulated stems from the nature of the attachment behavioral system itself, which is normally activated in the presence of fear or threat but which must be simultaneously inhibited in the case where the attachment figure *is* the source of the threat. A similar process is envisioned in adulthood at a representational level, where mental approaches to attachment-related thoughts and feelings may continue to be both activated and inhibited.

Fonagy (1991) advances a somewhat different intrapsychic theory of multiple models derived from clinical object relations theory. In object relations theory, unintegrated models of idealized and devalued versions of self and other have been viewed as based on the defense of splitting, a defense linked to the presence of particularly malevolent representations of important others (Kernberg, 1976). In Fonagy's view, the child's awareness of the malevolence of the caregiver is too painful to tolerate and leads the child to inhibit the ability to reflect on the mental states of self and other, leading to unintegrated and inconsistent representations of central relationships. Fonagy (1991), more explicitly than others, also stresses the lowered developmental level of the resulting mental representations.

A more radical and social constructivist view of the defenses, including splitting, is inherent in recent attachment research, however. Attachment researchers have demonstrated more dramatically than any other group the interactive basis for the deletions and distortions prominent in many implicit relational strategies. If negative affects, particularly hateful ones, produce hostile attack, intense devaluation, shaming, or withdrawal by the parent, they may be excluded from further discourse. Exclusion of negative affects from interaction also excludes these affects from the integrated developmental elaboration and understanding of anger-related behaviors, affects, and experiences that might come from more balanced acceptance and inclusion in interaction and discussion.

Attachment research has consistently grounded defensive maneuvers in infancy, such as infant avoidance, in the behavioral and affective responses of the caregivers, responses based on their own implicit models of relationships. These interpersonal defensive maneuvers have been viewed as interactive and adaptive in origin rather than purely intrapsychic in origin. Recent research on infants with disorganized attachment behavior has also tied these conflicted forms of infant behavior to fearful and hesitant or hostile and frightening responses of the caregiver (see Lyons-Ruth, Bronfman and Atwood, 1999; Lyons-Ruth, Bronfman, and Parsons, 1999). These disorganized attachment behaviors in infancy also predict later forms of role-reversal with the parent during the preschool years (Main, Kaplan, and Cassidy, 1985). These findings point to the parent's difficulty in attending to and balancing the initiatives of the infant with those of the self, with the ensuing collapse of intersubjective space so that only one party's subjective reality is acknowledged. This collapse of intersubjective space in the interactions between parent and child may also lead to the impaired capacity of borderline patients to integrate conflicting representations and to mentally reflect on the subjective states of self and other, as noted by Fonagy (1991).

This view of defenses as partially grounded in the structure of exchanges with important others is also congruent with the increasing awareness among analysts that interactions between patient and analyst instantiate the defensive exclusions or contradictions of the patient's implicit procedural knowledge. Currently, mutual reflection on "enactments" in the therapy is seen as a rich source of insight about these implicit procedural knowings, including the resort to defensive distortion or exclusion of information. Developmental research further establishes that many of the defensive deletions and distortions evident in enactments have "two-person" origins.

Part II: Enactive Relational Representation and the Process of Change

Because changes in the organization of meaning systems are what we are generally referring to when we talk about both developmental change and psychoanalytic change, accounting for changes in meaning systems is critical to both developmental and psychoanalytic theory. For developmental theory, in particular, change cannot be adequately described as simply making the unconscious conscious. Instead, new ways of being with others are being acquired. Yet no literature has grappled extensively with how "working models," "internalized objects," or "implicit procedural meanings" become either more articulated and complex over developmental time or reworked during psychoanalytic treatment. A sufficiently powerful model of change in implicit relational knowing is likely to require the synthesis of insights from both developmental science and psychoanalytic theory.

A Control Systems Model of Mind

What does current cognitive–developmental science have to offer a psychoanalytic theory of meaning? Findings from 30 years of cognitive-developmental research are converging with similar results from the neurosciences and from studies of adult cognition to yield the following general insights into the construction of meaning systems, insights that are also congenial to the clinical experience of mind and meaning.

1. The mind is naturally fractionated, with meaning systems often unintegrated with one another (e.g., Fischer and Granott, 1995).
2. Mental processing occurs at several levels in parallel, as well as in sequence (Marcel, 1983; Fischer and Granott, 1995).
3. All adapted activity expresses mental structure (Fischer, 1980).
4. All cognition is essentially re-cognition in that new learning automatically reorganizes old learning to some extent (Edelman, 1987; Freeman, 1990).

5. Meanings are co-constructed in interaction with the minds and artifacts of a particular culture (Vygotsky, 1962; Bruner, Olver, and Greenfield, 1966).
6. In domains of meaning with rich cultural investment (the provision of many minds and artifacts to assist in the mental articulation of a domain), meaning systems will develop through higher levels of organization, that is, will become articulated and integrated into higher-order coordinations and proceduralized to allow more elements into working memory more rapidly and completely than in domains without support (Bruner, Olver, and Greenfield, 1966; Fischer, 1980; Anderson, 1982).
7. Developmentally, constraints of working memory and processing speed set an upper limit on the level of organization in adaptive action that can be achieved, but up to this upper limit, level of organization realized will vary widely across domains, depending on the degree of support for elaborating the representational domain (Case, 1991; Fischer, 1980).
8. Even if an optimal level of complexity of thought can be demonstrated in a given domain, use of that optimal level may still vary widely with context (Fischer and Granott, 1995).

If these general features of thought are applied to implicit working models of relationships, we would expect to find that the flexible and integrated organization of implicit relational experience is particularly dependent on the quality and extent of participation by a relational partner. This dependence on the quality of the partner's participation also implies that implicit relational knowing is particularly vulnerable to fractionation and lack of integration among the implicit meaning systems governing relational behavior. That is, lack of mental integration may occur not only because of intrapsychic defensive processes, but also because of the absence of collaborative relationships within which to articulate and integrate relational understanding and ways of being. Areas of potentially conflicting enactive knowledge may remain unintegrated with one another, as occurs in splitting, and in addition, potentially conflicting symbolic and enactive knowings may operate in parallel without integration across modes of representation.

Recent cognitive–developmental theory (Fischer, 1980; Case, 1991; Fischer and Granott, 1995) offers the most powerful current model for how meaning systems and their associated adaptive skills for doing things in the world change with development. Modern cognitive–developmental theory sees development as involving the construction of progressively more complex control (or meaning) systems. These control systems are properties of both the person and the environmental context in which they develop. Cognition, action, and emotion are all interrelated products of these control systems. The best current description of how an enactive control system changes emphasizes the gradual microprocess by which single developed skills, or enactive relational procedures, are coordinated with other single skills or procedures to form second-level coordinated thought structures, which are, in turn, coordinated with one another. For each procedure one must learn to achieve a particular outcome reliably over a set of environmental variations and then coordinate that procedure with a related procedure. For example, after a conflict with his mother, a 2-year-old might learn to calm his distress from a variety of intensity levels, using a variety of supports (thumb, blanket, parental hug, shift of attention) and then coordinate this enactive procedure with a second set of procedures for engaging in playful games with the parent, leading to a set of coordinated second-level control structures for "making up," for moving from distress in relation to the parent to a calm state and ultimately back to positive engagement and play. This enactive relational procedure might then be coordinated with procedures for interacting with playmates rather than parents, so that a coordinated procedural control system develops for making up with playmates after a conflict.

It is important to note that, although words are used for the first time in the service of enactive relational procedures during toddlerhood, the embedding of words into procedures does not make the organization of the procedure itself available to reflective thought or verbal representation. The 3-year-old may be able to verbalize meanings of "good" and "bad," but he cannot represent consciously or verbally that he inhibits his impulse to reach out for comfort to his father because his father's physical withdrawal and cold voicetone communicate disapproval of comfort-seeking. The organizational structure of most relational behavior remains unconscious and implicit even though the child's new words and understandings may be incorporated into these implicit procedures.

Fischer (1980) and Case (1991) both detail this developmental process of gradual coordination of more complex, integrated, and inclusive implicit procedures or control structures through a series of developmental levels. The reader should consult Fischer (1980) and Case (1991) for their detailed expositions of how particular domains of procedural knowing are assembled component by component, during the years from infancy to adulthood. These theories have extended the older Piagetian framework in a number of ways that deemphasize his monolithic and hierarchical stage structures, replacing them with a set of more varied and context-responsive "skills" or modular meaning systems. These modular meaning systems require environmental support but operate within the general constraints of memory capacity and processing speed available at a given age.

In contrast to older views, there is no simple uniform progression through a series of stages, and people do not operate at a particular level across tasks. The series of levels and sublevels outlined by Fischer (1980) or Case (1991) represent, not epochs of development, but an analysis of task complexity, of the level of implicit mental articulation needed to accomplish a set of adaptive actions. The level of complexity of a given child's or adult's control systems typically varies widely across tasks. Development is viewed as a process of developing concurrently along a number of pathways that may be only loosely or not at all coordinated by level of articulation achieved. Even along a given pathway, level of complexity of thought and action will vary with contextual factors from day to day. To quote Fischer, "People do not have integrated, fundamentally logical minds. Instead, we have many control systems that are naturally separate, although potentially we can develop coordination and integration of many of them" (p. 153). This view is clearly consistent with clinical experience, in that an individual's relational repertoire for doing things with others may be quite discrepant from the person's skills in other areas.

These emerging context-sensitive and modular views of the development of meaning are congenial to many of the clinical insights of psychoanalysis. They emphasize the integral relations between meaning systems and adapted behavior; the fractionated and context-specific nature of both symbolic and procedural meaning systems, the importance of cultural partners in scaffolding or co-constructing representational systems to more flexible and inclusive forms; and the gradual, iterative, yet individually idiosyncratic process through which meaning systems become more articulated, integrated, and inclusive. More specifically than in the attachment literature, these researchers delineate the processing constraints on the elaboration of both procedural and symbolic meaning systems during particular developmental periods and delineate the gradual process through which components of a task or meaning domain are differentiated and systematically coordinated into more flexible and inclusive systems.

Although the language of cognitive science is often uncongenial to clinicians, a model of the slow articulation of a domain of meaning within a set of developmental constraints is likely to describe aspects of the construction of implicit and explicit relational knowing both during development and during psychoanalytic therapy. Contemporary neuroscience also describes mental organization as proceeding through a gradually accruing complexity of neuronal connections until a critical point is reached where higher level organization emerges spontaneously (Edelman, 1987). The neuroscience literature also stresses the individually idiosyncratic nature of the accruing neuronal organizations but the seemingly paradoxical convergence of these idiosyncratic pathways on species-typical behavioral outcomes. Somehow developmentally, we tend to arrive at a similar place through vastly different routes. These models of the increasing articulation and organization of both neuronal systems and relational procedures potentially provide support for a meaning-focused psychoanalytic enterprise from contemporary scientific views and create fertile ground for more collaborative dialogue across psychoanalytic and developmental disciplines.

Parallel Mental Processing

Recent awareness of the parallel nature of much cognitive activity and the sharp constraints on what can ever be the subject of sustained focal (conscious) attention has led to a more general realization that thinking progresses to highly complex, formal modes through the development of enactive procedures that are not easily, and never completely, translated into a verbal, explicitly retrievable medium (e.g., Fischer and Granott, 1995; Marcel, 1983). This enactive dimension is most obvious in the domains that do not easily lend themselves to verbal expression, such as musical composition or performance, complex artistic or athletic skills, and spatial or architectural expertise. However, the increased complexity of implicit knowing that comes with repeated exposure or repeated doing is also intrinsic to the most symbol-laden domains as well, such as the writing of scientific papers or the analysis of literature.

Knowing how to proceed in intimate relationships may be another domain in which complex knowledge is constructed outside a predominantly verbal medium, in which procedures for skilled interaction, incorporating a range of subtle affective cues, develop through a series of more articulated and integrated coordinations largely outside the domain of verbalized knowledge and conscious awareness. Clearly, as a species, we still have a very sparse systematic verbalized knowledge base for understanding how human interaction "works," even though we enact it daily at highly skilled levels. Even in the analytic literature, there is often a large gap between insights systematized in the literature and the subtlety and complexity of what the analyst implicitly knows and does clinically. Implicit clinical knowing, then, also proceeds to high levels of complexity outside the medium of words, even though systematized, verbalized knowledge is highly valued in the field.

In order to emphasize that the structure of thinking is inherent in action, Fischer (1980) calls his cognitive–developmental theory a theory of skill development. In his view, cognition at every level is fundamentally about learning to control a range of actions, whether physical or mental actions, in the service of achieving a particular outcome in the world, over a specific set of variations in environmental input. For example, at the sensorimotor level, between 9 and 12 months, the infant learns how to coordinate his focus of attention with the caregiver's, by using a variety of vocal sounds and gestures to redirect her focus of attention to coincide with his, no matter what her physical position or current focus of attention may be (see Bretherton, McNew, and Beeghly-Smith, 1981). A related, but much more complex, skill at the abstract level of thinking is to coordinate one's parenting and career identities over time with the parenting and career identities of one's spouse through joint negotiation and decision making (see Fischer, 1980). These examples point to the mentally organized structure of behaviors that are also imbued with strong affects serving basic survival needs. Both the cognitive–developmental and attachment research literatures, then, converge on the notion that implicit relational knowing is one realm where organized enactive or implicit procedural knowledge develops from the first months of life largely outside the arena of symbolic or verbalized knowledge.

Melvin Lewis (1995), in a related argument regarding amnesia and transference, also discusses the distinction between procedural and declarative memory and proposes a developmental shift hypothesis to account for infantile amnesia. According to his hypothesis, some early developmental structures, such as primary process and sensorimotor thought, are maintained as they are throughout development and would be manifested in preverbal, affective, sensory, and motoric memory patterns. In contrast, later memory functions, especially those involving language, would change extensively with development. He speculates that the concept of infantile amnesia as a result of repression may not be viable since nonverbal forms of memory can be recovered from infancy onward. He concludes, "The apparent lack of verbal access might have nothing at all to do with repression; it might simply be that early memories are encoded in a prelanguage form and that we have been looking for the wrong representation of very early memories—for words rather than for physiological responses, behavior and affect" (p. 410).

While his argument converges with the view advanced here that implicit relational representations are constructed from the first months of life, the model advanced here differs from this implied "developmental shift" view. In a developmental shift view, affective and behavioral representational systems that do not become more complex with development are contrasted with verbal systems that emerge during the second year and that *do* become more complex. A more powerful and general model is a parallel systems model, rather than a developmental shift model. In a parallel systems model, the affective and behavioral representations guiding interactions with others continue to become more articulated and complex with development, with newly acquired verbal capacity incorporated into interactive strategies, but the strategies themselves are not dependent on verbal articulation. This is clearly in keeping with the complexity of the transference phenomena that present clinically. In this view, affective and behavioral representations are not *preverbal*; they are simply not primarily verbal.

Following Bretherton (1991), Stern (1995), and others, these implicit relational procedures can be described as organized around a variety of local and superordinate goals and as including both interactive procedures and their associated webs of cognitive and affective meanings. These multivalent relational schemes would include not only verbal or verbalizable "cognitive" meanings if these are available, but also a rich web of imagistic "fantasies" and affect-related physiological sensations and the implicit relational knowing of how these meanings and fantasies are related to social actions. The integral connections between cognition and "valuation," or feeling, which is required in this model, have also been emphasized by Damasio (1994) and Edelman (1987) on the basis of recent neuroscience research. Stern (1995) has also recently delineated the multidimensional nature of early relational schemes as experienced in parent–infant psychotherapy.

If representations of "how to do things with others" integrate semantic and affective meaning with behavioral/interactive procedures, then a particular implicit relational procedure may be accessed through multiple routes, and representational change may be set in motion by changes in affective experience, cognitive understanding, or interactive encounters, without necessarily assigning privileged status to a particular dimension, such as interpretation. Stern (1995) has made a related point in relation to parent–infant psychotherapy, where the therapist's intervention may be targeted toward the parent's representation of her own experience, at the therapist–parent transference relationship, or at the parent–infant interaction itself. Mobilizing change across more aspects of these multidimensional thinking, feeling, and doing schemes at once will presumably enhance the effectiveness of the change process, assuming appropriate pace and timing so as not to overload the patient.

Task Structure in the Relational Domain:
A Common Element in Developmental and
Psychoanalytic Change

With the increasing influence of infant research, psychoanalytic theorists have struggled with the extent to which the parent–infant or parent–child dyad provides a useful analogy to the therapeutic dyad (e.g., Mitchell, 1988; Wolff, 1996). Following the work of Fischer and Case, I would propose that an essential common structuring element in developmental and psychoanalytic change is the task structure intrinsic to the process of getting to know another's mind. Both developmental and psychoanalytic change in how one conducts oneself in intimate relationships must be constrained by the series of differentiations and integrations required for the construction of collaborative procedures for acting in relationships. The continuing developmental construction of higher-order coordinations of mental entities that Case and Fischer have described in abstract terms have been systematically studied in relation to the child's progressively more complex ability to conceptualize the activity of other minds (see Hobson, 1993; Selman, 1980). The literature on the child's emerging "theory of mind" documents the child's evolving ability to think about thinking, including his own thinking. Self-reflective function, which Fonagy (1991) in particular has highlighted, is closely related to, but generally lags developmentally behind, reflection on the other's subjectivity (Landry and Lyons-Ruth, 1980).

Psychoanalytic discussions of representation usually involve the representation of subjective states, so the developmental emergence of a number of successive levels of "thinking about thinking" introduces a number of potential levels of "representation" of intersubjective events. Intersubjective awareness, then, is not best discussed in terms of whether conscious awareness or symbolic representation has been achieved per se. Instead, we must consider what level of "thinking about thinking" has been fluently achieved and procedurally integrated over which types of affective and relational contexts. Whether starting in early childhood or in adulthood, one must first elaborate an awareness of how one's own mental life is both similar to and different from that of others to elaborate further an understanding of how to make those similarities and differences explicit in dialogue and then to construct procedures for negotiating with the other in the face of differences. The same series of understandings must be elaborated by the developing child.

The essential features of both the verbal and the implicit procedural meaning systems constituting the domain of relational knowing are still poorly described and understood in both the developmental, cognitive, and psychoanalytic literatures. Developmental work on the child's emerging theory of mind (e.g., Carpenter, Nagell, and Tomasello, 1998; Hobson, 1993), work on the relational deficits characterizing autistic individuals (e.g., Hobson, 1993), and research on children's social understanding (Selman, 1980) contribute some detail from the research literature. The rich body of psychoanalytic descriptive work on severe character disorders also offers the potential for a theory of how the domain of intersubjective knowing is elaborated or remains unelaborated, under normal and abnormal conditions (e.g., Fonagy, 1991). This body of work first needs to be freed of prior untenable developmental assumptions, however (e.g., Westen, 1990; Lyons-Ruth, 1991).

Psychoanalytic work on the organization of the intersubjective worlds of child and adult patients and developmental research on the construction of intersubjective understanding are complementary lenses refracting a common underlying domain of knowing. In the "common structure" view offered here, the parent–child relationship is not a metaphor for the adult–patient relationship or vice-versa. Instead, both offer unique, but converging, routes to describing how human beings co-construct a set of procedures and understandings for negotiating the intersubjective field. Understanding how mind constructs the intersubjective field, whether during childhood or adulthood, is crucial to the further development of both psychoanalysis and developmental science. In this view both developmental and psychoanalytic change emerge from the dynamic interplay of the multiple constraints of intersubjective task structure, working memory capacity, and the quality and extent of participation of interacting partners. This complex constructivist view allows us to move away from a monolithic view of developmental sequence. It also allows us to see similarities in the processes of developmental and psychoanalytic change, not in terms of the adult's regression to or fixation at a stage of infancy or childhood, but in terms of the similarities through which humans of all ages approach and progress through the mastering of the complex task domain of negotiating with other minds.

Unique Features of Relational Control Systems

Analytic thinkers and infant researchers would both call for several additions to these cognitive models of meaning construction, however. Both analytic theorists and infancy researchers would call attention to the special problems presented by the need to know and be known by another mind, a condition that is a prerequisite for the construction of meaning systems regarding how to be with others. The elaboration of notions of intersubjectivity, or how two minds interface with one another, is an intrinsically collaborative process that depends on one mind becoming reasonably well known to at least one other mind. This necessary extended intersubjective collaboration can create unique and idiosyncratic contexts in which interpersonal meaning systems are elaborated, unlike the regularities and multiple examples more characteristic of commerce with the physical world. The availability of a learning context for elaborating intersubjective meanings is then highly constrained by the frequency and particular quality of the partner's participation in what Tronick (1998) has referred to as "the dyadic expansion of consciousness" (see also Sander, 1995).

Psychoanalytic thinkers in particular would also call attention to the powerful motive systems and accompanying strong affects that impact the elaboration of intersubjective meanings more strongly than they impact the elaboration of concepts of the physical world. The segregation of meanings associated with powerful negative affects has been a central insight of psychoanalytic observation since its inception. To date, cognitive researchers have not attempted to develop a thorough analysis of the meaning systems that guide intimate relationships. The cognitive term *sensorimotor intelligence* itself fails to acknowledge the existence early in infancy of an affective communication system served by an elaborate expressive facial musculature that is unique to the human species (Izard, 1978). In addition to the increasingly complex sensorimotor coordinations that are assembled over the first 2 years, there are also increasingly complex affective and interpersonal coordinations that are co-constructed, as delineated particularly in the attachment literature, as well as in related studies by Tronick, Sander, and Stern. These increasingly complex coordinations of interpersonal action and intersubjective awareness are likely to follow the microdevelopmental steps in the articulation of meaning systems explicated by Fischer and Case. That the first extended tutorial in intersubjective awareness is usually conducted with an attachment figure whose presence and participation are necessary for the child's survival further imbues these exchanges with powerful affects. How these affect systems organize, fragment, or distort the development of meaning systems has not been considered in any depth in the cognitive literature (but see Damasio, 1994).

Affective features, as well as cognitive features, are likely to be central to psychopathology, however. The *complexity* of one's verbal reasoning about others, and perhaps of one's implicit procedural knowing, has no simple relation to psychopathology. Verbal reasoning about others can be highly developed in the context of severe character issues and maladaptive behaviors (see work by Selman, 1980). Therapeutic work seems to be about identifying ways of proceeding, or assumptions about others, that are maladaptive outside the initial context of learning but may or may not be less complex. Instead, they may be more imbued with rage or fear, less integrated with other procedural knowings, less effective in modulating internal physiological stress responses, or more likely to involve fearful or hostile interpretations of others' behavior. Deconstructing complex, but maladaptive, ways of being with, while simultaneously co-constructing more adaptive but equally complex new ways of being together, is likely to involve a slow mutual journey through a series of intersubjective encounters that catalyze the construction of new control systems. A model that integrates motivational and affective processes with the increasing articulation and organization of relational control structures seems necessary.

Viewed developmentally, the domain of implicit relational knowing becomes more complex over normal development, largely through apprentice learning and participant observation rather than verbal instruction. Whether the gradual process of differentiation and coordination of components of meaning (or action) described in the developmental literature will prove useful to understanding the developmental construction or therapeutic reconstruction of implicit relational knowing remains to be fully explored. However, the question of how the meaning systems comprising the domain of implicit relational knowing develop and change needs to be grappled with by both developmental and psychoanalytic theorists.

Conflict, Negative Affect, and Fragmented or Dissociated Enactive Procedures

Procedural models for being with others are organized at first according to the developmental level of understanding available at the time they are taking form and may or may not become reorganized over time in accord with later levels of understanding. So an implicit relational procedure, along with its associated meanings and values, may remain at the initial level of representation or may be only partially updated from time to time, leaving coexisting variations at succeeding developmental levels (probably the norm for most areas of experience), or may have been repeatedly reaccessed and in the process reconstructed over time so that developmentally earlier versions have been largely replaced (see Edelman, 1987). Many such implicit procedures for how to negotiate affectively charged exchanges with others are a part of what is being brought to the psychoanalyst.

From the perspective of normal development, lack of articulation and integration of either implicit or explicit representational systems can have many origins, including developmental limitations in meaning-making at a particular age, implicit rules of family engagement that exclude particular ways of relating, implicit rules that include procedural action but refuse verbal acknowledgment, traumatic experiences whose implications threaten other survival-necessary "ways of being with," and the usual disjunctions of human life where somewhat contradictory implicit procedures may evolve governing, for example, public versus private life, sibling versus peer relations, or same-sex versus opposite-sex interactions.

Conflict at the level of implicit procedural representation inheres in the tension between the goals and needs of the child and the responses of the varied caregiving environments that are encountered developmentally. While other forms of discontinuity or limitation in procedures may exist, the ones most relevant to psychoanalytic theory are those associated with imbalanced interpersonal interaction, need frustration, and negative affect. Inadequate response to central goals and needs of the child creates both negative affects and areas of exchange that become foreclosed to further negotiation, articulation, and integration. Thus, disruptions or imbalances in interpersonal transactions are initially isomorphic with discontinuities or inadequacies in relational procedures and are associated with experienced conflict around the frustration of central goals. Conflict among the child's competing goals per se (such as to preserve a good relationship with the parent or to insist on one's own way; to do away with father or to love father) are unlikely to result in lasting difficulties in and of themselves unless corresponding conflicts between the goals of parent and child interfere with their developmental resolution (Fischer and Watson, 1981).

When flexible mental and emotional access to most levels of experience has been available within a development-enhancing dialogue, the resulting relational control systems will be reasonably well integrated, with both interpersonally contested issues and internally contradictory goals and meanings struggled with and resolved *to the extent necessary* to negotiate the world. If many of the patient's goals have been overridden and excluded from further interaction, negative affects related to the frustration of those goals will remain unresolved while caregiver negative affects toward the pursuit of those goals will also be represented. These points of unresolved conflict become internalized as discontinuities in implicit procedures, discontinuities often marked by strong conflicting emotions. Likewise, if relational goals have been enacted in relationships in forms that conflict with what is acknowledged or have been enacted in contradictory forms whose contradictions are never confronted, the resulting implicit procedural representations will be segregated, fragmented, or contradictory, with little opportunity to update, articulate, and integrate implicit "ways of being with" as new developmental capacities become available (see Bretherton, 1988). Therapeutic work will then be occurring around the fault lines where interactive negotiations have failed, goals remain aborted, negative affects are unresolved, conflict is experienced, and implicit procedural representations have become segregated from one another.

Viewing "internalized objects" or "transferences" as relational control systems governed by implicit procedural models makes clearer that segregated or fragmented implicit procedural maps will not only be imbued with conflicted affects but are likely to be underdeveloped in various ways compared to procedures that have developed in relationships characterized by more coherent communication. Alternately, one can view procedures developed under conditions of more restricted communication, not as "underdeveloped," but as differently developed under conditions where barriers to self-expression and the associated segregation and fragmentation of relational control procedures are valued and enforced.

Removing affective barriers to new ways of being with others is only one aspect of the change process, however; new procedures that are more articulated, integrated, and adapted to current reality must be developed. In traditional theory, the work after initial "insight" is achieved has proceeded under the rubric of "working through." If relational knowing is as much implicit and procedural as symbolic, the work of elaborating new implicit procedures for being with others must occur at enactive as well as symbolic levels.

A final subtle shift occurs in adopting a representational systems model of mind in that we must struggle with the issue of creating new representational structures. If representational systems are always in a process of reconstruction with every activation (see Edelman, 1987; Freeman, 1990), then analytic work is always involved in the creation of the new and the reworking of the old simultaneously. While "making the unconscious conscious" or verbalized may be one part of this co-constructive process, developmental research, in particular, suggests that the emergence of new implicit relational procedures developmentally is not simply about putting unconscious motivations or implicit procedures into words, but about new forms of organization emerging as new forms of "being with" are scaffolded between parent and child.

Nonlinear Models of Change: Increasing Elaboration and Emergent Properties

Analytic theory and practice have always recognized both the slow, incremental processes of forming an alliance and working through, as well as the observed major shifts in organization presumed to be attendant on a successful interpretation. Edelman's (1987) theory of neuronal group selection also points to the importance both of the small incremental processes by which certain neuronal groups gain articulation at the expense of other potential pathways and of the relatively sudden emergence of a higher-order organization once the number of reciprocal and recursive feedback loops reaches a critical point. Dynamic systems theory also draws our attention to the sudden emergence of new forms of organization with increased articulation of the constituents of the system (Thelen and Smith, 1994). Edelman's theory of neuronal groups further indicates that the small elaborations that occur as a neuronal group is slowly constructed or reconstructed with use *are* the engine of change, with a higher-order organization emerging as a function of the critical mass of new and overlapping articulated elements attained.

Applying the lens of these theories of self-organizing biological systems, what may need more emphasis is the extended period of intersubjective encounters between patient and analyst that have increased the complexity and organization of some aspects of the intersubjective field at the expense of others. This idiosyncratic and slow process of elaborating some aspects of neuronal organization at the expense of others—or, at another level of analysis, of slowly creating new implicit relational procedures—is the work that creates competing and destabilizing mental and behavioral structures. Viewed from a self-organizing systems perspective, as increasingly articulated competing organization emerges, the old organization is destabilized, with an increasing subjective sense of creative disorder and internal flux (Thelen and Smith, 1994; see also Stolorow, in press). At this point of increasing instability, the analyst (and the patient as well) may be able to crystallize the shift in mental organization and awareness to a new, and often more complex, form by making the additional re-cognitions needed through interpretation. Once this state of instability and flux is achieved, however, the reorganizing re-cognitions might also come about through an emotionally salient series of transactions with the analyst, as loosely captured by the term *corrective emotional experience*, or through a powerful transaction between the two participants when the analyst is forced somewhat out of role, as described under the rubric of enactment. The more distal source of change, however, is not the proximal crystallizing encounter or interpretation but the preceding long period of destabilizing patient–analyst encounters.

Such a model seems to capture well the feel of clinical work and is foreshadowed in much of previous analytic writing regarding the need to prepare for the interpretation. In the older literature, however, the focus was on elaborating the patient's symbolic representations via clarification and interpretation. The newer developmental and neuroscience literatures suggest that, in addition to conscious symbolic elaboration, patient and analyst must be working simultaneously at an implicit relational level to create increasingly collaborative forms of dialogue. Developmental research suggests that collaborative dialogue includes careful attention to the particular state of the other's intersubjective experience, open acceptance of a broad range of affects, active scaffolding to more inclusive levels of dialogue, and engaged struggle and intersubjective negotiation through periods when the other's mind is changing and new ways of relating are needed. Coherence of mind and perfectly collaborative communication are abstractions that will never be realized given the many simultaneous levels of human communication, the natural fractionation of representational systems, the constant process of new relational encounters, and the powerful affects that resist certain kinds of exchanges or insights. However, in developmental attachment studies, more inclusive, succinct, noncontradictory, and truthful forms of parent-child dialogue have been shown to yield more coherent internal working models of attachment and more flexible, integrated, and adaptive implicit relational procedures and to confer developmental advantages in "average, expectable" environments.

A corollary of this view of developmental process is that development is never "arrested" but takes different forms with different relational experiences. Thus, we must understand both the implicit and explicit relational meaning systems that *did* develop *and* the enactive relational procedures that *might have* developed under other circumstances and might serve the child or adult better in her current context. Patient and therapist are inevitably working simultaneously at affective, cognitive, and enactive levels to deconstruct the old, more limited, or more negatively toned procedures or meanings, while simultaneously constructing more integrated, flexible, and hopeful ways of making meaning and being together.

In the process of normal development, implicit relational procedures are continually being modified through new forms of dialogue that are more collaborative and inclusive, forms that achieve more specific recognition of the other's subjectivity and that allow the elaboration of new expressions of agency and affect. For an adult patient, more collaborative and inclusive dialogue may involve partially translating previously implicit procedural knowing into words, while for the young child the work may operate entirely at the implicit level through interactive play that is largely noninterpretation-based (see Ablon, 1996). For example, the therapist might engage with the child's fear of aggressive interactions by permissive and assertive moves in collaborative play that are never raised to the level of interpretation. The degree of verbalized self-awareness that is useful would depend on the usual level of verbalized self-reflective function characteristic of a child of a given age. In this conception any sharp distinction between insight-promotion and "corrective experience" or "developmental help" is not primary as long as there is a psychoanalytically informed engagement around the organization of the child's or adult's implicit and explicit relational meaning systems.

This conception of therapeutic process as the simultaneous deconstruction of maladaptive control structures and the increasing articulation of competing control structures offers a more general conceptualization of the several levels of process that are coming together in a new emerging organization at a moment of therapeutic change. If representational change involves not only cognition or "insight" but also changes in affectively rich "ways of being with," a shift in organization must also involve a reorganization of the analyst's and patient's ways of being together. Therefore, moments of reorganization must involve a new kind of intersubjective meeting that occurs in a new "opening" in the interpersonal space, allowing both participants to become agents toward one another in a new way. This "opening" between the two, which in this conception is part of a state of destabilization and flux created by an emergent new organization, allows new initiatives and spontaneous interpersonal actions to be applied toward constructing a new or different intersubjective arrangement (and representation). This new organization is not simply a product of the individual patient's intrapsychic work, however, but of the working out of new relational possibilities with the analyst. The analyst's specific participation as a new kind of relational partner is part of the "something more" that allows an integrated affective and relational change, in concert with the conscious insight that may or may not accompany the emergence of the new order. A more elaborated statement of this view of change in analytically oriented treatment is articulated in Stern et al. (1998).

Conclusions

A conceptual framework for understanding psychoanalytic and developmental change in implicit relational knowing is offered that is congruent with current developmental and neuroscientific research and congenial to the clinical "feel" of extended analytically oriented treatment. Three major shifts from previous analytic theory seem necessary to accommodate new research. First, developmental work makes clear that characteristics of the two-person dialogue make central contributions to the form of "internalized objects" or implicit relational procedures that are constructed by the child, as well as to the defensive deletions and distortions that mark those implicit procedures. Second, a theory of implicit or enacted procedural meaning is needed that is not isomorphic with previous conceptions of the dynamic unconscious. Third, a conception of how procedures for being with others become more articulated, adapted, and inclusive is needed that does not rely solely or primarily on translating procedural knowing into symbolic form. In summary, the analytically central concepts of motivation, affect, conflict, and defense need to be integrated with a theory of the development of implicit relational knowing to account more fully for both clinical and developmental phenomena.

References

Ablon, S. (1996), The therapeutic action of play. *J. Amer. Acad. Child & Adoles. Psychiat.*, 35:545–547.

Ainsworth, M. D. S., Blehar, M., Waters, E. & Wall, S. (1978), *Patterns of Attachment*. Hillsdale, NJ: Lawrence Erlbaum Associates.

Anderson, J. (1982), Acquisition of cognitive skill. *Psycholog. Rev.*, 89:369–406.

Baldwin, A., Cole, R. & Baldwin, C. (1982), Parental pathology, family interaction, and the competence of the child in school. *Monogr. Soc. Res. Child Develop.*, 47:197.

Beebe, B. & Lachmann, F. M. (1994), Representation and internalization in infancy: Three principles of salience. *Psychoanal. Psychol.*, 11:127–165.

Bollas, C. (1987), *The Shadow of the Object*. London: Free Association Books.

Boston Process of Change Study Group (1998), Interventions that effect change in psychotherapy: A model based on infant research. *Infant Mental Health J.*, 19:277–353.

Bowlby, J. (1969), *Attachment and Loss: Vol. 1. Attachment*. New York: Basic Books.

Bretherton, I. (1988), Open communication and internal working models: Their role in the development of attachment relationships. In: *Nebraska Symposium on Motivation: Socio-emotional Development*, ed. R. A. Thompson. Lincoln, NE: University of Nebraska Press, pp. 57–113.

———— (1991), Pouring new wine into old bottles: The social self as internal working model. In: *Minnesota Symposia on Child Development: Vol. 23. Self Process and Development*, ed. M. R. Gunnar & L. A. Sroufe. Hillsdale, NJ: Lawrence Erlbaum, pp. 1–41.

———— McNew, S. & Beeghly-Smith, M. (1981), Early person knowledge as expressed in verbal and gestural communications: When do infants acquire a "theory of mind"? In: *Infant Social Cognition*, ed. M. E. Lamb & L. R. Sherrod. Hillsdale, NJ: Lawrence Erlbaum, pp. 333–373.

Bruner, J. S., Olver, R. R. & Greenfield, P. M. (1966), *Studies in Cognitive Growth*. New York: Wiley.

Carpenter, M., Nagell, K. & Tomasello, M. (1998), Social cognition, joint attention, and communicative competence from 9 to 15 months of age. *Monogr. Soc. Research Child Develop.*, 63:1–174.

Case, R. (1491), *The Mind's Staircase*. Hillsdale, NJ: Lawrence Erlbaum.

Cassidy, J. & Berlin, L. J. (1994), The insecure/ambivalent pattern of attachment: Theory and research. *Child Develop.*, 65:971–991.

Claparède, E. (1911), Reconnaissance et moitie. (Recognition and me-ness.) *Arch. Psychol.*, 11:79–90. In: *Organization and Pathology of Thought*, ed. D. Rapaport. New York: Columbia University Press, 1951.

Clyman, R. (1991), The procedural organization of emotions: A contribution from cognitive science to the psychoanalytic theory of therapeutic action. *J. Amer. Psychoanal. Assn.*, 39:349–382.

Cohen, N. J. & Squire, L. R. (1980), Preserved learning and retention of pattern-analyzing skill in amnesia. Dissociation of knowing how and knowing that. *Science*, 210:207–210.

Craik, K. (1943), *The Nature of Explanation*. Cambridge, UK: Cambridge University Press.

Crockenberg, S. & Litman, C. (1990), Autonomy as competence in two-year-olds: Maternal correlates of child compliance, defiance, and self-assertion. *Devel. Psychol.*, 26:961–971.

Damasio, A. (1994), *Descartes' Error: Emotion, Reason and the Human Brain*. New York: Putnam.

Edelman, G. M. (1987), *Neural Darwinism*. New York: Basic Books.

Fairbairn, W. R. D. (1952), *An Object-Relations Theory of the Personality*. New York: Basic Books.

Fischer, K. (1980), A theory of cognitive development: The control and construction of hierarchies of skills. *Psychol. Bull.*, 87:477–531.

———— & Granott, N. (1995), Beyond one-dimensional change: Parallel, concurrent, socially distributed processes in learning and development. *Human Devel.*, 38:302–314.

———— & Pipp, S. (1984), Development of structures of unconscious thought. In: *The Unconscious Reconsidered*, ed. K. Bowers & D. Meichenbaum. New York: Wiley, pp. 88–148.

———— & Watson, M. (1981), Explaining the Oedipus conflict. *Cognitive Development*, 12:79–92.

Fonagy, P. (1991), Thinking about thinking: Some clinical and theoretical considerations in the treatment of the borderline patient. *Internat. J. Psycho-Anal.*, 72:639–656.

Freeman, W. (1990), Searching for signal and noise in the chaos of brain waves. In: *The Ubiquity of Chaos*, ed. S. Krasner. Washington, DC: American Association for the Advancement of Science, pp. 47–55.

Grice, H. P. (1975), Logic and conversation. In: *Syntax and Semantics III: Speech Acts*, ed. P. Lole & J. L. Moran. New York: Academic Press, pp. 41–58.

Gunnar, M., Brodersen, L., Nachmias, M., Buss, K. & Rigatuso, R. (in press), Stress reactivity and attachment security. *Devel. Psychobiol.*

Hertsgaard, L., Gunnar, M., Erickson, M. & Nachmias, M. (1995), Adrenocortical response to the strange situation in infants with disorganized/disoriented attachment relationships. *Child Devel.*, 66:1100–1106.

Hobson, P. (1993), The intersubjective domain: Approaches from developmental psychopathology. *J. Amer. Psychoanal. Assn. Suppl. Research*, 61:167–192.

Hoffman, L. (1992), Some practical implications of a social constructivist view of the psychoanalytic situation. *Psychoanal. Dial.*, 2:287–304.

Izard, C. E. (1978), Emotions as motivation: An evolutionary-developmental perspective. In: *Nebraska Symposium on Motivation*, ed. R. A. Dienstbier. Lincoln, NE: University of Nebraska Press, pp. 163–200.

Jacobs, T. (1991), The interplay of enactments: Their role in the analytic process. In: *The Use of the Self*, ed. T. Jacobs. Madison, CT: International Universities Press, pp. 31–49.

Jacoby, L. L. & Dallas, M. (1981), On the relationship between autobiographical memory and perceptual learning. *J. Exper. Psychol.: Gen.*, 110:300–324.

Kernberg, O. (1976), *Object Relations Theory and Clinical Psychoanalysis*. New York: Aronson.

Kihlstrom, J. (1987), The cognitive unconscious. *Science*, 237:1445–1452.

Kobak, R. & Sceery, A. (1988), Attachment in late adolescence: Working models, affect regulation, and representations of self and others. *Child Devel.*, 59:135–146.

Landry, M. & Lyons-Ruth, K. (1980), Recursive structure in cognitive perspective-taking. *Child Devel.*, 51:386–394.

Lewis, M. (1995), Memory and psychoanalysis: A new look at infantile amnesia and transference. *J. Amer. Acad. Child Adol. Psychiat.*, 34:405–417.

Lichtenberg, J. (1989), *Psychoanalysis and Motivation*. Hillsdale, NJ: The Analytic Press.

Lyons-Ruth, K. (1991), Rapprochement or approchement: Mahler's theory reconsidered from the vantage point of recent research on early attachment relationships. *Psychoanal. Psychol.*, 8:1–23.

——— (1998), Implicit relational knowing: Its role in development and psychoanalytic treatment. *Infant Mental Health J.*, 19:282–289.

——— (in press), "I sense that you sense that I sense . . .": Sander's recognition process and implicit relational knowing in the psychotherapeutic setting. *Infant Mental Health J., Festschrift Issue in Honor of Dr. Louis Sander*.

——— Alpern, L. & Repacholi, B. (1993), Disorganized infant attachment classification and maternal psychosocial problems as predictors of hostile-aggressive behavior in the preschool classroom. *Child Devel.*, 64:572–585.

————— Bronfman, E. & Atwood, G. (1999), A relational diathesis model of hostile-helpless states of mind: Expressions in mother-infant interaction. In: *Attachment Disorganization*, ed. J. Solomon & C. George. New York: Guilford, pp. 33–70.

————— —————, & Parsons, E. (1999), Maternal disrupted affective communication, maternal frightened or frightening behavior, and disorganized infant attachment strategies. In: *Atypical Patterns of Infant Attachment: Theory, Research and Current Directions*, ed. J. Vondra & D. Barnett. *Monographs of the Society for Research in Child Development*, 64.

————— & Zeanah, C. (1993), The family context of infant mental health, Part I: Affective development in the primary caregiving relationship. In: *Handbook of Infant Mental Health*, ed. C. Zeanah. New York: Guilford, 1993, pp. 14–26.

————— & Jacobvitz, D. (1999), Attachment disorganization: Unresolved loss, relational violence, and lapses in behavioral and attentional strategies. In: *Handbook of Attachment Theory and Research*, ed. J. Cassidy & P. Shaver. New York: Guilford, pp. 520–554.

Main, M. (1993), Discourse, prediction, and recent studies in attachment: Implications for psychoanalysis. *J. Amer. Psychoanal. Assn., Suppl. on Res. in Psychoanal.*, 61:209–243.

————— & Goldwyn, R. (1994), Adult Attachment Rating and Classification System. Unpublished coding manual, Department of Psychology, University of California at Berkeley, Berkeley, CA.

————— & Hesse, E. (1990), Parents' unresolved traumatic experiences are related to infant disorganized attachment status: Is frightened and/or frightening parental behavior the linking mechanism? In: *Attachment in the Preschool Years: Theory, Research and Intervention*, ed. M. Greenberg, D. Cicchetti, & E. M. Cummings. Chicago: University of Chicago Press, pp. 161–184.

————— Kaplan, N. & Cassidy, J. (1985), Security in infancy, childhood and adulthood: A move to the level of representation. In: *Growing Points of Attachment Theory and Research. Monographs of the Society for Research in Child Development*, ed. I. Bretherton & E. Waters. 50:66–104.

————— Tomasini, L. & Tolan, W. (1979), Differences among mothers of infants judged to differ in security of attachment. *Devel. Psychol.*, 15:472–473.

Malatesta, C. Z., Culber, C., Tesman, J. R. & Shepard, B. (1989), The development of emotion expression during the first two years of life. *Monogr. Soc. Res. Child Devel.*, 54.

Marcel, A. (1983), Conscious and unconscious perception: Experiments on visual masking and word recognition. *Cognitive Psychol.*, 15:197–237.

McLaughlin, J. (1991), Clinical and theoretical aspects of enactment. *J. Amer. Psychoanal. Assn.*, 39:595–674.

Mitchell, S. (1988), *Relational Concepts in Psychoanalysis*. Cambridge, MA: Harvard University Press.

Ogden, T. (1994), The analytic third: Working with intersubjective clinical facts. *Internat. J. Psycho-Anal.*, 75:3–19.

Oster, H., & Eckman, P. (1977), Facial behavior in child development. In: *Minnesota Symnposium on Child Psychology*, Vol. 11, ed. A. Collins. New York: Thomas A. Crowell, pp. 231–376.

Piaget, J. & Inhelder, B. (1973), *Memory and Intelligence*. New York: Basic Books.

Prigogine, L & Stengers, I. (1984), *Order Out of Chaos: Man's New Dialogue with Nature*. New York: Bantam Books.

Rumelhart, D. E., & McClelland, J. L. & the PDP Research Group. (1986), *Parallel Distributed Processing*, Vol. 1. Cambridge: MIT Press.

Sander, L. (1987), Awareness of inner experience: A systems perspective on self-regulatory process in early development. *Child Abuse and Neglect.* 11:339–346.

——— (1995), Thinking about developmental process: Wholeness, specificity, and the organization of conscious experiencing. Invited address, annual meeting of the Division of Psychoanalysis, American Psychological Association. Santa Monica, CA.

Sandler, J. & Sandler, A. (1994), The past unconscious and the present unconscious: A contribution to a technical frame of reference. *The Psychoanalytic Study of the Child*, 49:278–292. New Haven, CT: Yale University Press.

Schacter, D. L. & Buckner, R. L. (1998), Priming and the brain. *Neuron*, 20:185–195.

——— & Moscovitch, M. (1984), Infants, amnesia and dissociable memory systems. In: *Infant Memory*, ed. M. Moscovitch. New York: Plenum, pp. 173–216.

Seligman, S. (1995), Applying infant observation research to psychoanalytic clinical work: A contemporary perspective. Plenary presentation to the Congress of the International Psychoanalytic Studies Organization of the International Psychoanalytical Association. San Francisco, July.

Selman, R. F. (1980), *The Growth of Interpersonal Understanding*. New York: Academic Press.

Spangler, G. & Grossmann, K. E. (1993), Biobehavioral organization in securely and insecurely attached infants. *Child Devel.*, 64:1439–1450.

Stern, D. (1998), The process of therapeutic change involving implicit knowledge: Some implications of developmental observations for adult psychotherapy. *Infant Mental Health J.*, 19:300–308.

——— (1985), *The Interpersonal World of the Infant: A View from Psychoanalysis and Developmental Psychology*. New York: Basic Books.

——— (1995), *The Motherhood Constellation*. New York: Basic Books.

——— Sander, L., Nahum, J., Harrison, A., Lyons-Ruth, K., Morgan, A., Bruschweiler-Stern, N. & Tronick, E. Z. (1998), Non-interpretive mechanisms in psychoanalytic therapy: The "something more" than interpretation. *Internat. J. Psycho-Anal.*, 79:903–921.

Stolorow, R. (in press), Dynamic, dyadic, intersubjective systems: An evolving paradigm for psychoanalysis. *Internat. J. Psycho. Anal.*

Thelen, E. & Smith, L. B. (1994), *A Dynamic Systems Approach to the Development of Cognition and Action*. Cambridge: MIT Press/Bradford Books.

Trevarthen, C. (1980), The foundations of intersubjectivity: Development of interpersonal and cooperative understanding in infants. In: *The Social Foundations of Language and Thought*, ed. D. Olson. New York: Norton, pp. 316–342.

Tronick, E. (1989), Emotions and emotional communication in infants. *Amer. Psychol.*, 44:112–119.

——— (1998), Dyadically expanded states of consciousness and the process of normal and abnormal development. *Infant Mental Health J.*, 19:300–308.

Tulving, E. (1972), Episodic and semantic memory. In: *Organization of Memory*, ed. E. Tulving & W. Donaldson. New York: Academic Press, pp. 382–403.

van IJzendoorn, M. H. (1995), Adult attachment representations, parental responsiveness, and infant attachment: A meta-analysis on the predictive validity of the Adult Attachment Interview. *Psychol. Bull.*, 117:387–403.

Vygotsky, L. S. (1962), *Thought and Language*. Cambridge: MIT Press.

Westen, D. (1990), Towards a revised theory of borderline object relations: Contributions of empirical research. *Internat. J. Psycho-Anal.*, 71:661–694.

Wolff, P. (1996), The irrelevance of infant observations for psychoanalysis. *J. Amer. Psychoanal. Assn.*, 44:369–391.

Wood, D., Bruner, J. & Ross, G. (1976), The role of tutoring in problem-solving. *J. Child Psychol. & Psychiat.*, 17:89–100.

Part III

Social and Cultural Dimensions of Relationality

The most intricate, dynamic, and creative work in the inaugural years of the relational perspective focused on the clinical situation, on the complexity of dyadic interactions and the deep engagement and interpenetration of subjectivities in systems. But, almost from the beginning, some intrepid writers and thinkers were trying to widen our gaze to take in intersubjectivity and interaction in wider, more complex contexts.

The emergence and evolution of having and being a body requires thinking about the powerful intersect of public and private in sexuality, examining the meaning of class consciousness, cultural identity, and racial subjectivities. All these complex situations require subtle attunement to a dexterous balancing of multiple fields of inquiry. All four writers in this section manage these theoretical balancing acts while staying grounded in the clinical situation.

Here four relational thinkers consider subjectivity and intersubjectivity in complex social, political, and ideologically tinged contexts, and our collective theoretical vision is appreciably widened.

Psychoanalysis and the Urban Poor

(1993)

Neil Altman

▼ ▼ ▼ ▼ ▼

Editors' Introduction

Relational psychoanalysis is inherently a contextual psychology placing the self within an intersubjective field. Within the American interpersonal tradition, Sullivan and his followers, along with the American "cultural school," took the lead in reformulating Freudian theory in social terms. Following the 1960s cultural challenge of authority, the civil rights movement, feminism, and the women's movement, as well as the impact of postmodernism in academia, foundational values and assumptions have been questioned across disciplines. Developments in American relational theory must be understood against this historical backdrop, allowing for a more critical examination of the place of psychoanalysis within our culture and society.

Relational psychoanalysis is marked by the strong impact of feminism on its theories and values. Neil Altman has been the trail blazer in taking psychoanalysis to the margins: to those excluded by traditional theory and practice, to those made peripheral by our society. Altman's (1995) book *The Analyst in the Inner City* (The Analytic Press) examined issues of race, class, and culture by focusing on the clinical problems of conducting psychoanalysis with inner city and poor populations and within public clinics.

In an effort to bridge the gap between psychoanalysis and social theory, Altman argues that racial, cultural, and social-class divisions reflect the splits that accompany the consolidation of an individual self. Following Mitchell, Atman draws on object-relational notions of splitting and projective identification as well as the Sullivanian concept of the "not-me" in order to develop his own integrative relational theory. According to Altman, the "disowned other" is unconsciously constructed to embody those psychic qualities unacceptable to the self. Societal polarization along racial and class lines, in public and private sectors, supports this psychic process by delineating groups that reinforce splitting. Altman demonstrates that psychoanalysis has its own value-laden and culturally embedded framework, which goes unchallenged so long as psychoanalysis excludes large segments of the population. By limiting itself to affluent private-practice settings, psychoanalysis maintains a homogenous American suburban environment with respect to culture, class, and race. Altman, who spent many years working in inner-city clinic and hospital settings and who, as one of the founders and the first president of the Section on Psychoanalysis and Social Responsibility of the Division of Psychoanalysis (39) of the American Psychological Association, has been a leader and pioneer activist in the application of psychoanalysis to social issues.

Altman's focus moves back and forth between such microcosmic levels as therapist–patient interaction, the relations among the mental health disciplines, staff relations within a clinic, and macrocosmic social forces as wide-ranging as capitalism, the mental health system, the dominant philosophy of science. In Altman's work, social, cultural, and critical theory come together with clinical theory and practice to illuminate the difficult problems of contemporary life and to keep psychoanalysis central to any discussion of the modern world.

Psychoanalysis and the Urban Poor*

Although there have been efforts in Europe (Jacoby, 1983) and Latin America (Langer, 1989) to apply a psychoanalytic approach to people from a lower socioeconomic class background, in this country there have been few such attempts. In the United States, psychoanalytic treatment has generally taken place in a private practice setting where the lower-class patient cannot afford the fee. Yet economic factors do not fully

* Originally published in *Psychoanalytic Dialogues*, 3:29–49. © 1993 The Analytic Press, Inc.

explain the traditional exclusion of the lower-class patient. Even in low-fee training clinics attached to universities, institutes, and hospitals, lower-class patients have often been "selected out" if they applied for treatment. Criteria of "analyzability," to be discussed further below, were often cited. Psychoanalysis came to be a treatment for the educated, middle-to-upper-class patient, as documented by Hollingshead and Redlich (1958) in their empirical study of social class and mental illness in New Haven of the 1950s.

In recent years, there has been some degree of reversal of this tendency to exclude the lower socioeconomic status patient from psychoanalytic treatment. As fewer people seek out psychoanalysis, patients from lower-class backgrounds have sometimes been accepted in training clinics out of necessity. Moreover, clinicians with psychoanalytic training often spend part of their professional time in public clinics where such patients are increasingly the vast majority, no matter where the clinic is located.

As psychoanalysts embark on work with inner-city people in public clinics, they often wonder about the extent to which the psychoanalytic treatment model is applicable or adaptable in this context. The purpose of this paper is to argue that, beyond being thus applicable and adaptable, the psychoanalytic model is essential to work with such patients. Further, I attempt to demonstrate that a psychoanalytic model is necessary to understand the impact of the institutional context on work with these patients. In these ways, my effort is to breach the polarity that has developed in psychoanalysis between work with relatively affluent patients and work with the poor and between work in private practice and work done in public clinic settings.

Any attempt to understand the meaning of what an inner-city patient presents in treatment must take account of the institutional context of that work, as well as the patient's and analyst's ethnicity, culture, and socioeconomic status. Therefore, I will take a moment to describe the community in which the clinical work was done that forms the basis of this paper. I will provide the reader with relevant data regarding the ethnic groups in the community, the poverty in which they live, and the unexpected sources of strength and richness to be found there.

The clinical work discussed in this paper was done in a community mental health center associated with a large inner-city hospital in New York City. The community in which this hospital is located, in the early-to-mid-20th century, was home to working-class and middle-class people of Jewish, Irish, and Italian descent. They were first-and-second-generation immigrants who had recently escaped the poverty and over-crowded conditions of the Lower East Side of Manhattan. The construction of expressways in the 1950s and 1960s had a profound impact on the area. One expressway cut through the heart of the community, causing one side to become "the other side of the tracks," an undesirable place to live. At the same time, the expressways stimulated the development of suburbs, which drained this community of many of its upwardly mobile people.

As middle-class people left this area, other social forces led to the immigration into the community of new groups of people. The industrialization of Puerto Rico, other Caribbean islands, and the southern part of the United States led to the displacement of many rural Puerto Ricans and Afro-Americans from the South and the Caribbean who came to New York in search of new opportunities. When they found such opportunities, these immigrants, like upwardly mobile people of the previous generation, tended to move "uptown" or to the suburbs. Those who did not find the opportunities they sought had no choice but to stay. The community sank into ever-deeper poverty. Landlords began abandoning their properties, which often burned, leading to a massive depletion of the housing stock in the 1960s. Blocks that once housed middle-class people were turned to rubble in an astonishingly short period of time.

The community has nonetheless remained a culturally rich and dynamic center of New York life. New immigrants have continually reinforced the cultural diversity of the area, bringing with them new hopes and aspirations. In the last ten years there have been immigrants, some of whom entered this country legally and some of whom did not, from the Dominican Republic and from the war-torn countries of Central America. Those who are not here legally often do not seek out social services for fear of being revealed and deported. The first generation of these immigrants generally consists of people who do not speak English and who live in close proximity to family members or people from the same country, even the same town or village. The traditional emphasis on family life is reinforced by the need to have sustaining human connections in an alien environment. The second generation, the children and adolescents, learn to speak English in school and from their peers and begin to become acculturated. Much family conflict is stimulated when second-generation adolescents begin to rebel against the traditional values of their parents, demanding more freedom and autonomy, for example. Some adolescents fall in with a drug- and crime-prone subculture that, with its expensive cars and clothing, is easily noticeable on the streets, further alienating them from their parents.

At present, the social class of the people who live in this community is somewhat diverse within a limited range. By all the indicators of social class cited by Hollingshead and Redlich (1958), that is, residential address, education, and occupation, the people of this area are in the lowest social classes. There are working-class people who do blue-collar or clerical jobs. Many other people in this community have found themselves lacking skills for the available jobs in a service economy; as a result, welfare rolls have swelled in the community, and there are a large number of families who subsist on public assistance, some for three or more generations. School dropout rates are high, although a significant number of female heads of households (at least second generation in this country) attempt to go back to school in their 20s and 30s, once their children are in school. Many families are single-parent families, usually headed by females. The absence of men reflects a process of marginalization that began with the undermining of their traditional breadwinning role when unable to find jobs. Adolescent pregnancy and childbirth are very common, reinforcing the school dropout rates and, in many cases, resulting in the raising of young children by grandmothers. The death of some young parents from AIDS or their inability to parent due to crack abuse further increases the role of grandparents in child care.

The ethnicity of the people in this community creates a complicated mosaic. Not only are there people from many different countries and cultures, but there are various levels of acculturation to North American industrial and postindustrial society. The first-generation people brought with them a culture born in a rural, agricultural context, with traditional values related to family life, religion, and so on. Further social changes in this community are aspects of the so-called feminization of poverty, alluded to previously.

For purposes of dealing with a manageable level of complexity in this paper, I attempt to deal with social class as a variable in psychological work in some degree of isolation from culture and ethnicity. The reader should bear in mind that this is an artificial isolation, which results in some degree of oversimplification.

The Theoretical Background of this Paper

As mentioned previously, there is a polarity in psychoanalysis between work with the poor in public clinics and work with the well-to-do in private practice. This polarity has been reinforced, it seems to me, by two traditional currents in psychoanalytic thinking. The classical Freudian model, with its emphasis on creating a "blank screen" context for psychoanalytic work, is not adaptable to work in a public clinic in which the therapist is often called upon to fill multiple roles, for example, advocate with other social welfare agencies, in addition to one's primary role as therapist. Second, the ego psychological approach, with its tendency to define pathology in terms of defect or deficit, lends itself to a stratification of patients according to "ego strength" that often mirrors stereotypes based on class, ethnicity, or race. Concepts of what constitutes ego strength are context-bound. Frustration tolerance, for example, or ability to delay gratification, is seen as an ego strength in a particular culture heavily influenced by Calvinism. In another cultural context, affiliativeness, quite at odds with Calvinist individualism, can appear as a prominent ego strength. Such context-bound judgments find their way into classical theory and technique in their requirement that the "analyzable" patient be able to tolerate the abstinence of the analyst. One can thereby be led to find lower-class or culturally different patients unsuitable for psychoanalytic work or to address their ego "deficits" with a modified technique. The result is a two-tiered psychoanalysis unwittingly reflective of the social class differential between lower-class patient and higher-class patient or between lower-class patient and higher-class analyst. As pointed out by Sennett and Cobb (1972), social class differences are often interpreted as reflecting "questions of character, of moral resolve, will, and competence" (p. 256). That is, in a society in which everyone is presumed to have equal opportunity to advance socially, one's lower-class standing is easily seen as evidence of personal failure. The two-tiered psychoanalysis that may result when ego psychology is applied to psychoanalysis colludes with and reinforces this view of such patients as inferior.

I hope to demonstrate in this paper that a psychoanalytic approach based on object relations theory avoids this tendency toward stratifications of patients and nicely accommodates the influence of a public clinic context on psychoanalytic work. With respect to the stratification of patients, let us consider, for example, contrasting views on "analyzability." A classical/ego psychological approach, in which insight is the sole mechanism of analytic change, naturally places a premium on verbal intelligence in the selection of patients (Bachrach and Leaff, 1978). The ability to tolerate frustration without "acting out," specifically, the ability to tolerate the analyst's abstinence, is also crucial. Such criteria clearly favor the relatively highly educated and sophisticated patient, thus introducing a bias against many lower-class people who are less likely to have had the same educational background as a middle- to upper-class patient. By contrast, in many object relations approaches in psychoanalysis, the patient-analyst relationship is presumed to carry the therapeutic impact. Analytic anonymity and reserve per se are not considered essential to a neutral stance (Greenberg, 1986). Object relations approaches, as I argue later, do not necessarily draw a hard and fast line between verbalization and so-called acting out. The patient's nonverbal actions can be seen as having useful communicative value. Therefore, verbal intelligence becomes a less central prerequisite for analytic work. Criteria of analyzability thus become considerably more flexible (see Green, 1986 for such a reconsideration of analyzability). In general, the relational emphasis on the interconnectedness of people easily accommodates the focus on the family or the social group embedded in the cultures of many inner-city patients.

In developing an object relational approach to the issues that commonly arise in work with lower-class patients, I draw heavily on the concepts of W. R. D. Fairbairn (1952, 1958). Fairbairn was a Scottish psychoanalyst contemporary with Melanie Klein and D. W. Winnicott. His work elaborated on Klein's concept of "internalized objects." Specifically, he elaborated on the nature of the "bad" internalized object; he also developed a concept of linkages between self- and object representations that formed one of the bases of the work of Kernberg. I compare this object relational approach with the work of Fred Pine (1985) with inner-city patients, from an ego psychological perspective. I focus on how the approaches vary in their views of analyzability and in the understanding and clinical management of such issues as missed appointments, crises, and concrete advocacy (e.g., help with socioeconomic problems).

The Case of Linda

Let us begin with a clinical vignette. A patient, Linda, is referred to a public mental health clinic because she has been feeling nervous. She was brought into an emergency room the previous night by her sister after losing her temper and throwing dishes at her boyfriend. She is angry because she suspects that he has another woman. Linda's sister, on her behalf, says that she needs pills for her nerves. Linda has several times in the past received prescriptions for "nerve medicine." She tends to take them irregularly, regardless of how they are prescribed. The emergency room resident, having seen Linda before and knowing that she tends not to follow up on treatment, decides not to give her a prescription that night and to send her to the outpatient clinic the next morning. She is seen there by a psychology intern who talks with her for a long time. The intern hears a story of parental abandonment as a child, of numerous betrayals by parents and boyfriends. The patient expresses a great deal of anger at many people in her life. The intern points out that the latest betrayal, by her boyfriend the previous night, is only the latest in a long series of previous events and so strikes a very raw nerve. The patient acknowledges the intern's comment and promises to return the next week to talk with her again, without asking for medication. She says that talking to the intern has made her feel much better.

The next week, Linda does not show up, much to the disappointment of the intern, who felt she had established a strong and meaningful connection with her in their first meeting. Since Linda has no phone, the intern writes her a letter. There is no response for two weeks from Linda. In the third week, however, the intern is called by the receptionist to say that Linda is in the waiting room to see her. She knows she has no appointment but would like to see her for just a moment. The intern feels confused, irritated, worried. When Linda comes into her office, she apologizes for not returning to the clinic, explaining that she has been getting the runaround from welfare and that she has decided to apply for SSI (Supplemental Security Income; a Social Security program to provide money to people who cannot work because of a physical or mental disability) on the basis of her mental condition. Would the intern please send her medical records to the Social Security Administration on her behalf?

The intern feels quite disoriented. Linda's actions seem to be an indirect, yet powerful, communication of hostility and despair, provoking similar feelings in the intern. She had thought that this woman could benefit from psychotherapy. Linda seems to be settling for crumbs from life. Why accept the status of a mentally disabled person so easily? Is she trying to exploit the system? Perhaps, in her world, there are no options. You either find a secure source of income from the "system," or you do not eat. And, anyway, what should a would-be psychotherapist say to Linda? The intern feels caught between rejecting her, on one hand, and colluding with her exploitativeness, hostility, and despair, on the other. Should she go along with Linda's request as a temporary expedient to establish a relationship with her? Would a rejection undermine any chance that Linda would come back? Would acceding to Linda's request be a collusion with Linda's devaluation of herself and her exploitation of the system? Which course of action would less seriously undermine a therapeutic relationship? Besides all that, Linda really does not seem to want psychotherapy. Should the intern urge it on her? After all, Linda does not come from a background where people go for therapy when they are in trouble. Perhaps the intern needs to start with her where she is and work toward being a therapist. But along the way, how does one avoid foreclosing one's ability to take a therapeutic stance in the future? The intern, trying to deal with all these thoughts, not to mention her feelings and her anxiety, asks Linda about the experiences that led up to her decision to apply for SSI and about whether she sees herself as being able to work. She inquires as to how the patient would feel if she got SSI. She also conveys her opinion that the patient could benefit from psychotherapy and that perhaps psychotherapy would lead Linda to see other options in her life. Linda agrees to give it a try and leaves with another appointment.

Theoretical Perspectives

This vignette contains elements common to work in public clinics with lower-socioeconomic status patients. Missed appointments, presentation in crisis, and a focus on assistance with concrete, bread-and-butter issues are typically encountered in this context. From a classical psychoanalytic or ego psychological point of view, this clinical situation is highly problematic in terms of a psychoanalytic treatment model. The patient is seen as having very limited tolerance for anxiety (defined in relation to the emerging awareness, in treatment, of repressed drives and their derivatives) and frustration (defined in relation to the "abstinence" of the classical psychoanalytic situation). These ego "defects" result in the patient's attempt to break the frame in a very disruptive way by missing appointments. Her conscious motivation in relation to her would-be therapist is to obtain concrete help in a way that would compromise the therapist's neutrality and abstinence. Although she seems potentially psychologically minded, there appear to be major obstacles to the establishment of a viable therapeutic alliance. Are these obstacles insurmountable from a classical/ego psychological point of view?

Fred Pine (1985),[1] drawing on his work supervising trainees with inner-city patients, whom he describes as "socioeconomically distressed" and from "destructive familial and social backgrounds," attempts to

---

[1] Pine's work is characterized here as classical and ego psychological in its theoretical orientation. I recognize that in his latest work (Pine, 1990) he attempts to integrate the four psychologies of drive, ego, object relations, and self. However, I believe that, while he has moved toward assimilating an object relations psychology in his theorizing, he remains essentially rooted in classical and ego psychological theory. For example, he (1990) writes, "I propose repetition in the effort at mastery of the strain trauma in old object relationships as a primary and the most distinct motive force in the domain of the object relations psychology at the clinically relevant level" (p. 84). This is actually an ego psychologically-based approach to object relations. An approach that stresses the primacy of object seeking per se, not in an effort at mastery of trauma, is more properly spoken of as an "object relations" theory. Pine moves in this

adapt classical theory and technique to patients such as Linda. He frames the basic problem in work with such patients as adapting to their limited tolerance for anxiety and frustration. Pine believes that such patients require support from the therapist in one form or another in order to tolerate the anxiety attendant upon interpretation. For example, he might warn a patient a moment in advance that he was about to say something that would be difficult to hear, in order to give the patient an opportunity to orient to the stressful situation. Or he might refrain from interpreting a transference wish or feeling while it is active in relation to the therapist, commenting on it only in retrospect some days later, when the anxiety level is lower. Pine calls this technique "striking while the iron is cold."

Pine finds that he can offer such support to patients who need it, without compromising the basic goal of analytically oriented treatment, which, for him, is insight through interpretation. In summarizing his position, he challenges the traditional notion that supportive therapy and insight-oriented therapy are mutually exclusive. Instead, he says that a distinction can be made between interpretation in the context of abstinence and interpretation in the context of support. Patients with limited tolerance for anxiety and frustration, for Pine, can be reached only through interpretation in the context of support.

This polarity between abstinence and support rests on culture-bound notions of ego strength and creates a two-tiered psychoanalysis, as noted above. The polarity arises within the context of drive-theoretical concerns about gratification's interfering with the emergence of transference and leading to nonanalytic cures based on suggestion. Within a classical context Pine begins to breach the polarity between "analyzable" and "nonanalyzable" by sacrificing analytic purity and rigor in favor of a pragmatic attempt to impart insight effectively to those who are considered otherwise unreachable. Pine defends the "analytic" nature of this sort of work by a far-reaching reworking of classical theory and technique. Taking off from his perception that some patients need support from the therapist, he then develops a conception of curative factors in the analytic situation based on a parent-child model (Pine, 1985, chaps. 10–12). The therapist's reliability, nonjudgmental attitude, and ability to recognize, distinguish, and name feelings, for example, are seen as potentially curative factors in themselves. Just as such qualities in a parent

---

direction elsewhere in the same book when he writes, "Significant for the clinical relevance of the object relations psychology is the tendency to repeat these old family dramas, a repetition propelled by efforts after attachment or after mastery or both" (p. 35).

facilitate growth in children, in the therapist, they facilitate growth in patients. In essence, Pine adds the relationship with the therapist per se not only as the context for the development of insight but as a curative factor aside from the development of insight. He believes that these relational factors are operative in all analyses. A polarity is reintroduced, however, when Pine states that in patients with "strong egos" these relational factors operate in the background of the analysis. In work with patients with "weak egos," that is, with a history of early deprivation and poor capacity to tolerate anxiety and frustration, the analyst's "parenting" qualities are in the foreground as curative factors. Pine gives as an example his work with a young woman whose anxiety about the therapeutic work with him led her to miss a large number of sessions. Pine made an arrangement with her in which a certain hour would be available to her whether she used it or not. (Although he does not discuss the fee, it appears that the patient was not charged when she did not use this hour.) This was an hour in which he did administrative work at his hospital office. She came regularly, but very infrequently. If Pine were to be away at the time of her hour, he would inform her, even if she had not used her hour for many weeks or months. Under these conditions, Pine felt that his reliability and availability were facilitative of growth and change in his patient, aside from any insight through interpretation in the sessions that did occur.

In considering a patient such as Linda, then, Pine would see a picture of impaired ego functioning. Missed sessions, presentation in crisis, and focus on concrete help would be the reflections in treatment of this impaired ego. Insofar as relational, preoedipal issues predominate in the clinical picture, Pine would likely believe that relational, "parent-child" issues would be prominent in the transference. Insight through interpretation would be in the context of support rather than abstinence. The behavior of the analytically oriented therapist working with Pine's model would likely be less frustrating and more welcoming, supportive, and engaging with a patient such as Linda than with a patient seen as better able to tolerate anxiety and frustration.

The polarity between ego strength/abstinent analytic stance, on one hand, and ego weakness/supportive analytic stance, on the other, is further undermined by Mitchell's (1988) concept of the "developmental tilt." Such a "tilt" occurs when relational needs are seen as relatively early developmentally or as primitive, in comparison with drive-defense conflicts. One is easily led, thereby, to an emphasis on the deficits of a patient such as Linda, at the expense of her strengths and resources. When the "parent-child" model of treatment is reserved for those with "ego weaknesses," which are only too readily associated with lower-class membership, the result, again, can be a paternalistic/maternalistic atti-tude that reflects and perpetuates our society's class structure.

The issues raised by work with a patient such as Linda can be approached from a different angle—from the point of view of object relations theories. Interactions such as occurred with Linda and the intern are reframed, such that they can be understood and handled in an uncompromisingly analytic manner. When a therapist working from this point of view sits down with a patient, the question he is likely to ask himself is, Who am I in this patient's object world? That is, the therapist assumes that the transference will involve his being seen by the patient through the template of the patient's internalized objects. For Fairbairn (1952), for example, the transference involves the patient's see-ing the analyst as an exciting (i.e., tempting, promising) or a rejecting object. The technical problem that arises for people working from this point of view is, How does one open up the closed system of the patient's internalized object relations? How does one get seen as a new object, rather than simply a new version of an old object?

Greenberg (1986) points out that the problem is more complicated than that. The therapist must first enter the patient's world, must become a new version of an old object, in order to attain significance in the patient's life. The problem then becomes striking a balance between being seen as enough of an old object to be significant and being seen as enough of a new object so that there is room for change. From this point of view, the issues with Pine's patient, discussed just above, no longer revolve around the support that she needs. The question now is what sort of object the analyst is for her and how to strike the proper balance between new and old object to facilitate analytic work.

The issue of analyzability is now also strikingly different. The crite-ria from this point of view no longer have to do with intelligence or ver-bal ability, with qualities that facilitate the attainment of insight through interpretation. The criteria now have to do with a capacity to experi-ence multiple realities in the analytic situation, with what Mitchell (1988) and Winnicott (1971) would call the capacity to play in the inter-action with the analyst. As Green (1986, p. 36) points out, the criteria for analyzability may have more to do with the analyst's instrument than with the capacities of the patient.

With this object relations point of view in mind, let us return to the issues raised by work with poor patients. I begin with some typical rela-tional configurations that tend to get established with such patients in the context of a public clinic. I emphasize the role of this context on the way in which the therapist is viewed by the patient.

When a patient of lower socioeconomic status walks into a public clinic, from her point of view she enters another of the institutions that control crucial aspects of her life. A frame is already established for the therapy that is about to occur. A hospital or a hospital clinic is part of the network of institutions and bureaucracies that include public assistance, Medicaid, and Social Security. These institutions both provide and frustrate. At least, they are the potential source of provision. In fact, a person dealing with one of these systems is likely to encounter an overworked, harassed clerk whose mandate is not to provide benefits to anyone who cannot demonstrate impeccable qualifications of need. Could there be an external situation better calculated to evoke Fairbairn's inner world of exciting (that is, tempting) and rejecting (that is, frustrating) objects? In Fairbairn's picture of the inner world, the self is seen as split into two, a needy, desirous self (the libidinal ego) attached to the exciting object and a self that rejects need (the antilibidinal ego) attached to the rejecting object. Thus is depicted the combination of desperate need and hatred of both self and other that is felt by many poor patients as they apply for, or are asked to come for recertification of their need for, public assistance.

An object relations approach can thus lead us to re-conceptualize the relationship that economically deprived patients have to the institutions in their lives, including mental health clinics. Such relationships can be described as transferential, that is in object relations terms, as evocative of internalized object relationships, in the same way that Joseph (1988) discusses transference as a reaction to the "total situation" of the analysis. The nature of the institution in which psychoanalytic work takes place helps establish the relational context of that work. The relationship to the therapist and to the institution in which their work takes place allows patients to maintain and to elaborate their internal object worlds on an external stage. Fairbairn's depiction of that object world seems particularly apt in elucidating the sort of internalized object relationships likely to be elicited by the sort of stage that is presented to the patient in public clinics.

Recall now the intern and her patient, Linda. As Linda requests help from the intern with SSI, the intern finds herself identified, despite their conversation about her life, with the entire tantalizing social welfare system. In principle, is this situation different from any other transferential situation? Perhaps there are echoes here of what we would presume was Linda's experience with a parent. As one considers the therapeutic possibilities in this situation, Linda herself becomes a sort of exciting and rejecting object. A would-be therapist would like to engage her in an examination of these issues, but she is so elusive. Countertransference is induced, which, as Bollas (1987) points out, can be the analyst's entree into the patient's inner world.

Let us examine one likely transference-countertransference configuration that can be created by a patient such as Linda when she misses appointments. Particularly when there has been a session that stimulates some hope for productive work together, such a patient can leave the therapist feeling rejected, abandoned, angry. The therapist in a public clinic may, after many such experiences, bypass such feelings and say to herself, in effect, "Good. Now I have time to relax or catch up on my reading." She may hesitate to call the patient, if it seems too much like pursuing her. On the other hand, she may feel that she is abandoning the patient, perhaps in a retaliatory way, if she does not pursue her.

From an object relations perspective, what we are dealing with here can be seen as the patient's way of processing her own experiences of unreliability on the part of important people in her life. As the therapist feels rejected, despairing, or angry in relation to the patient, the therapist is sampling the patient's own experience. The situation provides the opportunity to feel one's way into the patient's object world, into her experience. This is a process described by Bollas (1987) as follows: "The analysand not only talks to the analyst about the self; he also puts the analyst through intense experience, effectively inviting the analyst to know his self and his objects" (p. 250).

Sometimes there is an added twist to this scenario. After missing several weeks, perhaps after the case is closed in the clinic, the patient may show up without an appointment, as Linda did. The patient may, in addition, be in crisis. With some patients, this pattern can become the modus operandi in the clinic. In extreme cases, patients may come only in crisis, without appointments, and rarely, if ever, keep the appointments that are offered to them. From an object relations perspective, one can find in such a situation the patient's attempt to maintain contact, a connection, with people who are experienced as basically rejecting, unreliable, and ungiving. That is, a crisis coerces a response. A crisis dramatizes the need of the patient to such an extent that a caretaking response is virtually guaranteed. Ogden (1986) makes a similar point in stating that self-other boundaries are blurred in a crisis. For Ogden, crises are a way of reestablishing the "unmediated sensory closeness" characteristic of Melanie Klein's paranoid-schizoid position. In the later depressive position, whole object relatedness is associated with a sense of isolation, which can be reversed when a crisis brings people together. Ogden writes: "Crises are not events which occur between separate people. They are events in which patient and therapist are 'in it together'" (p. 123). In responding to crises, the therapist experiences the patient's way of maintaining or attempting to maintain object ties in a depriving environment.

The therapist is in a very uncomfortable position as she begins to empathize with and sample the patient's experience of abandonment and despair. The "burnout" with which therapists in public clinics struggle is akin to a generalized "burnout" that can be observed in poor patients. In other words, one is tempted to withdraw, to give up, in the face of the anxiety, sense of futility, and despair that are engendered both by the patient's psychological situation and by the overwhelming social problems that impact on him or her. One way of coping with these feelings is to question the suitability for psychoanalytic therapy of inner-city patients. One may thereby justify not engaging the pain of these patients' lives, while taking the focus off one's own sense of helplessness and futility.

Problems such as missed appointments and presentation in crisis are formidable therapeutic obstacles; how are we to approach the issue of the feasibility of dynamically oriented therapy with patients such as Linda? I hope to have demonstrated in this paper that these clinical phenomena can also be seen to have a communicative function that is potentially therapeutically useful. Linda's behavior can be received and processed by a dynamically oriented therapist in the service of understanding the patient's experience. This is so even when there are many missed appointments; in fact, from an object relations point of view, one might say that missed appointments, crises, and requests for concrete help are necessary for the therapist to begin to feel his or her way into the patient's world. By contrast, from an ego psychological point of view, as presented and expanded by Fred Pine, such clinical phenomena are evidence of ego deficits, rather than modes of induction into the patient's inner world. These deficits then call for supportive measures and attention to the so-called nonspecific therapeutic factors, such as the analyst's reliability and nonjudgmental attitude, rather than an examination of the internalized object relationship that is being replayed.

Can one intervene in a therapeutic way under these conditions? Pine, as we saw, provides us with a rich array of supportive measures so as to make the situation less anxiety-provoking to the patient, while increasing the ability of the patient to manage anxiety-provoking experiences.

From an object relations perspective, missed appointments, crises, and so on are the ways in which the therapist becomes what Greenberg calls an "old object," a modern representative of an internalized object. The therapeutic issue is whether the therapist can also be enough of a new object for the patient to allow for change to occur in the patient's inner world as a consequence of the analytic work. In Fairbairn's (1958) terms, can the analyst avoid being "press-ganged" into the patient's internal object world, like everyone else in the patient's life?

This is a knotty problem with any patient. It is not easy to find the proper balance between being an "old" and a "new" object in the patient's world. In the case of a patient from the lower socioeconomic classes, I submit that there is an additional complication, which is that deprivation is an ongoing and real factor in the patient's life. The therapist's position as a modern version of the internalized exciting and rejecting object is reinforced by the socioeconomic differential between patient and therapist, by his or her position as part of the social service network, and by the real power he or she potentially has as an advocate. Some of these issues can be illustrated now with a second vignette.

The Case of Nancy

An 18-year-old woman, Nancy, from a lower-class family now in its third generation on public assistance, was in her second year of once-a-week treatment. She reported a dream to her male therapist in which she surreptitiously put her hand in his pocket and found a $100 bill. This session was the first in which the therapist had asked Nancy for dreams. Her associations explicitly to the dream had to do with thinking that perhaps she was about to come into some money, but she had no idea how the therapist might be involved. She went on to talk about feeling resentful that the father of her year-old baby was failing to provide financial support as promised. She said that she hoped to be able to locate her father, who had been released from prison, she thought, and might be somewhere now in the community. He had always been supportive when she was a little girl, she said with tears in her eyes, but every man in her life who was ever supportive let her down sooner or later.

At the end of this session, the therapist wrote out a slip for Nancy that allowed her to receive bus fare from the clinic receptionist. Patients such as Nancy who are on Medicaid are entitled to reimbursement for their travel expenses to medical appointments. On this occasion, Nancy took the slip and then asked the therapist if he would write out slips for two of her younger brothers, who had accompanied her to the clinic and were sitting in the waiting room. The therapist hesitated. The therapist was in the habit of writing a slip for one of her brothers who accompanied her, because Nancy said she never ventured out alone in the neighborhood where she lived. The therapist felt some justification, but he also felt uneasy about giving bus fare at all. One of Nancy's brothers, who lived at home, was a daily drug user, despite having no visible source of income. The two other brothers probably used drugs as well, at least occasionally. Was it right to give money for bus fare to her brother, knowing that he was probably spending considerable sums on drugs? With these thoughts in mind, the therapist said he could give a slip for bus fare only to Nancy and one brother. Only after Nancy left did the therapist note the parallel between the dream and the request for extra bus fare at the end of the session.

How are we to understand this dream, along with the ensuing events in the session? On one hand, they suggest that the patient sees the therapist quite literally as a source of money to be exploited. What are the deeper resonances of this view of the therapist? A drive-based view might give primacy to a sexual element, insofar as she is putting her hand into the therapist's pocket to find money. Perhaps the money can be seen as a symbolic representation of the therapist's penis, and a sexual wish is being portrayed in the dream. An ego psychological perspective might call attention to the patient's difficulty with frustration tolerance. The frustration involved in the therapeutic situation leads to an attempt to get the therapist to gratify the patient in a concrete way, whether the gratification is seen in sexual or monetary terms. This attempt could be seen as "resistance" to an analysis of the underlying wish as a manifestation of an ego weakness that must be managed in order to make interpretive work possible, or as both. There might be seen here evidence of an antisocial personality structure, perhaps based on defenses against underlying feelings of deprivation.

A Fairbairnian perspective would call our attention to the way in which the therapist is portrayed in the dream as an exciting object. The exciting quality can be linked to the therapist as the bearer of money, as a sexually exciting object, or both. The dream, in fact, seems to imply an identification of sexuality and money, or nurturance, more broadly. The therapist as rejecting object also seems inherent in the dream. Why else would Nancy need to take the money from the therapist surreptitiously? The way in which the session ended, in fact, seems to leave the therapist in the role of depriving object. From this perspective, then, the bus fare issue has provided a focus for the manifestation of the patient's internal object world in the therapeutic setting. The therapist has become an "old object." The therapeutic problem is how to shift one's position away from enacting the internal drama with the patient, to examining with the patient the nature of the dream and the ways in which the script is written.

I would like to call attention at this point to the way in which the administrative structure of this clinic plays a role in this vignette. The fact that the therapist fills out the bus fare slip means that he is put in the role of deciding who gets the reimbursement and who does not. From one point of view, the therapist's neutrality and anonymity are compromised when he is in the role of dispensing or withholding money. The transference becomes uninterpretable because the therapist has taken action in reality. From this perspective, the bus fare decisions should be made by clerical or administrative staff to preserve the therapist's neutral position, so that the patient's transference fantasies can be properly analyzed.

From a relational perspective, the administrative issue brings us back to the question of how the therapist can strike the proper balance between being an old object and being a new object for the patient. As with Nancy, when the therapist manages the dispensing or withholding of money, the stage is set for the therapist to be seen as an exciting and rejecting object by the patient. A focus is provided. Is this a desirable development from the point of view of the treatment? In some cases, it may be so. The bus fare issue may provide a focus for the analysis of these transference issues when the therapist is being seen primarily as a new object by the patient. In other cases, the therapist may already be seen, in an excessively concrete way, as an exciting and rejecting object. The socioeconomic differential between patient and therapist makes it quite likely that the therapist will be seen in this way by many patients. In these instances, the therapist's involvement with bus fare may "heat up" the transference feelings further and work against the development of a view of the therapist as a new object. It may become difficult to find any sort of detached perspective from which to view, with the patient, the transferential perceptions that have developed.

Administrative Issues

Moving beyond the specifics of Nancy's case, I would now like to conclude with some further observations on the administrative structure of public clinics, based on the need to think psychoanalytically about the context in which we work. In particular, I would like to focus on how administrative policies and structures may have an impact on the therapist's attempt to find the optimal new object-old object balance for facilitating analytic work. I focus on three ways in which I think that administrative factors are conducive to the perception of the therapist as exciting and rejecting object. For some patients, the result may be that the closed system of internal reality is reinforced; the therapist does not become sufficiently the new object for therapeutic work to proceed.

Medicaid, that is, public funding for medical care for poor people, is a source of two problems at present. One problem is that patients on Medicaid pay nothing for their treatment; the second is that missed appointments are not reimbursable.

When patients pay the therapist for their treatment, an egalitarian element is added to the situation. The therapist is being hired to provide a service. While transference tends to put the therapist into a parental role, the economic arrangements provide some degree of counterpoint. When Medicaid pays, the therapist and the psychotherapy itself become a benefit. How could the therapist be more effectively set up as an exciting object? Requiring at least token payments would facilitate the therapist's assumption of new object status.

In private practice, the therapist is able to tolerate some missed appointments as long as the patient is willing to pay for them. Whether missed appointments are seen as defensive or as the reflection of an internal object situation, they can become part of the therapeutic work. When Medicaid does not pay for them, the therapist comes under administrative pressure not to continue treatment when appointments are not consistently kept. With deprived patients one is most likely to be drawn into their inner world through their missed appointments. If missed appointments endanger the treatment, the therapist is put in the position of becoming an unreliable, if not retaliatory, object. It would facilitate the work, then, if Medicaid allowed for some missed appointments. Aside from the rationale presented here, there are reasons to do so even from within a medical model. Insofar as compliance with treatment is an issue within medicine, it would make sense for physicians to be able to work on an ongoing basis with initially noncompliant patients.

Next, let us consider the way in which public clinics deal with emergencies. Emergency situations often lead to hospitalization, which is a very expensive treatment modality. In an attempt to minimize cost, there have recently been established "crisis teams" to do intensive crisis intervention on a short-term basis. When the crisis is past, the patient is returned to her therapist or referred to one. Insofar as crises and emergencies are the way in which some patients attempt to establish contact with a depriving object, however, it is critical that the therapist who does crisis intervention be able to follow the patient beyond the crisis. If the patient comes to an emergency room or a crisis team and is transferred out as soon as he or she is stable, the likelihood is that stability will become associated with loss and further deprivation. In this way one encourages a crisis-based approach to establishing contact with caregivers. As crisis manager, the therapist becomes like the parent who is not available to a child unless the child can foment an emergency. It would facilitate the work, then, if crisis intervention were integrated, as far as possible, into the usual clinical responsibilities of the staff in a clinic.

Lately, insurance companies and Medicaid have been moving toward putting caps on the length of treatment. Behavioral goals are set up, and treatment must be rejustified if it continues beyond a fixed number of sessions, if it is reimbursed beyond that point at all. From any psychodynamic point of view, such arrangements are problematic therapeutically. Symptom relief, whether it is seen as "transference cure" from a Freudian perspective or "compliance" from Winnicott's point of view, leaves unchanged the less tangible psychopathological situation. From a parent-child model, it would be as if economic considerations determined when children had to grow up. From an object relations perspective, the economic factors potentially put the therapist in the position of reinforcing the patient's expectation of abandonment. As society becomes less willing to pay for psychotherapeutic treatment, the opportunity to work with the patient's inner object world diminishes. In order to work effectively with a patient such as Linda, then, the length of treatment needs to be based on the patient's need. I want to emphasize that I am not thereby advocating long-term treatment for everyone, since I believe that patients need to leave treatment, as well as to be able to stay in it for a period of time. We should be free, however, to adapt to our patients' need to stay and to leave, as they see fit.

In conclusion, at this historical moment, the influence of psychoanalysis on work in public clinics seems to be on the wane. I mean to buck this trend in this paper, to argue for more, rather than less, influence for a fully psychoanalytic approach to lower socioeconomic-status patients in public clinics. I hope to have demonstrated that the psychoanalytic perspective is necessary for a full and rich understanding of the influence of the institutional context of the work, for an enlightened approach to mental health administration, and for the clinical management of many events that tend to occur in therapy in this context. I further hope to have demonstrated that an object relations-based approach potentially counteracts the common tendency toward a two-tiered psychoanalysis, in which lower-class patients are often shunned or treated in a "modified" fashion.

References

Bachrach, H. M. & Leaff, L. A. (1978), Analyzability: A systematic review of the clinical and quantitative literature. *J. Amer. Psychoanal. Assn.*, 26:881–920.
Bollas, C. (1987), *The Shadow of the Object*. New York: Columbia University Press.

Fairbairn, W. R. D. (1952), Endopsychic structure considered in terms of object relationships. In: *Psychoanalytic Studies of the Personality*. London: Routledge & Kegan Paul.

———— (1958), On the nature and aims of psychoanalytical treatment. *Internat. J. Psycho-Anal.*, 39:374–385.

Green, A. (1986), *On Private Madness*. Madison, CT: International Universities Press.

Greenberg, J. R. (1986), Theoretical models and the analyst's neutrality. *Contemp. Psychoanal.*, 22:81–106.

Hollingshead, A. B. & Redlich, F. C. (1958), *Social Class and Mental Illness: A Community Study*. New York: Wiley.

Jacoby, R. (1983), *The Repression of Psychoanalysis*. New York: Basic Books.

Joseph, B. (1988), Transference: The total situation. In: *Melanie Klein Today, Vol. 2*, ed. E. Bott-Spillius. London: Routledge, pp. 61–72.

Langer, M. (1989), *From Vienna to Managua: Journey of a Psychoanalyst*. London: Free Association Press.

Mitchell, S. A. (1988), *Relational Concepts in Psychoanalysis*. Cambridge, MA: Harvard University Press.

Ogden, T. (1986), *Matrix of the Mind*. Northvale, NJ: Aronson.

Pine, F. (1985), *Developmental Theory and Clinical Process*. New Haven, CT: Yale University Press.

———— (1990), *Drive, Ego, Object, Self: A Synthesis for Clinical Work*. New York: Basic Books.

Sennett, R. & Cobb, J. (1972), *The Hidden Injuries of Class*. New York: Vintage Books.

Winnicott, D. W. (1971), *Playing and Reality*. Middlesex, England: Penguin.

Afterword

A decade after the publication of this paper on working psychoanalytically in public clinics, the public sector is being dismantled, starved of resources, so that psychotherapy of anyone who hasn't the resources for private treatment is unlikely to be available. Yet I am as glad as ever that this paper exists as a beginning effort to think about how psychoanalytic perspectives can be as relevant for those with limited economic resources in public clinics as for people who can afford to be seen in private practice. Part of the raison d'etre of this paper is contrarian—to counter the trend within psychoanalysis and within society as a whole to marginalize the economically impoverished and people of "Third World" background. The more such people are marginalized, the louder I want this paper to speak.

On the other hand, I am not entirely comfortable with the clarity that is obtained from a contrarian stance. Such clarity may be helpful politically; it lends itself to strong positions and to decisive action. Yet, the very same contextual thinking that informs this paper leads to suspicion of polarized structures of any sort. A case in point is the way the clarity and forcefulness of my argument in favor of object relations theory in public clinics seems augmented by the contrast with an ego-psychological approach and with elitism in general. Does elitism not reemerge in this use of an elitist position as a counterpoint? Is such a development inevitable, the return of the repressed elitism, as it were? Or might there have been a way to put my object relations approach in a historical perspective, into conversation with ego-psychological perspectives, without creating an oppositional structure? While taking an oppositional position may make one feel differentiated and alive, oppositionalism is still in part a "false self" (Winnicott, 1965) organization inasmuch as one is still controlled by that which one is opposing (Altman, 2004).

Despite these reservations, I have taken my critique of ego psychology further. I argue that European psychoanalysts and psychoanalysis sought white privilege (Macintosh, 1998) in the United States, as other European immigrant groups sought white privilege, by joining up with the capitalist and medical establishments through ego psychology. In the process, connections with African Americans have tended to be sacrificed; thus, psychoanalysis became a "white thing" (Leary, 1997), sacrificing a potential ability to speak to nonwhite and nonprivileged people. Botticelli (1997), in his critique of the book (Altman, 1995) that grew out of this paper, defended polarizing thinking when faced with an oppressive and established power. I agree with him, yet I find it important not to forget the underlying mutual dependence of opposites, the way one can be haunted and defined by what one disavows.

Going on to fill in some gaps from this paper. I developed some psychoanalytic perspectives on race, social class, and culture, including some ideas about how these social factors can structure transference and countertransference both in clinic settings and in private practice (Altman, 1995). Perhaps what I feel most pleased about, looking back at this paper, is the way I found to link up intrapsychic, dyadic, and social/contextual/institutional factors in an expanded and integrated notion of transference–countertransference. In my book, I went on to call the larger social factors a "third," following the lead of Ogden (1994) and Benjamin (1998) who used this term to capture the sense of something operative in the psychoanalytic situation that is both beyond the intrapsychic and the interpersonal, and also immanent in and transforming of the intrapsychic and interpersonal.

Thus, in this paper, we have Fairbairn's picture of the intrapsychic situation as organized by attachments to "exciting" and"rejecting" objects; we also have the interaction between patient and analyst organized this way; then we have the structure of the social welfare system that is conducive to this form of transference–countertransference. The effort here is to find a way, clinically and theoretically, to keep all these levels in mind simultaneously and nonreductionistically, that is, without making one level primary and the others secondary. If we can do that we will have come a long way toward transcending the polarizing forms of thinking that this paper fell prey to in some ways.

References

Altman, (1995), *The Analyst in the Inner City: Race, Class, and Culture through a Psychoanalytic Lens*. Hillsdale, NJ: The Analytic Press.

———— (2004), History repeats itself in transference and countertransference. *Psychoanal. Dial.*, 14:807–815.

Benjamin, J. (1998), *The Shadow of the Other*. New York: Routledge.

Botticelli, S. (1997), Theorizing the social in psychoanalysis: Review of *The Analyst in the Inner City: Race, Class, and Culture through a Psychoanalytic Lens* by Neil Altman. *Psychoanal. Dial.*, 7:535–546.

Leary, K. (1997), Race, self-disclosure, and "forbidden talk": Race and ethnicity in contemporary clinical practice. *Psychoanal. Quart.*, 66:163–189.

McIntosh, P. (1998), White privilege: Unpacking the invisible knapsack. In: *Revisioning Family Therapy*, ed. M. Goldrick. New York: Guilford, pp. 147–152.

Ogden, T. (1994), *Subjects of Analysis*. Northvale, NJ: Aronson.

Winnicott, D. W. (1965), Ego distortion in terms of true and false self. In: *The Maturational Processes and the Facilitating Environment*. New York: International Universities Press.

Perversion Is Us? Eight Notes

(2001)

Muriel Dimen

Editors' Introduction

For over a decade Muriel Dimen has been crafting a deep new vision of sexuality within a relational context. This work is creative in two distinct ways. She is involved in a powerful experiment with writing and communicating ideas and clinical process. And, working out the limenal, enigmatic, contradictory phenomenal meaning of sexual life, she always keeps close tabs on the power of politics and culture to write deep constituting marks on our deepest and most private experiences.

This work in psychoanalysis sits on a rich bed of intellectual and political life, first as an anthropologist and then in feminism.

Dimen's work illuminates how close the ethnographic impulse and the psychoanalytic one can be. In both practices, a keen and acute observation is required. But in both cases, this observation done too rigidly colonizes the other. Done well these practices can mix identification and difference with respect and openness. Dimen's characteristic mode of operation whether at work clinically or at work on theory, is to court surprise, to be willing to get deeply stirred up and transformed by what she hears and experiences and to keep her eye carefully on the various police actions—cultural, local, personal, unconscious—that bedevil our modes of living and interacting.

Her latest book, in which there is a 25 year range of essays and theoretical investigations, is called *Sexuality, Intimacy, Power* and there you can see how much for Dimen the term relational always includes a complex interweaving of relational matrices, that are both large cultural and intimate and interpersonal. In this way she participates and innovates in what has been a longstanding project both in psychoanalysis and anthropology, that is, the study of the impact/interpenetration of culture and psyche. It is her understanding and clinical practice to require that one sits in many spots to do such work, always with a clear-headed view that any answer to the question of how and why desire and excitement and creativity or malignancy flows in any individual is provisional.

As an inextricable part of Dimen's project to understand and work with the impact of sexuality on interpersonal and intrapsychic experience in analytic treatments and in culture, she has opened a creative vein in the matter of clinical and theoretical writing. She is interested in innovative forms of expression in both communicating her ideas and in developing them. New modes of thought entail and respond to new forms of writing and communication. Memoir, fiction, disruptions of the obvious, live in a Dimen essay alongside trenchant theoretical work done in the usual way with mind and reason and argument. But, in the Epilogue to her book, Dimen describes what it means to work as a psychoanalyst on problems of sexuality and desire. You must work, she argues, with heart, mind, and body, knowing that however fully you engage, your subject exceeds you.

In unique style Dimen brings the living experience of analytic work into theoretical writing. Reading Dimen is often like being in an analytic session, where a surprising, unexpected word opens up new vistas, and an old familiar word, as in this essay on "perversion," takes on new life and colors. In this essay Dimen is experimenting with ideas, forms of writing, ways of engaging her readers, and ways of bringing into active play the deeply private experience and the inexorably powerful force of history and culture and power, and the excesses of sexual life. She does this by drawing her readers into a personally engaged encounter.

Perversion Is Us? Eight Notes*

▼   ▼   ▼   ▼   ▼

Note 1. How to Talk About This: Anxiety and Disgust

"Just signed the contract for *Flesh and the World*," writes Michael
Bronski, a culture theorist. "We had talked about my writing about
blood and cutting. . . . Am I ready for this? Usually I have no trouble
writing about anything in my sexual history—s/m, public sex, intimate
moments with a lover, piercing, sex as a salve for death, jerking off on
death beds, piss, violence. . . . It's a great subject—and the essay is sure
to be mentioned in the reviews as, well, cutting edge." Ten days later, he
writes, "I have no idea what tone to strike—lurid, medical, religious,
psychological, confessional? . . . Assume an honest, open tone and simply describe the experiences. Don't forget to mention that it was the most
potent sexual stimulation I have ever encountered. Leave out the fact
that we were on drugs (you wouldn't want to give cutting and blood
sports a bad name)" [Bronski, in press a].

What tone to strike indeed? I was glad to find in Bronski (in press
b)—a man who practices what (he agrees) would surely be named a perversion—the uneasiness that I, whose perversities do not run in this particular direction, feel too. This essay was not easy to write. In fact, it
isn't an essay at all. It is a set of notes, excerpts from clinical reports of
my own, literary essays, psychoanalytic theory, notes accompanied by
commentary, free association, developed thoughts, fragments of theory—
a form that will mirror and predict my topic. Perversion in the context
of multiplicity and discontinuity is a discursive construct that, when
examined, begins to fall apart so that we must wonder: why do we still
talk about it?

In a way, notes make an end run around anxiety. And anxiety shows
up a lot around sex. You may not agree with Bronski's (in press a) assertion that "everyone likes . . . slasher films where sex and anxiety are
bound together and released in the spattering of red fluid," but hundreds
of millions of box-office dollars can't be all wrong. As Sallie Tisdale, a
Buddhist whose *Talk Dirty to Me* (1994) made *Newsweek* headlines several years ago, wrote, "the merging of two into one in orgasm, this

---

*Originally published in *Psychoanalytic Dialogues*, 11:825–860. © 2001 The
Analytic Press, Inc.

blending of identity, combines bliss and anxiety in a strange stew" (p. 281). Anxiety, Harry Stack Sullivan is said to have said, is like a blow on the head—it stops you from thinking. To write a coherent essay, you have to think in a straight line. To write notes, you jig and jog, zig along until you meet anxiety and then zag away in another direction, hoping to come back to that anxious spot from another angle, sparking this thought here and that feeling there and that idea way over there, hoping that this little bit of fireworks will end in a pattern of power and significance. Anyway, it is more my mode to open questions up, not to answer them. "Psychoanalysis," L. Jacobson (personal communication) said, "is not an answer, it's a question." Unanswered questions court anxiety. Anxiety, discovered a friend just embarked on the psychoanalytic journey, is a tool for change.

Perversion is a topic rife with anxiety. Tisdale (1996) was probably right when she said, "We all have an edge, a place where we are bothered." We can see this anxiety in Bronski's writing, which, itself note-like, combines excerpts from his journal with excerpts from his essay-in-progress. Puzzled by anxiety's presence, Bronski (in press a) reminded himself and us about his participation in other transgressions, "s/m, public sex, intimate moments with a lover, piercing, sex as a salve for death, jerking off on death beds, piss, violence." This anxiety shows up in psychoanalytic writing too. I have in mind here some of the most significant recent thought about perversion, the work of Bach, Chasseguet-Smirgel, Kernberg, and Khan—thought that I want to use, historicize, and critique. Sometimes this anxiety is handled by demonizing the pervert on behalf of Western civilization, as in Chasseguet-Smirgel's (1985) *Creativity and Perversion*. Sometimes it is stilled by bringing perversion into the safe precincts of matrimony, as in Kernberg's (1995) *Love Relations*, or love, as in Bach's (1995) *The Language of Perversion and the Language of Love*. And always, even in Khan's (1979) extraordinary essay on foreskin fetishism, the anxiety is relieved by exclusion, so that however empathically the pervert patient is comprehended, the pervert is still the other guy doing alien and even disgusting albeit (or therefore) fascinating things. Perversion may be defined, after all, as the sex that you like and I don't.

Cutting and bloodletting. Are these perversions perversions—transgressions to end all transgressions, *la crème de la crème?* Do sexual blood sports carry the anxiety and shame, the stigma and danger, the horror and *frissons* formerly associated with your run-of-the-mill perversion? Maybe stigma leaps from practice to practice just as genes in certain species of corn jump from chromosome to chromosome (Keller, 1983). Homosexuality, for example, came off the diagnostic books a long time ago, even if in the minds of some people, including analysts, it remains a perversion. Maybe, as the stigma lifts from one marginal sexual practice, it doesn't disappear but alights on another—from homosexuality to b&d, from b&d to bloodletting, from bloodletting to . . . Do visions of slippery slopes enter your minds?

Throughout these notes, I am noting anxious moments, and this is one: Stigma lurks.

Our collective cultural relationship to perversion is, we might put it, one of projective identification. Perhaps perversion brews anxiety because, as Stoller (1975) sympathetically suggested during the "sexual revolution," we depend on it to hold what we cannot bear to remember about ourselves. It fascinates endlessly because it serves psychic and social functions. For the individual, Stoller opined, perverse practices redress the ancient humiliations of childhood. For the family, perversion siphons off aggression, serving as a scapegoat by containing the cruelty and hatred threatening family integrity and security. By thus preserving the family, it conserves a cultural cornerstone and, therefore, society itself. At the same time, Stoller contended, perversion, by soaking up the anxiety and aggression brought on by oedipal rigors, safeguards heterosexuality and, therefore, the species. Absent a sponge for the anger, resentment, and hostility generated by oedipal competitiveness, these agonistic affects fester, contaminating the desire for the opposite-sexed other required by reproductive sexuality. Does what Ferenczi (1933) darkly dubbed "the hate-impregnated love of adult mating" (p. 206) require sanitizing?

What sex was to the 19th century, perversion is to us now. Once upon a time, sex situated taboo, transgression, stigma, shame, excitement, dangerous pleasure, anxiety. A century of revolutionary sexual thought and a generation of revolutionary sexual practice later, sex is at least officially disarmed. If Barney Frank is in Congress, where can the frontier lie? Now the kids pierce noses, tongues, and eyebrows (forget earlobes!) and tattoo everything—an intimate erotics of body and rebellion, the dark side of which shows up in the self-mutilations that some deem adolescent self-hatred.

A moment of anxiety. Don't mention children and perversion in the same breath.

Note 2. Pathology and Suffering, Shame and Pain

When, three years ago, I asked Dr. MH whether I might use material from our work together for this paper, he consented. Two days later, he said that, while he still felt comfortable with my writing about him, he found himself in a bit of shock. That I had included him as a pervert opened his eyes: "I had thought it was OK, depathologized. But now . . ." He trailed off, and I filled in: "It says something is wrong."

How do shame and suffering become one? When Dr. MH, with whom I have worked three times weekly for slightly more than five years (three years at the original time of writing), said "I had thought it was OK, depathologized. But now . . . ," his anxiety registered, in part, the ambiguous power of diagnosis. In the matter of mind—as opposed to body—to pathologize is simultaneously to identify the illness that needs cure and to stigmatize the badness that causes shame. From a Foucaultian perspective, this doubled power inheres in all disciplinary institutions. Schools and the education system, government and its manifold activities, prisons and the correctional system, hospitals and the medical system, the mental health care system and what the French call *les psy*—all these organized practices have a doubled power, the power to name and the power to blame.

Think how often your patients express the anguished fear that "there is something wrong with me." Some of us had it too when we were patients—the fear that you are a fundamentally and irreparably damaged human being, damaged goods, not even human in fact, something unwholesome and decaying at your core. "There is something wrong with me" is a cry of shame, the narcissistic injury for which there are no words—the injury that, because it inhabits the Real and lacks representation, often turns concrete, mutating into psychical or physical harm to self or others. Dr. MH complains of frightening fantasies of violence, of occasional outbursts of rage in the dangerous neighborhoods to which his clinical work takes him.

What is the "it" that Dr. MH (whose initials and sexual interests I have altered) thought had been pathologized? This "it" is, at least on the face of it, not singular but plural. Included are erotic fantasies and practices of beating; fetishes, including shiny belts, especially those of patent leather, and photographs; the payment of money (itself possibly a fetish) for beatings as well as for massages and handjobs; secrets and deceptions (the enlistment of putatively unwilling partners into beating scenarios); exhibitionism and voyeurism while cruising; the photographing of consenting and unsuspecting subjects whose body type, rarely found, meets Dr. MH's needs; the secret touching of a shiny belt worn by someone with just such a special body. When, upon first consulting me, Dr. MH told me he was a pervert, he did not have in mind his overeating and overdrinking, although he was nearly as ashamed of these practices as he was of the others—and we might want to think of them as what Louse Kaplan (1990), writing in the feminist tradition, called "female perversions."

How can Dr. MH remember that something is wrong without feeling bad about himself? He entered treatment having self-pathologized. A mental health professional, he knows a sexual perversion when he sees one. He also knows full well what people in general but also psychoanalysts in particular think about perversion—the uneasy mix of clinical and moral evaluation, the cloud of shame in which perversities are practiced and studied, the anxieties they provoke. He hasn't read Chasseguet-Smirgel's (1985) *Creativity and Perversion* and probably never will—even my paper was, he complained, too dense for him—but he would find right there a mirror for his self-hate. For Chasseguet-Smirgel, "perversion is the equivalent of Devil religion" (p. 9). Dr. MH came of age in the 1970s, during that decade's sexual free-for-all—an epoch against which *Creativity and Perversion* must be read. Saving civilization by reinforcing traditional signs of purity and danger (Douglas, 1970), this near jeremiad sounds a clarion call for a certain personal and moral sanity—and, I would hazard, purity, if we recall that the Latin *sanitas* means "cleanliness"—in the face of a presumed cultural degeneration.

In Chasseguet-Smirgel's (1985) view, perversion degrades psyche and culture alike. Out of de Sade's texts, she distilled a definition: The pervert wishes to obliterate the distinctions on which psychic structures and social orders depend. The pervert makes a double erosion, of the difference between the sexes and of that between the generations. Chasseguet-Smirgel pointed out that sex, in the Sadean texts, takes place not within the heterosexual adult couple but all over the place—between males and females, between males, between females, between adults and children. Disorder is created, and, as borders are violated, pollution prevails. Things out of place soil, Douglas (1970, passim) maintained in her ethnographic treatise on pollution, and Chasseguet-Smirgel in turn deemed such soiling the goal of perversion, which, in its confusion of the sexes and generations, lives defiantly in the anal phase. It chews everything up, reduces everything to excrement, and thus embodies "a system of values [that] is only the first stage in an operation whose end is the destruction of all values"(p. 10).

Ouch. I do not doubt the hatred that wants to obliterate, the despair that annihilates. As a literary effort, *Creativity and Perversion* succeeds quite well: It riles you up and thereby captures perversion's intensity. At the same time, however, its formulations do not do much beyond demonizing perverts and amplifying self-disgust. There is a glitch, a contradiction, at the book's core. The theory of perversion advocated by it departs boldly from classical formulations, but the theory of the clinical subject by which it implicitly abides lags behind. In its view, not oedipal but narcissistic dilemmas generate the perverse solution. The inability to sustain loss, inadequacy, castration, and death; troubles of identity, of the fusion of ego and non-ego, of the differentiation of self and other—these issues, unresolved, may find expression in perverse sexual practices.

Although this argument sounds sympathetic to the narcissistic patient—we are all, Chasseguet-Smirgel (1985) announced early on (p. 26), open to the perverse solution because it soothes wounded narcissism—*Creativity and Perversion* speaks as superego to id. Distilling its definition of perversion from the Sadean corpus produces an odd clinical picture: The crippled narcissist, whether hero or villain, is a mature adult who is and can be held to account for his ignorance of shared values. The patient is deemed responsible in a way that, Mitchell (2000) argued, contravenes the request that analysts, who agree to hold up the side of reason, make of their patients—to surrender "to love and hate with abandon" (p. 133). In *Creativity and Perversion* (e.g., p. 34), narcissistic perverts always fall short when compared with neurotics. When perverts tell examination dreams, for example, they hear interpretations of their wish to escape the law, never their wish for unconditional acceptance (pp. 30–34). Here patients are not said to seek recognition or selfhood or connection. Rather, they are driven by sex and aggression, especially the wish to ruin the parental coupling.

In *Creativity and Perversion*, intersubjectivity begets no explicit clinical or theoretical attention. Chasseguet-Smirgel (1985) felt speechless, ground up—experiencing, one might propose, a sort of annihilation anxiety in the countertransference (p. 112). With pervert patients, who take the analyst's words as seduction or attack but never interpretation, there lacks, she justifiably claimed, a space, a depth, a third dimension—what Winnicott termed *intermediate space*. "In such a situation," Chasseguet-Smirgel wrote, "there are not three persons—the analyst and the 'normal' part of the analysand, investigating, and taking care together of the sick part of the analysand" (p. 111). Instead, there is an excremental mess made of parts of both analyst and patient—a mess that can paralyze the analyst's mind.

But consider Chasseguet-Smirgel's (1985) take on her countertransference. It is as though the unsettlement is induced, solely the patient's fault. Or at least Chasseguet-Smirgel neither entertained the utility of a two-person psychology to illuminate this impasse nor allowed that she had brought any feeling or idea or history of her own to it. Yet, if the message of her book holds—that perversion shakes civilization to its core—then the analyst herself must feel some uneasiness even before she meets the pervert patient. Perverse sexual practices challenge just those fundamental cultural values that orbit on the procreating couple and, in Chasseguet-Smirgel's view, anchor Western civilization. And it is very clear that her clinical philosophy centers on these values: Hating life, perverts do not accept the primal scene as likely to produce a child and therefore cannot "form . . . a couple with the analyst so as to give birth to a child that would be themselves, re-created" (p. 116).

Yet what of the analyst's hatred? Or love? What of the analyst's reflection on these inevitable emotions? They do not show up in *Creativity and Perversion*. This absence creates a knot of affect, subjectivity, inter-subjectivity, and the meaning of perversion. In Chasseguet-Smirgel's account, the bounded, cogitating, omniscient analyst stands front and center. Nowhere to be found, however, is the analyst who reflects on the personal and clinical (not to say cultural) meaning (Chodorow, 2000) of her feelings, who in the chaotic clinical mix of part-selves might be able to identify with the patient. Absent these dimensions of the analyst's sub-jectivity, the patient's subjectivity finds no purchase. Subjectivity is a shared state of mind. Residing not only in each being, but also in the space between, it is evoked in each person by the other. Benjamin's (1998) proposal that recognition of that other subject is the point of the psychoanalytic process seems spot-on.

That this recognition takes place through affect (Stein, 1991; Spezzano, 1993) complicates matters. Affects, to come at the problem from the other side, are by nature intersubjective. As Mitchell (2000) and Morrison (1989) see it, they are highly contagious. Lacking floors and ceilings, walls and doors and windows, they cannot but be interpersonal. Constituting the atmosphere of early object-relational life, affects chal-lenge the separateness of "I" on which conventional constructions of subjectivity, and the personal and cultural values associated with them, depend. In, for example, "anxiety, sexual excitement, rage, depression, and euphoria," Mitchell (2000) wrote, it is often impossible to say which person started what. So when the pervert patient is said to be hateful, might it be hard to tell in whom the hatred first arose?

The analyst needs her theory of perversion (if this is a concept she requires in order to think about sexuality), but she also needs to know both what she feels about perversion—its affective meaning to her and the values embedded in that meaning—and what those perverse prac-tices mean to her patients. And then she needs to know how these two subjectivities together produce and reproduce the transference neurosis through which the analytic cure, such as it is, takes place.

Certainly Chasseguet-Smirgel's patient enjoyed grinding her up, but what, one might have asked, is this enjoyment all about? If chewing can be destructive, it can also be creative (Winnicott, 1969a, b): If you want to grind someone up, you may want to kill them, but you may also wish to take them in so as to metabolize their identity and thereby grow an identity of your own. Not to concern yourself with what perversion means to a particular patient is, in fact, to enact a perversion of your own—to reduce your patient to a non-entity by annihilating his or her subjectivity, to confuse what the patient means to you with what the patient means to himself or herself, and thereby to violate the patient's (emergent) boundaries. This is an act of power and knowledge not without its own pleasures (Foucault, 1978).

To think in the way I am proposing requires a therapeutic balancing act. Maybe you don't like perverse sexual practices, but that's not your business. Assuming that no work gets done when an inclination, practice, or pleasure is cloaked in shame and disgust—when the superego shames the id, inciting further resistance—my initial clinical goal with Dr. MH was to question the self-loathing that clings to his practices like a stink. Trying to hold all my responses in mind, I negotiate between acceptance and rejection, attraction and repulsion, curiosity, disgust, and boredom—a sort of guarded neutrality, if what we mean these days by neutrality is some point of balance (see Greenberg, 1993 for a related idea). Neutral in the *I Ching* sense of "no blame:" I try to stay the Zen course of accepting what exists because it exists. Guarded in the sense of analytic caution: ultimately this congeries of shame, disgust, and excitement, which no neutrality of mine can ever excise from either a patient's or analyst's psyche or their culture, must itself be explored.

But you can't do this condescendingly, as though one day your patient will scale the heterosexual heights. You really have to believe that his solution—the body type, the nongenital erotic practices, the sexual contact acquired on the sly and through commerce—is, other things being equal, viable. Dr. MH needs to have his practices and preferences and affects protected and guarded, kept safe and whole, until he can decide whether he wants to keep them or change them or let them go. But he can't explore his shame until he feels safe enough to find out what's wrong, until he feels sufficiently acceptable to look at it without becoming it, to stand in the spaces (Bromberg, 1998), between his shamed and shaming states of mind.

Note 3. What Is a Perversion?

Another difficulty arises from the circumstance that there is so often associated with the erotic relationship, over and above its own sadistic components, a quota of plain inclination to aggression. The love-object will not always view these complications with the degree of understanding and tolerance shown by the peasant woman who complained that her husband did not love her any more, since he had not beaten her for a week [Freud, 1930, p. 105, n. 3].

Now I don't suppose that anyone has previously taken this footnote as relevant to perversion. You would more likely use it as Freud meant you to—as an example of the "quota of plain inclination to aggression" bedeviling us all. Aggression is not, however, a found object, a plain natural phenomenon; it is as constructed as we now understand sex to be. As Freud told the story, aggression has, to my mind, a rather perverse distribution. A woman waits for a man to exercise aggression, which to her signifies love. To turn this formulation around, the man agents aggression, and the woman receives it—he the subject and she the object. For him to love is to give aggression; for her to be loved is to get it. He is active, she is passive. He does, she is done to. Sound familiar? Why are we not surprised?

I will hold off on the obvious gender implications of this construction of aggression and power in Freud's thought. I want first to pull out another thread. When I began work with a supervisee whose problem was a difficult countertransference to a patient's sexual perversion, I asked what the perversion was. The supervisee missed a beat, then replied as though the answer was self-evident: "Sadomasochism." Specifically, the patient engaged in practices of bondage and domination and had as well elaborate fantasies of torture dramatized in photographs and videos. As we know that versions of perversion exist, however, we need to ask why perversion is often equated to sadomasochism as a matter of course.

A signifying chain links perversion, sadomasochism, gender, and power. Let me put this differently. In keeping with the *fin de dixneuvième siècle* discovery that the abnormal reveals the normal, Freud (1905) begins his *Three Essays on the Theory of Sexuality* with "The Sexual Aberrations." What he did not see, and what the second wave of feminism, especially psychoanalytic feminism, did, is that the sexual order to which the aberrations and perversions were central is equally a gendered order. In psychoanalytic feminist view, gender is "no longer a consequence" (Goldner, 1998) of mind or body or culture but a principle informing all; it is "everywhere and nowhere" (Chodorow, cited in Goldner, 1998). Produced by patriarchy and heterosexuality, it is also always a matter of power—an argument too long and complicated for me to make here (Firestone, 1970; Millett, 1970)—but a fact that certain psychoanalytic applications of gender theory tend to forget.

Returning to Freud's "joke" about the peasant woman and her complaint, we may wonder whether sadomasochism and, next to it, aggression, as constructed in both psychoanalysis and culture, are always and everywhere gendered. I am not the first to indicate the paradox: All Freud's case examples of feminine masochism are men. As Kaplan (1990) put it: "The sexual perversions . . . are pathologies of gender stereotyping" (p. 196). Look at it this way: If gender as an elemental structure of dominance and subordination is so critical to psyche, soma, and culture, is it any wonder that we think of perversion as inevitably sadomasochistic?

Listen to the mix of sex, gender, and power in Dr. MH's fantasy: "I really am a ninny, a squirmy little faggot. . . . I am having a fantasy of the heat pipe as a penis going into the ceiling. I am thinking of men butt-fucking each other. Then I think of Romans with helmets on." I say, "They wouldn't be ninnies, would they?" "I hadn't thought of that." "The wish to have those desires and not feel like a ninny, to feel like a warrior." "Wanting to be taken care of is to be a ninny. That's part of men's attraction to women, cuddling up, being taken care of, but real men take care of women." So are real women ninnies? In a power structure, someone has to be the ninny. In a power structure, weakness and longings for closeness—call them ninniness and tenderness—tend to fuse. In his transferential longings for care, does Dr. MH feel like a ninny with me? Does he think I think his need for me makes him a squirmy little faggot? I shall return to Dr. MH's longing for tenderness, which is so crucial to current thinking about perversion (Benjamin, 1988).

Is wife battering a perversion? Like Freud's peasant woman, Ms. K, a sculptor, described the most satisfying sexual intercourse as what she's had after her lover has beaten her up. Perhaps, she wonders, the combustion of sex and violence originates in the beating she got as a six-year-old at her mother's hands—a punishment for making mud pies in her room. Or possibly it stems from her father's denied lust for her—manifested in his humiliating attack on her teenage sexuality (one day he tried to pull her tank top down in front of her brothers). The influence of feminism on psychoanalysis, mused culture theorist Apter (1992), "may be shifting . . . what qualifies as perverse. Whereas traditionally attention has been devoted to determining the epistemological boundaries between, for example, sadism and masochism . . . , rape, abuse, incest and other forms of violence . . . may now increasingly come to be theorized psychoanalytically as forms of perversion" (p. 313). If, as Goldner (n.d.), cofounder of the Intimate Violence Project at the Ackerman Institute, told us, "one-third of all [heterosexual] women will, at some point in their lives, be physically assaulted by an intimate male partner—slapped, kicked, beaten, choked or attacked with a weapon" (p. 6), that makes physical abuse almost normative for the culture in general and for heterosexuality, marriage, and (given that abuse is no stranger to homosexual households either) even attachment in particular. If aggressive sex and eroticized aggression are so at home in the nuclear family, can we say that the abnormal is at home in the normal?

Freud's joke about wife battering is a joke about power that also performs power, and the performance is patriarchal. Is it perverse of Freud to illuminate a shady sexual pleasure by attributing it to his social inferiors? Why else would he think it funny to tell a joke about a peasant woman waiting to be beaten? Yes, we all know that Freud was a man of his time, but, you know, he is also a man of our time. And I do know that television host Bill Maher would lampoon me—that is, if these notes were of any interest to the Nielsen ratings—for political correctness. Why couldn't Freud tell that joke about one of his bourgeois patients instead of a stereotypical woman from an Austro-Hungarian village? That she lacks an ethnicity is probably part of the humor. She is an "other," one of "them" as opposed to "us," which is a binary we see frequently in the psychoanalytic discourse on perversion; recall Chasseguet-Smirgel's (1985) distinction between the pervert and "ourselves" (p. 34). And she is subordinate. And she is a woman, the butt of, and buttfucked by, not only her husband's aggression but Freud's.

Caution: regulatory practice at work. That's how Foucault (1978, passim) would put it. After the Catholic church, psychoanalysis is, in his thought, perhaps the exemplary disciplinary power—its pronouncements routinely enforcing social injustice through the apparent neutrality of objective science. Psychoanalysts are routinely caught in the clinical dilemma that I indicated earlier: The power to name is also the power to blame and to shame. It is not far-fetched to think that Freud, for example, was using this anonymous couple as a rhetorical device to needle the sexually uptight Europeans who constituted his audience. One job of psychoanalysis is, after all, to reveal to the suffering the thing that, denied, sickens them. Doing it at the expense of those who can't talk back is, however, the ultimate in bullying. How tenacious Freud's misogyny is, how on the beaten track is his class pride, and how truly ambivalent is his attachment to sexuality. When he says to his readers, "Look, you may think that this perverse desire is beneath you, you may think only lower types like peasants engage in it, but the truth is that you, the civilized, want it too," he simultaneously liberates and imprisons, frees by naming and binds by shaming.

Note 4. Accepting/Disowning the Perverse in the Normal

No healthy person, it appears, can fail to make some addition that might be called perverse to the normal sexual aim [Freud, 1905, p. 160].

It is difficult to comprehend the idea of perversion otherwise than by reference to a norm [Laplanche and Pontalis, 1973, p. 306].

Well, you can't say it much more loudly or clearly than that. Perversion is culturally constructed. By this, I do not mean the crude misapprehension that psyche is culture's clone. Rather, perversion links with a set of meanings and practices that render each other intelligible and habitable. To label something a perversion is simultaneously to identify something else not perverse. The normal, what does not need to be said because it goes without saying, serves in this discourse as a residual category. In *Three Essays*, for example, Freud (1905) defined his somewhat coy but ubiquitous and textually crucial locution, "the sex act," only once and nearly by the by, about 10 pages into his first chapter: We may think of the "normal sexual aim . . . as . . . the union of the genitals in the act known as copulation" (p. 149). On the next page, after pointing out that kissing is not a perversion even though it does not involve the sexual apparatus but rather mucus membranes that constitute the portal to the digestive tract, Freud defined *perversions* as "sexual activities which either (a) extend, in an anatomical sense, beyond the regions of the body that are designed for sexual union, or (b) linger over the intermediate relations to the sexual object which should normally be traversed rapidly on the path towards the final sexual aim" (p. 150).

There's no way around it. Freud argued with but ended up joining Krafft-Ebing, who said, "Every expression of [the sexual instinct] that does not correspond with the purpose of nature—i.e., propagation—must be regarded as perverse" (cited in Davidson, 1987, p. 39). The normal is the heterosexual, the coital, the reproductive. Abelove (1991), a European historian covering the topic of sexuality, called it "cross-sex genital intercourse" or "intercourse so-called": "penis in vagina, vagina around penis, with seminal emission uninterrupted" (p. 337). I call it PIV—penis in vagina.

Perversion and that inadequately specific term *normality* construct each other. Perversion is necessary in more ways than Stoller (1975) imagined. How do you know what's normal unless you know what's not, unless you have a boundary? How do you know what's not normal unless you know what is? In the discourse of psychosexuality, perversion and heteronormality constitute each other's limits. Perversion marks the boundary across which you become an outlaw. Normality marks off the territory that, if stayed inside, keeps you safe from shame, disgust, and anxiety.

The binary thus formed is, however, only illusorily clear. Even people who engage in normal sexuality, Freud said, tend to include a perverse moment or two in their ordinary sexual practice—a position that, we shall see, Kernberg shared, sort of. And they don't even find it a problem: "Everyday experience has shown that most of these extensions, or at any rate, the less severe of them, are constituents which are rarely absent from the sexual life of healthy people, and are judged by them no differently from other intimate events" (Freud, 1905, p. 160). Do you recognize yourself here? Routinely, Freud said, the sexual instinct enjoys overriding disgust. Perhaps, suggested de Lauretis (1994, p. 24), Freud deemed the perversions positive; after all, the perverts, like the woman in "A Case of Paranoia" (1915) or "Leonardo da Vinci" (1910) or the unnamed homosexual woman whom Freud (1920) said was "in no way neurotic" (p. 158), were not ill. Indeed, they lived functional if not happy lives (remember "ordinary unhappiness"), in contrast to the neurotics and hysterics who came to him because they could not live at all. "Neuroses are, so to say, the negative of perversion" (1905, p. 165).

Note 5. Fixity and Flexibility

If, in short, a perversion has the characteristics of exclusiveness and fixation—then we shall usually be justified in regarding it as a pathological symptom [Freud, 1905, p. 161].

Not only civilizations, psychology, too, has great difficulty, where borderline cases are concerned, in distinguishing with confidence what is still part of normal sexuality, what is perverse and what is neurotic or psychotic. . . . For instance, is it normal or not to demand that the love object must be tall or petite, fair or dark, very bright or rather simple, domineering or submissive, and so on? Perhaps we may accept the conditions just quoted as normal; when they exact that a woman limp or even have a false leg, or that the man wear spectacles, or that the woman wear black underwear during coitus, the difficulty of drawing the boundary becomes greater [Balint, 1956, p. 20].

Is it normal or abnormal to insist that the love-object be only one gender or another? I remember during psychoanalytic training some two decades ago a discussion of a homosexual woman being treated by one of our male candidates. He was professing his liberalism: "I have no problem with her being a lesbian. [You can already hear the excess of protest, of course.] It's just that she's restricting her choices." I don't think anyone mentioned what Balint (1956) had noticed two decades earlier—that those who are exclusively heterosexual restrict their choices too.

Now that psychoanalysis has welcomed into the fold of mental health the homosexual as well as the heterosexual, how will we define illness in the sexual domain? Many have fixed on the criterion of flexibility.

Khan (1979) observed "the limited nature of the fantasies of the fetishist" (p. 143). Kaplan (1990) and McDougall (1995) argued also for flexibility as a criterion of mental health. This criterion makes sense. Kaplan remarked on "the inherent flexibility" (p. 506) of our sexual nature—a flexibility that, according to Lacan (1977), defines desire. Lacan would contrast desire with need: Need, like hunger, must have one thing and one thing only, food. Desire thrives on substitutes. It may be satisfied or deferred—turned into pleasure or babies or buildings or bombs. It may accept a blowjob or PIV or a beating, a fantasy or a body, a belt or a breast or a picture, a male or a female or a transvestite.

Truth to tell, though, human beings aren't the only flexible sexuals, and they are not all that flexible either. The Bonobo chimpanzees' sexuality is far more versatile, serving not only as a source of pleasure, a means to procreation, or a tension-release mechanism, but a tool of social cohesion and an expression of dominance and subordination (de Waal and Lanting, 1997). On the other hand, human sexual limits are notorious. In the 1960s, we said, "If it moves, fuck it." Most of us, of course, didn't do that at all, or, if we did, it was for about five minutes. Balint (1956), among others, noticed that sexual preference is really not catholic, hardly ecumenical at all. Person (1980) maintained that most adult fantasies are rather fixed. Our "sex-prints" (Person, 1980, p. 618; see also Stoller's, 1979, idea of sexual scripts) are not only individualized but quite unvarying and as such ground identity in a fluid society.

Are we all a little bit perverse? Well, so some argue, though not always in the most charitable way. Let's return to Chasseguet-Smirgel (1985) here, and put off an evaluation of Kernberg's contribution just a little bit longer. Chasseguet-Smirgel (1985) said, "Perversions [are] a dimension of the human psyche in general, a temptation in the mind common to us all" (p. 1). As we have seen, however, her "we" is not so ecumenical as it sounds. Unlike "us," for example, perverts hate the truth. "The perverse solution," she insisted, "tempts us to replace the love for truth with 'a taste for sham'"(p. 26), a temptation to which "they" yield. I would have her consider Bronski's (in press a) struggle between his wish to represent the sexiness of cutting and . . . well, hear him out:

> Journal entry of two days ago is complete shit. I know perfectly well what is missing from the essay: honesty and truth. . . . What am I leaving out? That as much as I loved Jim, I thought he was fucked up about sex and his own sexual desires? That his s/m practices, including cutting, were mostly vain attempts to break through the crushing repression of his southern boyhood and his horrible feelings about himself? That for the first year we were together (out of five) he would have to leave the

room after coming, so he could be alone? That some of these times he cried?. . . The romanticism of our blood games—and my presentation of it—is countered by the fact that there was often blood dripped all over the floor and furniture from other men he brought home.

A moment of anxiety. "Blood, mother, blood," cried Norman Bates in *Psycho* in 1960. "Blood and AIDS!" we scream in 2001.

Well, but who doesn't lie about their sexual pleasure? Bill Clinton's not alone here, you know. A patient once allowed that she liked being fucked from behind while in a forward bend. I asked her what she liked about it. She didn't answer. "Sex is funny that way," was all she wanted to say. Is there nothing you are ashamed of? As Tisdale (1994) put it, "Tongues loosen during orgasm, things get said that would never be said otherwise" (p. 280). Remember Gordon Lightfoot's verse about the room where you do what you don't confess? Shame, excitement, pleasure, the overriding of disgust. And why *should* you confess?

Still, viewed from another angle, Chasseguet-Smirgel's (1985) diagnosis may contain a truth that her truth cannot encompass. Replying to a commentary on my discussion (Dimen, in press) of "Dr. Fell," Bronski (in press b) referred to my criticism of her assertion, shared culturally, that "perverts hate the truth." Surprisingly, however, Bronski retorted, "this phrase to me is delicious for, ironically, as a pervert, I believe it to be completely true." Perverts do hate the truth, he insisted, but what truth is that? Chasseguet-Smirgel's idea works, Bronski suggested, because the pervert is always on the outside, always the other: "The 'truth,' as it is so carefully and lovingly called, is almost always what is held as a cherished belief by those in the dominant culture: those with power, those who have the power to name—and, as it follows, to name-call." Truth, in Foucauldian view, is an effect of power, a form of domination that *les psy* embody in characterizing perversion. There is, you could say, a bit of projection going on: The contempt and arrogance that Chasseguet-Smirgel (1985) or, in fact, Kaplan (1990), who remarked that the pervert's self-regard is as "the one with secrets of Great Sex" (p. 41), identified in the sexuality of perverts shows up also in the psychoanalytic discourse about perversion. So often when "we" are all said to be perverse, what is really meant is, "There but for the grace of God go I." We may be merely tempted, but they, poor wretches, give in. Dr. MH may use his hatred of his sexual desires as a form of hate speech, as an expression of his self-loathing, but so does psychoanalysis. Psychoanalysis prescribes sexual convention even as it subscribes to sexual liberation, but, in the fashion of projective identification, it splits this contradiction in two and then denies having done so—a disavowal that on occasion shows up as a bit of hate speech itself.

Indeed, it may be the details of desire, the particularities of pleasure, that most incite disgust, challenge sexual conventionality, set off the alarm. I could elaborate on Dr. MH's beating fantasies and practices, his furtive touching of belts, his Peeping Tom photography, his veiled invitations to a beating. But, I submit, these somewhat expectable instances and aspects of perversion discomfit less than what actually turns him on. Dr. MH has a very particular preference. The object of his desire is a man possessed of a strong but severe face, twinkly eyes, and white hair; a belly that protrudes just a little bit under the belt line; and thighs that spread out when he sits down, forming a lap. In a culture of thinness and fitness, I wonder whether a taste for poochedout bellies and full thighs on elderly men is more transgressive than all the bondage and domination in the world.

A moment of anxiety. Taboo, in Douglas's (1970) view, neighbors on pollution. Shame isn't far away, either.

Perversion and normality construct each other. It is only relative to a desire like Dr. MH's that heterosexuality and homosexuality look like models of normality. Dr. MH's desire tests flexibility as a criterion for mental health, or, rather, his very specific tastes remind psychoanalysis, and the culture that embeds it, of what is projectively identified away from the norm into the marginal—the restriction of desire that, so necessary to civilization, causes "modern nervousness," as Freud (1908) put it. Dr. MH is anxious when we discuss his taste and the photographs he takes of men who fit his fantasy. "But you can't get what you need otherwise" is his plaint. Advertisements and, for that matter, erotica and pornography are full of thin young people, not softly paunched seniors with full thighs. You could, as Dr. MH does, make a case for the bellied woman in the body of the man he desires. But can you also feature this? Maybe it's Dr. MH who is on the side of health. The rest of us, who hate the signs of age in ourselves and others—the softening flesh, spreading bellies, graying hair—defend against our certain death by fixating on the billboarded thin young people whom we would be so happy to resemble. To rewrite Laplanche and Pontalis (1973) as quoted at the beginning of note 4, "It is difficult to comprehend the idea of the norm otherwise than by reference to a perversion."

The discourse on perversion, I have been contending, seethes with moralism, my own included. I want to ask for a moment of cultural relativism, that moralistic discourse par excellence. Suppose Dr. MH had lived in 19th-century Euro-America, in which men's portliness, a form of conspicuous consumption, signaled prosperity. As L. Jacobson (personal communication, 1999) asked me, if Dr. MH had lived there and then, would he have been turned on by emaciation? Consider the following. While conducting graduate archival research, a patient, Elizabeth, lived in an inexpensive, immigrant quarter of Paris. A white woman of some 250 pounds (which, we figured out, she unconsciously hoped would keep her from being an object of desire), she was troubled by the evident delight of North African men who gasped, in patriarchal pleasure, "Une grosse femme." Sexism is sexism, no? or No? In *Reconstructing Gender: A Multicultural Anthology* is Haubegger's (1997) essay, "I'm Not Fat, I'm Latina." Or, as someone responding to this paper said, is this comparison racist?

Anxiety. You will think me a moral relativist, someone for whom all bets are off, no law applies, anything goes, from bloodletting to child abuse to . . .

Note 6. Fetishism and the Paradigm Shift

> [The] meaning and purpose of the fetish . . . is [to] substitute for the woman's (the mother's) penis that the little boy once believed in and—for reasons familiar to us—does not want to give up [Freud, 1927, pp. 152–153].

> Fetishism is a state of omnipotently but precariously controlled mania. Hence it is at once intensely pleasurable and frightfully vulnerable [Khan, 1979, p. 165].

Perhaps because we are all fetishists in one way or another, as Balint (1956) suggested, fetishism occupies an ambiguous place in the psycho-analytic theory of perversions. Sometimes it belongs, sometimes it is excluded. In the classical view, fetishism is not a perversion, because the fetish is what enables a man to be heterosexual, not homosexual. The fetish, symbolizing the mother's penis, demonstrates that castration does not happen: Mother still has her penis. With his fetish close at hand, then, he need not flee women for the imagined safety of another man and his penis. Rather, standing in for the destructive, uncannily penis-less vagina so feared by the boy is, say, a leather boot the man insists his wife wear before they have sex, or a bit of fur he caresses, or the car about which he fantasizes, or the dress he wears at the kitchen sink.

This definition of fetishism held, in principle, as long as homosexuality remained a perversion. If sexual preference no longer separates the perverse from the normal, however, what happens to our understanding of fetishism? Even Balint (1956), writing 17 years before the removal of homosexuality as a diagnosis from the Diagnostic and Statistical Manual of Mental Disorders, argued that homosexuality is not a perversion. Why is that? His explanation is illuminating. For Balint, what determines normality is not sex but love—a stance that epitomizes the sea change that psychoanalytic thought underwent over the course of the 20th century. What drives human beings and binds them together is, to use slightly different language, attachment—not the amoral, impersonal, imperious libido. Because homosexuals, Balint argued, experience "practically the whole scale of love and hatred that is exemplified in heterosexuality" (p. 17), because "all the beautiful, all the hideous, all the altruistically loving and all the egotistically exploiting features of heterosexual love can be found in homosexual love as well" (p. 17), we cannot argue for the perversity of their desire. (I could riff on the way that, even in this prescience, heterosexuality still measures mental health: Exactly what does "practically" mean? How do homosexuals fail? But never mind.)

As what we may call the *relational turn* has taken place, a new psychoanalytic and probably cultural normality has been erected and, along with it, a new clinical goal—not the derepression of forbidden desire but the healing of the mutilated capacity to love. As a oneperson psychology has given way to, or at least moved over to accommodate, a twoperson psychology, fetishism, like perversion, becomes interpretable in intersubjective space. Khan's (1979) remarkable essay, "Fetish as Negation of the Self: Clinical Notes on Foreskin Fetishism in a Male Homosexual," encapsulates the paradigm shift in psychoanalytic thinking about fetishism in particular and perversion in general. This exceptionally moving and theoretically interesting piece of writing comprises two parts. The first, a 30-page section, is severely difficult and is based on the first, five-year phase of an analysis. The second, which reads like a spare eight-page short story, arose from the second phase, which took place a decade later.

The story behind the story told in this essay is that of the relational turn. The first part is a Tower of Psychoanalytic Babel. It attempts to have it all—to retain the classical model of fetishism and sexuality while incorporating the language and findings, most notably and rather surprisingly, of ego psychology, as well as those of object relations. The range of concepts includes: "ego pathology," "the (breast) mother," "internal objects and early ego development," "transitional object phenomena," "separation anxiety," "pathological body-ego development," "disintegration," "bisexual primary identifications," "flight from incest," and "defence against archaic anxiety affects."

In the second section, the struggle to integrate theories of attachment and narcissism with drive theory has vanished. This herculean effort is no longer necessary because in the 15 years between the two writings, from 1965 to 1979, the paradigm had shifted. By 1979, it was possible to dispense with references to the classical oneperson model of genitality and drive and to focus on matters of narcissistic integration and damage and of broken and restored interpersonal relatedness, and so it was possible to tell a simple, accessible story, a story of the negation and recovery of self. As Khan (1979) wrote, "The title of this paper reflects largely the understanding of the fetishistic reveries and practices as we began to comprehend them in the second phase" (p. 139).

Fetishism, in Khan's (1979) view, is not about sex; it's about a state of mind. Things, or body-parts, are used to regulate not sex but psychic equilibrium, which in turn is primally dependent on the quality of object relations. "What the patient had sought from his treatment was the assimilation of this manic sexual fetishistic excitement and affectivity into an ego-capacity that could be related to the self, the object, and the environment" (p. 165). The manic defense against psychic deadness, an idea Khan drew from Winnicott, defines fetishism. For this patient, it patched together the fragmentary psychic structure constituted by an idealized attachment to a highly narcissistic mother whose marital instability and depression pockmarked his early life with a series of losses. In arousing uncircumcised working-class boys against their will and ejaculating into their foreskins, Khan's patient was simultaneously repairing his mother, binding her to him, and reintegrating himself. Classically, Khan wrote, the fetish is an auxiliary means serving heterosexual gratification and defending against perversions, especially homosexuality. Postclassically, however, we could do worse than cite McDougall (1995, p. 174), even though she denied anything as disjunctive as a paradigm shift: Fetishism is a "technique . . . of psychic survival . . . required to preserve the feeling of subjective identity as well" (p. 237).

Note 7. Relatedness, Aggression, and Social Control

I feel like I'm not getting into the meet [!] of anything [Dr. MH].

I have deliberately widened the issue of perversion from one of sexual identity to one of identity in general in order to include character perversions and also perverse relationships, where the other person is used as a functional or part-object. Perversion in this larger sense is a lack of capacity for whole-object love [Bach, 1995, p. 53].

What makes a good life? A good psyche? So often the answer to this question seems to depend on what a person thinks comes first. Your idea of elemental human nature determines your idea of mental health. With the early Freud, we postulated that sex comes first, attachment second, and therefore the derepression of sexuality became the clinical telos, achieved by the authoritative if not authoritarian doctor pronouncing on the patient. Now, with the relational turn, we have flip-flopped. As Domenici (1995) argued, drive theory sees affective and interpersonal needs as "an overlay upon a more basic template of sexuality and aggression" (p. 34). In contrast, objectrelations theory (to name but the most influential and general of the new psychoanalytic schools) reverses the matter, making sexuality the secondary precipitate of a desire for connection and intimacy—a desire entailing, presupposing, creating, and regulating a narcissistically intact self. Now the relationship of analyst and patient, opened up for intersubjective construction and deconstruction, becomes a key clinical tool, object of knowledge, a goal.

"Perversion," wrote Bach (1995) "is a lack of capacity for whole-object love" (p. 53). A moment of anxiety, at least for me. Perversion isn't about sex?

The new psychoanalytic vision of mental health, I have suggested, matches a new cultural norm, which means really a new morality. Specifically, it needs to be contextualized in the "family values" ideology that came to the Euro-American fore in the late 1980s and early 1990s as a sort of backlash against the 1960s and 1970s. The tangle of values and theory and therapy backgrounds everyday psychoanalysis. Sex brings it out, but perversion inflames it. Perversion is so disturbing, so challenging of received and ordinarily unquestioned norms. Its power to pollute the normal reveals the sanctity with which the normal is endowed, provoking a defense of normality, sometimes with a flare of outrage, as in Chasseguet-Smirgel's (1985) *Creativity and Perversion*, and sometimes with a canny redefinition of it, as in Kernberg's (1995) *Love Relations*. Both these major works have been influenced by the relational turn. Chasseguet-Smirgel, as we have seen, switched the etiology of perversion from Oedipus to Narcissus, even though clinically she kept the classical faith. Kernberg made a somewhat different move. If Chasseguet-Smirgel's account includes unnoticed inconsistencies between theoretical and clinical stances issuing from the *décalage* of theory we have already seen in Khan's (1979) study of foreskin fetishism, Kernberg intentionally tried to meld the relational turn with the founding paradigm. *Love Relations* inscribes a developmental trajectory in which psychosexuality evolves as a complicated weave of corporeality, psychodynamics, and intersubjectivity. In a tour de force, Kernberg whipped up a multiply twinned solution, an integration of two capacities—for body pleasure and for "total object-relation." Kernberg (1976) wrote that, at maturity, genital pleasure organizes body-surface erotism into the matrix of total object relation and complementary sexual identification (p. 185).

In this new, widely shared model, love and intimacy are the new signs and critieria of health, if not health itself. If you don't have them, there's something wrong. Across the entire analytic spectrum, attachment and its vicissitudes are what we look at and look for as we sit with our patients. I am alert to it with Dr. MH. Perhaps in response to my being away one August, Dr. MH said, "I feel like I'm not getting into the meat of anything." But what I wrote down in my notes was not *meat*, I wrote *meet*. As I was thinking both about this essay and about a feeling of impasse in our work, I decided (inspired by Gerson's, 1996, disclosure of his transcription errors) to tell Dr. MH of my slip of the pen and to propose an interpretation. Consciously he may have wanted his flesh, his meat, beat, so to speak, but unconsciously he wished to meet me, to encounter and engage me—and, further, this was an idea that did not yet seem safe to him, and so he needed me to hold it for him. To my surprise, Dr. MH agreed. He had (as of the first writing of this essay three years ago) been complaining the preceding six months that therapy had plateaued for him. He did not want to come to session. Nothing seemed to be happening. His sexual appetite had fallen off. Following my interpretation, we began speaking of his mistrust of me, of his doubt that I can hold him in mind. Now we approached the possibility of tenderness. We entertained the possibility that his fear of my pathologizing him is also a wish for me to be more critical of his sexual practices— somewhat, we thought, the way he wants to be spanked—to show him not that he is wrong but that something is wrong and needs fixing.

But I am trying to decipher what sense it makes to call Dr. MH's difficulty with love and intimacy a perversion—for that is how Bach and, I think, Kernberg too would label it. Interpreting sexuality in object-relational terms is now an indelible part of our view and technique. Consider Ogden's (1989) choice to "use the term 'perverse' to refer to forms of sexuality that are used in the service of denying the separateness of external objects and sexual difference, and thus interfere with the elaboration of the depressive position" (p. 166, n. 11). Perversion here still denotes sexuality, but only the sexuality that defends against object-relational dangers. What is really wrong in a perversion, then, is not sex but relatedness and, by implication, development if not character itself.

Caution: regulatory practice still at work. When perversion relocates from sex to relatedness, its moral baggage comes along. If psychoanalysis once carved heterosexual order out of the polymorphously perverse jungle, now it fashions a model of mature total object relation as the criterion of mental health. Yet who among us can claim to have achieved that? Wholeness and totality in relatedness are as intimidating as a heterosexuality untroubled by the homosexuality it has renounced (Butler,

1995). Bronski (in press a), tricking with Jim, lived with Walta, "the love of my life," whom he might tell of sex on the side—as many gay men do—but not of the cutting. Do you, by the way, tell your lover everything? Vital questions of cultural value pop up here. Does whole-object love mean telling all? Some? Does the idea of whole-object love replace heterosexuality as the unachievable ideal to which we must, in aspiring, submit?

Yikes. I feel like I'm criticizing motherhood. I respect the intent of Bach's (1995) revisionism. The "capacity for whole-object love" is surely a good thing. But surely it's also a case of new wine in old regulatory bottles. "There's something wrong" still turns into "There's something wrong with me," though the referent shifts from sex to love. Sure, for most of us, it's awful not to be able to love and be loved. But why call this absence, this suffering, this failure, a perversion? All that assigning this diagnosis accomplishes is to preserve a traditional discourse, perpetuate an oppression, and make people feel bad.

Must there always be stigma? "It's my body" is the claim made regarding parent-mortifying adolescent body practices like piercing or, in the 1970s, the long hair guys sported or the bras women didn't. But adolescent rebellion may be equally cultural critique or, if you will, symptom. Perhaps kids mark themselves to remind their elders that, in our culture, stigma never disappears. In the new family-values psychoanalysis, stigma hops from sex to relatedness, from abjected forms of sexual desire to the impaired capacity to love. Sex recedes, and relatedness steps forward—a relatedness that has its perverse and, implicitly, normal forms, a clinical as well as theoretical happenstance not without its puritan underpinnings (Green, 1996) and cultural contouring (Dimen, 1999).

We return to Stoller's (1975) argument about perversion and aggression. Does psychoanalytic preoccupation, like stigma, jump from sex to love because of an uncontainable aggression? Where, that is, does aggression lie in this model of mature caring? Oh, yes, I know that you can get angry and repair and so on, but somehow the family values version of intimate struggle doesn't quite capture the intensity and ruthlessness of fear and anger and rage marking long-standing intimacy. Let me remind you of a scene from *Taxi*, the old television sitcom. Latka, an immigrant from some unnamed Balkan state, has married Simka, his fiancée recently arrived from their homeland. In order to get a green card, Simka has to prove to the immigration officer that she and Latka are married. Naturally, the day they are to appear, she has PMS and (what else?) forgets the marriage license. Of course, when she arrives without it, Latka gets angry at her. The officer helps them out by posing a series of questions designed to let them show that they live together on a regular basis. Question after question, they fail. Finally, he asks them to name the last movie they saw together. Latka answers one thing, Simka another, they begin to disagree, they begin to fight, they lapse into Ruritanian, and the next thing you know they have spiraled into a vindictive, hate-filled screaming match that is, of course, hysterically funny—at which point the officer interrupts them and says, "Okay, okay, I believe it—you're married. Only married people fight like that."

K. Leary (personal communication) has observed the short clinical shrift given aggression in the literature during these relational days. Particularly in the context of the two-person psychology that is so rapidly becoming the new psychoanalytic convention, aggression might seem a bit incongruous (perhaps in part having to do with the maternal dimensions of the two-person model and the psychocultural divorce of aggression and femininity). Yet, as Freud's joke goes, aggression is ubiquitous, showing up not only between analyst and patient but between psychoanalysis and its customers. I am concerned, as I said earlier, with psychoanalytic participation in domination—in naming, blaming, truth framing, and shaming. You might think of this psychoanalytic re-creation of the cultural morality producing it as a sort of aggression.

This participation tends to be quite invisible and therefore all the more powerful, as revealed by an inspection of Kernberg's (1995) take on perversion in *Love Relations*. On this view, a healthy sexual relationship in fact encompasses occasional sexual engagements in which one uses the other "as a pure sexual object" (p. 58). This permission for part-object exploitation in sexuality corrects the drift toward purity that, I have been suggesting, infuses the new familyvalues psychoanalysis. In an act of liberation, it admits aggression into the sanctum of sanity. Proposing the Kleinian integration of love and hate as signaling mature object-love, it does us all a favor by reintroducing Freud's recognition of perversion's ubiquity and giving it an object-relational place.

At the same time, this redefinition of normality is an act of imperialism. Speaking from the center of psychoanalytic power, of disciplinary authority, it colonizes the sexual margins, allowing the conventional to own the unconventional without any of the risks of unconventionality. In a royal co-optation of the sexual revolution, *Love Relations* renders perverse erotics acceptable, but only under the condition that it be practiced by that guardian of nonconformity, the heterosexual, married couple: "If a couple can incorporate their polymorphous perverse fantasies and wishes into their sexual relationship, discover and uncover the sado-masochistic core of sexual excitement in their intimacy, their defiance of conventional cultural mores may become a conscious element of their pleasure" (Kernberg, 1995, p. 96). That heterosexual couples might readmit pregenitality to their bed, that they might acknowledge the erotics of pain, that, like adolescents who pierce and tattoo, they might get off on sexual rebellion—what a daring vision.

But then comes the stretch: "It is in the very nature of conventional culture to attempt to control the basically rebellious and implicitly asocial nature of the couple as it is perceived by the conventional social environment" (Kernberg, 1995, p. 96). Here I must protest: the couple's "basically rebellious and implicitly asocial nature"? Unnoticed here is the absolute legitimacy conferred by heterosexual matrimony and the corresponding marginalization and denigration of other forms of intimacy, as told by the absence of homosexual coupledom from the model of mental health in *Love Relations*. Kernberg (2000) recently indicted psychoanalysis' neglect of ideas beyond its perimeters—not only those of science but of history and sociology as well. If, however, he himself had consulted the critique of psychoanalysis found in those disciplines in the latest generation (e.g., Weisstein, 1970; Kovel, 1981), his own idealization of the marital unit would not have escaped his ordinarily critical eye. Maybe radical notions of all sorts flit like fireflies in the matrimonial darkness. But, in Kernberg's own oeuvre, the procreating couple still reigns as the navel of the psychoanalytic universe—a stable center of sanity and social responsibility. I don't understand, then, how it can also situate rebellion and asociality.

Talk about a moment of anxiety. This time, though, it's not the anxiety of stigma or pollution or shame—it's the anxiety of domination.

These mystifying, double-binding pronouncements incarnate the Foucaultian nightmare. They exemplify the worst tendencies toward domination; toward naming, blaming, truth framing, and shaming; in effect toward stigmatizing and the participation of psychoanalysis in the cultural morality governing it. *Les psy*, argued Foucault (1978), belong to a new form of power, "a technology of health and pathology" (p. 45) that constantly attends to and scrutinizes its subject, becoming itself a domain of pleasure. The body is a principal route to the subject—hence, the centrality of stigma to this power structure and its operation. This theory may be paranoid but is not on that account wrong; at the same time that the maneuver proposed by *Love Relations* unlocks one ball-and-chain by authorizing aggression on the sexual side of intimacy, it snaps another one on. You read *Love Relations*, and you think you can't possibly get it right; Kernberg knows, and you don't. Either you love the wrong way, or you can't love at all.

You enter the "perpetual spirals of power and pleasure" that Foucault (1978) argued inhere in the technology of desire in contemporary society (p. 44). This spiraling finds itself in the knowledge that psychoanalysis creates and exercises, knowledge in which power is sensualized and pleasure therefore enhanced. Power, knowledge, and pleasure are, to use Butler's (1990, passim) neologism, interimplicated. Always suggesting, engaging, triggering, or in fact constituting one another, they form a psychopolitical gyroscope, in which "an impetus [is] given to power through its very exercise; an emotion reward[s] the overseeing control and carrie[s] it further" (Foucault, 1978, p. 45). As I read Foucault, I begin to imagine his two paradigmatic models of social control, the confessional and the couch, and think about the one I know. I think about pleasures and powers and knowledges of the psychoanalytic encounter. "Pleasure spread[s] to the power that harrie[s] it; power anchor[s] the pleasure it uncover[s]" (pp. 44–45). And now listen to the darker side of the transference–counter-transference embrace, a psychoanalytic sadomasochism that may glue the analytic couple, as well as the writer-reader couple: "the pleasure . . . of exercising a power that questions, monitors, watches, spies, searches out, palpates, brings to light" (the analyst's pleasure at probing, asking, knowing, helping) and, "on the other hand, the pleasure that kindles at having to evade this power, flee from it, fool it, or travesty it" (the patient's pleasure at resisting, the erotics of the repetition compulsion). Following Foucault, we must conclude that sadomasochism is the principal psychodynamic animating the desire and struggle for power fueling the infrastructures of contemporary society, and it shows up everywhere authority and hierarchy are found (Chancer, 1992), including, need I say, in psychoanalysis.

Anxiety.

Note 8. Shelter from the Storm?/Rabbit in a Briar Patch

I like deep massage, I like being beaten, I like catharsis [Dr. MH].

He is just an alienated isolate in human society and lives from that stance [Khan, 1979, p. 170].

As if by will alone a single drop of crimson, scarlet, carmine blood forms and runs down my chest. It stops, and I stare at it in the mirror. I don't feel like a saint, I don't feel beautiful, I don't feel sexy. I just feel alive and begin to cry [Bronski, in press a, p. 14].

The label of perversion is as clinically superfluous as we now understand the label of homosexuality to be. It is not a diagnostic category; it does not tell us what to do. Now we take our clinical cue not from disorders of desire but from struggles of self and relationship—splits in psyche, maladies of object love, infirmities of intimacy. My strategy of detoxification has had some success with Dr. MH. Focusing on his discomfort with his being, with his self and his obese body, we have checked, if not eliminated, the depredations and degradations of his shaming self, and cleared space for the possibility that he might after all be an acceptable person. We have opened a channel through which might flow his longing just to be, to feel, to be a held baby.

Glimmers of self-acceptance come and go. Recently he was able to dance without embarrassment for the first time in many years. His self-loathing is occasionally less virulent, at times quiescent. We explore in a widening spiral the range of Dr. MH's sexual practices and fantasies, thereby rendering them not much more toxic than the other dilemmas of his life—those of work and family, for example. As we explore, however, we must survive the periods of deadness that accompany the diminution of the manic defense.

Psychoanalysis offers shelter from the storm, but it is not without its dangers. We have to be careful, E. Ghent (1986, personal communication) said to me once in supervision. He recapped the end of *Long Day's Journey into Night*, when, following Hickey's false promises of peace after sobriety, the punch leaches from the whiskey: "Bejees," says Hope, "what did you do to the booze, Hickey? There's no damned life left in it" (O'Neill, 1940, p. 154). Evaluating his patient's and his own accomplishments, Khan (1979) suggested that we be mindful of "the great hazard of the analytic cure of a pervert's self-cure" (p. 176). Khan's foreskin fetishist emerged from biphasic analysis "a person real in himself, creative in his intellectual pursuits, unharrowed by that ungraspable anxiety in himself, and beginning to live a life which to him is meaningful, sentient and true, and has a purpose as well as a direction in terms of its future" (p. 176). At the same time, however, he "lives a life which, by ordinary standards, is extremely lacking in human contact. . . . He is just an alienated isolate in human society and lives from that stance" (p. 170). Of another patient, Khan wrote that the glow was gone: When the manic defense collapses, when the perversions cease, a certain liveliness, an "instinctual fervour and dynamism" vanish too (p. 176).

I wonder, though. A great absence in Khan's clinical account is of his own concordant countertransference to perversion. Had he been able to empathize, might he have found a way to help his patients keep the glow or create it elsewhere? V. Bonfilio (1999, personal communication) said that unless he thinks about how he lost his glow and found a new one, he cannot be of much help to his patients who are risking all with the throw of those analytic dice. There are good reasons, based on the internal structure of Khan's arguments, to think that, theoretically speaking, the only acceptable glow is that produced by conventional forms of intimacy. Certainly Khan enjoyed his homophobia; Godley (2001), writing in the *London Review of Books* of his disastrous treatment with Khan, recounted a telephone call from Winnicott that Khan took in session, in which the two men shared "a giggly joke about homosexual fellatio" (p. 6). The "spiral of degradation" (p. 5) that constituted the treatment, as well as his posttreatment relationship with Godley, suggests, however, that Khan's own glow derived as much from cruelty as from married intimacy.

With Stoller (1979), I wonder about the link between the glow and aggression, even the imbrication of sex, death, and life. If Khan's countertransference problem was, you might put it, love, then mine is perhaps hate or, at least, aggression, which I know is one reason that anxiety has dogged this paper. And it is not clear whether fear of aggression is my problem, Dr. MH's, or ours; we'll see. The effort of loving him, even as he wards me off with gestures and sentiments soaked in hatred, echoes my struggle to negotiate between the love speech of naming and the hate speech of blaming; the depressive position being always in precarious balance, love and hate are never far apart, and intimacy is always both challenged and made possible by aggression.

If you domesticate desire, take the hate away from love and the aggression from sex, whence the glow? In "More Life," an essay whose title is borrowed from a speech by Prior in Tony Kushner's *Angels in America*, Corbett (2001) proposed a new developmental theory of multiplicity: There are many routes to sanity, maturity, sexuality. Probably this is another of our jobs, to midwife more life. "I like deep massage, I like being beaten, I like catharsis," said Dr. MH. Certainly his manic defense fuses elements of both connection and sexuality. At the same time, his pleasure in the deathlike shattering of self born in the crucible of catharsis (Bersani, 1988) sounds familiar to many of us. Chodorow (1992) wisely connected perversion and liveliness: "If we retain passion and intensity for heterosexuality, we are in the arena of symptom, neurosis, and disorder; if we deperversionize heterosexuality, giving up its claim to intensity and passion, we make it less interesting to us and to its practitioners" (p. 301). Of his final selfcutting, Bronski (in press a) wrote in the last line of his penultimate paragraph, "I just feel alive and begin to cry." He wrote here in the midst of death, the plague of AIDS that stole his lovers from him. Pain and blood are signs of life. Perhaps he struggled with psychic death too. In any case, is life after deadness not a decent goal? Certainly, Ogden (1997) would agree. Perversion, Ogden argued, shows up in analysis as a defense against deadness, even if his prescription was the family-values usual: "In a healthy development, a sense of oneself as alive is equated with a generative loving parental intercourse" (p. 143). Are

there no other ways to represent life, exuberance, passion, and pleasure besides reproductive heterosexuality?

How can we prescribe health when we cannot know, going forward,
what produces illness? There needs to be a way to back off from the
authoritarian and dominating inclinations that psychoanalysis shares
with other regulatory practices. Remembering doubt is one route; writing disruptively is another. As Kaplan (1990) wrote, the anorexic was
once a smart and compliant child who surrendered all "for the safety
and self-esteem of becoming a narcissistic extension of Mother. Yet from
a prospective view, . . . no sensible clinical observer would predict from
observations of a girl's relationship to her mother during infancy and
childhood an anorectic solution to the dilemmas of adolescence" (p.
458). Freud (1920) said it earlier, in *The Psychogenesis of a Case of
Homosexuality in a Woman:* "The synthesis is thus not so satisfactory
as the analysis; in other words, from a knowledge of the premises we
could not have foretold the nature of the result" (p. 167). Notice the
judicious contingency of his formulation, which Khan, for all his
grandiosity, in fact shares. How different from the certitude of marking
Love Relations, a seamless narrative that seems to wrap everything up
in the service of truth but also hides all the loose ends.

Notes pull on those threads, rupture the surface coherence, or at least
I hope they do. In this presentation both clinical and rhetorical, I have
taken the liberty of leaving you with many open questions alive in both
clinic and culture about our diagnostic categories, our standards of
health and illness, of morality, and of truth—a strategy that I think is
true to the passion of psychoanalysis past and present, theoretical and
clinical. Something has gone wrong for Dr. MH, and he suffers because
of it. In order to make it better, he and I need to find out what that is.
It may be that, once we find the answer, we will discover that the books
had been telling the truth and the answer was there all along. Then,
again, maybe we will create a new truth, one that works for him, or for
us, or maybe even for others. We just don't know right now. I am
reminded of what Pete Seeger said about his daddy's vision of truth: "It's
like a rabbit in a briar patch. You know it's in there somewhere, but you
can't ever get at it."

Perversion, even in Freud's understanding, let alone in light of the
cultural revolution that has taken place since the 1960s, challenges our
intellect, our passion, our practice. My study group read this paper and
worried that Dr. MH might be recognizable in the psychoanalytic community. They wanted me to disguise him more. I was surprised. Although
he is a mental health worker at a very high level, he is not a psychoanalyst, does not run in psychoanalytic circles, does not read psycho-

analysis. He and I thought it important that he be identified by his title so as to say to the readers of this essay that he is, if not of them, at least among them. This is, of course, a rhetorical strategy and, I hope, a performative one. If Chasseguet-Smirgel and Kernberg are right, then let us acknowledge their moral, perhaps even moralistic, but finally routine, familiar, and ancient point: Perversion is us.

What, after all, is pathology? If perversion can coexist with health, if its status as illness varies with cultural time and place, then, conversely, any sexuality may be symptomatic—or healthy. If all sexualities may claim wholesomeness, if all have a valid psychic place, then all are subject to the same psychic vicissitudes. Put yet another way, sexuality has nothing inherently to do with mental health or mental illness. You may be ill if you are heterosexual and healthy, if you are homosexual, bisexual, transvestite, or . . . whatever. By the same token, you, like Khan's fetishist or like Barbara McClintock, Nobel laureate in medicine and discoverer of jumping genes, may live alone, without the trappings of conventional intimacy (Keller, 1983, p. 205). And who's to say that there's something wrong . . . something wrong with that . . . something wrong with you?

References

Abelove, H. (199), Some speculations on the history of "sexual intercourse" during the history of the "long eighteenth century" in England. In: *Nationalisms and Sexualities*, ed. A. Parker, M. Russo, D. Sommer & P. Yaeger. New York: Routledge, pp. 335–342.

Apter, E. (1992), Perversion. In: *Feminism and Psychoanalysis: A Critical Dictionary*, ed. E. Wright. Oxford, England: Blackwell, pp. 311–313.

Bach, S. (1995), *The Language of Perversion and the Language of Love*. Northvale, NJ: Aronson.

Balint, M. (1956), Perversions and genitality. In: *Perversions: Psychodynamics and Therapy*. New York: Random House, pp. 16–27.

Benjamin, J. (1988), *The Bonds of Love*. New York: Pantheon.

——— (1998), *The Shadow of the Other: Intersubjectivity and Gender in Psychoanalysis*. New York: Routledge.

Bersani, L. (1988), Is the rectum a grave? In: *AIDS: Cultural Analysis, Cultural Activism*, ed. D. Crimp. Cambridge, MA: MIT Press, pp. 197–222.

Bromberg, P. (1998), *Standing in the Spaces: Essays on Clinical Process, Trauma, and Dissociation*. Hillsdale, NJ: The Analytic Press.

Bronski, M. (in press a), Dr. Fell. In: *Bringing the Plague: Toward a Postmodern Psychoanalysis*, ed. S. Fairfield, L. Layton & C. Stack. New York: Other Press.

——— (in press b), Sex, death, and the limits of irony. In: *Bringing the Plague: Toward a Postmodern Psychoanalysis*, ed. S. Fairfield, L. Layton & C. Stack. New York: Other Press.

Butler, J. (1990), *Gender Trouble: Feminism and the Subversion of Identity*. New York: Routledge.

——— (1995), Melancholy gender—refused identification. *Psychoanal. Dial.*, 5:165–180.

Chancer, L. (1992), *Sado-Masochism and Everyday Life*. New Brunswick, NJ: Rutgers University Press.

Chasseguet-Smirgel, J. (1985), *Creativity and Perversion*. New York: Norton.

Chodorow, N. (1992), Heterosexuality as compromise formation. *Psychoanal. Contemp. Thought*, 15:267–304.

——— (2000), *Psychoanalysis and the Search for Personal Meaning*. New Haven, CT: Yale University Press.

Corbett, K. (2001), More life: Centrality and marginality in human development. *Psychoanal. Dial.*, 11:313–335.

Davidson, A. I. (1987), How to do the history of psychoanalysis: A reading of Freud's *Three Essays on the Theory of Sexuality*. In: *The Trial of Psychoanalysis*, ed. F. Meltzer. Chicago: University of Chicago Press, pp. 39–64.

de Lauretis, T. (1994), *The Practice of Love: Lesbian Sexuality and Perverse Desire*. Bloomington: Indiana University Press.

de Waal, F. & Lanting, F. (1997), *Bonobo: The Forgotten Ape*. Berkeley: University of California Press.

Dimen, M. (1999), Between lust and libido: Sex, psychoanalysis, and the moment before. *Psychoanal. Dial.*, 9:415–440.

——— (in press), The disturbance of sex. In: *Bringing the Plague: Toward a Postmodern Psychoanalysis*, ed. S. Fairfield, L. Layton & C. Stack. New York: Other Press.

Domenici, T. (1995), Exploding the myth of sexual psychopathology: A deconstruction of Fairbairn's anti-homosexual theory. In: *Disorienting Sexualities*, ed. R. Lesser & T. Domenici. New York: Routledge, pp. 33–64.

Douglas, M. (1970), *Purity and Danger: An Analysis of the Concepts of Pollution and Taboo*. New York: Penguin.

Ferenczi, S. (1933), The confusion of tongues between adults and the child. *Contemp. Psychoanal.*, 24:196–206, 1988.

Firestone, S. (1970), *The Dialectic of Sex*. New York: William Morrow.

Foucault, M. (1978), *The History of Sexuality, Vol. I*. New York: Vintage Books, 1980.

Freud, S. (1905), Three essays on the theory of sexuality. *Standard Edition*, 7:135–248. London: Hogarth Press, 1955.

——— (1908), "Civilized" sexual morality and modern nervousness. *Standard Edition*, 9:177–204. London: Hogarth Press, 1957.

——— (1910), Leonardo da Vinci and a memory of his childhood. *Standard Edition*, 11:59–130. London: Hogarth Press, 1957.

——— (1915), A case of paranoia running counter to the psycho-analytic theory of the disease. *Standard Edition*, 14:261–270. London: Hogarth Press, 1957.

——— (1920), The psychogenesis of a case of homosexuality in a woman. *Standard Edition*, 18:145–172. London: Hogarth Press, 1955.

——— (1927), Fetishism. *Standard Edition*, 22:152–157. London: Hogarth Press, 1957.

———— (1930), Civilization and its discontents. *Standard Edition*, 21:64–146. London: Hogarth Press, 1961.

Gerson, S. (1996), Neutrality, resistance, and self-disclosure in an intersubjective psychoanalysis. *Psychoanal. Dial.*, 6:623–645.

Godley, W. (2001), Saving Masud Khan. *London Rev. Books*, February 22:3–7.

Goldner, V. (1998), Theorizing gender and sexual subjectivity. Presented at annual meeting of the Division of Psychoanalysis (Division 39) of the American Psychological Association, Boston.

———— (n.d.), Violence and victimization: Enactments from the gender wars. Unpublished manuscript.

Green, A. (1996), Has sexuality anything to do with psychoanalysis? *Internat. J. Psycho-Anal.*, 76:871–883.

Greenberg, J. (1993), *Oedipus and Beyond*. Cambridge, MA: Harvard University Press.

Haubegger, C. (1997), I'm not fat, I'm Latina. In: *Reconstructing Gender: A Multicultural Anthology*, ed. E. Disch. Mountain View, CA: Mayfield, pp. 177–179.

Kaplan, L. (1990), *Female Perversions*. New York: Anchor Books.

Keller, E. (1983), *A Feeling for the Organism: The Life and Work of Barbara McClintock*. New York: Freeman.

Kernberg, O. (1976), *Object Relations Theory and Clinical Pychoanalysis*. New York: Aronson, pp. 185–214.

———— (1995), *Love Relations*. New Haven, CT: Yale University Press.

———— (2000), A concerned critique of psychoanalytic education. *Internat. J. Psycho-Anal.*, 81:97–120.

Khan, M. M. R. (1979), Fetish as negation of the self: Clinical notes on foreskin fetishism in a male homosexual. In: *Alienation in Perversions*. New York: International Universities Press, pp. 139–176.

Kovel, J. (1981), *The Age of Desire: Notes of a Radical Psychoanalyst*. New York: Pantheon.

Lacan, J. (1977), The subversion of the subject and the dialectic of desire in the Freudian unconscious. In: *Écrits*, trans. A. Sheridan. New York: Norton, pp. 292–325.

Laplanche, J. & Pontalis, J-B. (1973), *The Language of Psychoanalysis*, trans. D. Nicholson-Smith. New York: Norton.

McDougall, J. (1995), *The Many Faces of Eros*. New York: Norton.

Millett, K. (1970). *Sexual Politics*. New York: Simon & Schuster.

Mitchell, S. (2000), *Relationality: From Attachment to Intersubjectivity*. Hillsdale, NJ: The Analytic Press.

Morrison, A. (1989) *Shame: The Underside of Narcissism*. Hillsdale, NJ: The Analytic Press.

Ogden, T. (1989), *The Primitive Edge of Experience*. New York: Aronson.

———— (1997), The perverse subject of analysis. *J. Amer. Psychoanal. Assn.*, 44:1121–1145.

O'Neill, E. (1940), The Iceman Cometh. In: *Best American Plays*, Third Series 1945–51, ed. J. Gassner. New York: Crown, 1952, pp. 95–172.

Person, E. (1980), Sexuality as the mainstay of identity. *Signs*, 5:605–630.

Spezzano, C. (1993), *Affect in Psychoanalysis*. Hillsdale, NJ: The Analytic Press.

Stein, R. E. (1991), *Psychoanalytic Theories of Affect*. New York: Praeger.

Stoller, R. (1975), *Perversion: The Erotic Form of Hatred*. Washington, DC: American Psychiatric Press.

———— (1979), *Sexual Excitement*. New York: Pantheon.

Tisdale, S. (1994), *Talk Dirty to Me*. New York: Anchor.

———— (1996), Lecture. Open Center, New York.

Weisstein, N. (1970), Kinder, küche, kirche as scientific law: Psychology constructs the female. In: *Sisterhood Is Powerful*, ed. R. Morgan. New York: Random House, pp. 205–220.

Winnicott, D. W. (1969a), Creativity and its origins. In: *Playing and Reality*. New York: Basic Books, 1971, pp. 76–93.

———— (1969b), The use of an object and relating through identification. In: *Playing and Reality*. New York: Basic Books, 1971, pp. 86–94.

Afterword

This Afterword might well be a Foreword. In it, I would alert the reader to the point and purpose and motive of this essay. The existence of a Foreword, however, might suggest that I knew what I was doing when I wrote the essay. Which is only partly true.

Tensions. "Perversion is Us? Eight Notes" culminates two decades' worth of thinking and writing about sexuality. Looking back on this work (collected and transformed into *Sexuality, Intimacy, Power*, 2003), I notice a tension. Old ideas were seeking new expression. New concepts jumped out and begged for new ways of putting things. Experiments in form led to experiments in thought. Old questions found new answers, and these led to new queries.

Intimacy of form and content—or telling by showing—became my method starting in 1979. Performativity—the text doing what it says—become my guide. Thus, in "Perversion Is Us? Eight Notes," form intensifies content, conveying multiplicity, dialectics, and provisionality through a set of alternations: the call and response of notes and exposition, repartée between academic tones and everyday palaver, psychoanalysis in antiphony with social theory. I certainly didn't plan my modus operandi in advance. But it didn't just happen either. Only by reviewing its evolution (see "Prologue," Dimen, 2003) can I see how it might have come to be. Much as in a psychoanalysis or a life, you know how you got where you got only afterwards, hence this Afterword.

Two main problems underlay this methodological solution: the existence of dualism and the search for a Third. Philosophers, says feminist philosopher Naomi Scheman, use the term dualism to denote
the idea that "some part of the world is divided into two kinds of
stuff" (personal communication, November 25, 2001). You might sum
up this notion with the phrase "either/or." Descartes, for example,
posited two incommensurable realms of existence, *res cogitans* and
res extensa (Scheman; Paul Stepansky, personal communication,
October 11, 2001). "Either/or," and neither the twain shall meet. But
dualism is also a problem that, according to Scheman (1993), sets the
core modern epistemological task: to identify, and then bridge, gaps,
such as those between mind and body, masculine and feminine, psyche and society. My approach to this task is deconstructive, my form
of argument is dialectical, and my perspective is one of contingency
(See Rorty, 1989).

Thirds. You need something—a "both/and" beyond the "either/or"—
to bridge the gaps. You need a third term, toward whose creation (or
discovery) I take two routes. One is conceptual. Hence the three
polarities, each pair potentially confronted by a third, that circulate
throughout my work, as is evident in "Perversion Is Us? Eight Notes":
mind/body, body/culture, culture/mind. The other route is structural,
or formal. It is not only what you say that changes things, it's how
you say it. Like Sándor Ferenczi (1933), who found that his use of
obscenity enabled patients to retrieve dissociated memories, I hope
my experiments in voice and form will have produced a third voice
in the reader's response, be it consternation, a feeling of reward, or
a dream. Indeed, out of my own and others' thirding to this work
have emerged new projects. In "Sexuality and Suffering, or the Eew!
Factor" (Dimen, 2005), I delve into the darkness of abjection, humiliation, embarrassment, and lonely shame that infuses and indeed
intensifies sexual joy. I am very interested in the paradox of *jouis-
sance*, "a form of pleasure so intense as to be barely distinguishable
from pain" (Dean, 2001, p. 271).

Psychoanalysis has begun to embrace this "complexity, ambiguity,
ambivalence, impurity" (Scheman, personal communication, November
25, 2001). For some time now, psychoanalysis has been at the crossroads where two conceptual roads meet: a one-person psychology
and a two-person psychology (Greenberg and Mitchell, 1983; Ghent,
1989). Figuratively, a crossroads is a turning point. When you reach
it, you make a decision: you choose to go left, right, or straight ahead
(or, I suppose, back). Often enough, however, a crossroads proves just
the right place to set up shop or settle down. Many a rural market

412 | *Muriel Dimen*

has grown into a big city at just such a spot. Settlers are joined by newcomers, new ideas variegate the old, inventions follow by accident or design.

Intersubjectivity. Psychoanalysis, at the either/or crossroads of a one-person and a two-person psychology, has decided to stop where it is, at the site of intersubjectivity. Interesting questions now populate the growing community. Ghent (1989), in fact, insisted that it is in the tension of this meeting point—this "both/and"—that analysts now need to work, and, if their writings are any evidence, others seem to agree.

The multiple voices in "Perversion Is Us? Eight Notes" speak, I hope, to intersubjectivity, which functions, in turn, as a third, registering the veridicality of the two psychologies. Philosophers traditionally theorize the third through the dialectic, which locates polarities in dynamic contest, not in a static stand-off. Contemporary psychoanalytic thought interprets dialectical method variously. Hoffman (1998) defines the dialectic as "interdependence and interweaving" (p. xxi). Ogden (1998) emphasizes the tension of contradiction: "Dialectics is a process in which opposing elements each create, preserve, and negate the other" (p. 14).

Dialectics. The result of dialectics is unstable. Hoffman's interweaving goes on forever. In Ogden's metatheoretical explication, "Dialectical movement tends toward integrations that are never achieved. Each potential integration creates a new form of opposition characterized by its own distinct form of dialectical tension" (p. 14). Such movement toward unfinished integrations is "the analytic third," experiencing, comprehending, and narrating the shifting nature of the analysand's and the analyst's mutual creation and destruction of the other. Ogden persuasively claims, in fact, that psychoanalytic conceptions of the subject, as well as of technique, are fundamentally dialectical (p. 7): for example, consciousness and unconsciousness each serve as an empty set to the other—neither makes sense without the other's existence.

Let us say that we are persuaded that old-fashioned, either/or thinking does not suit our analytic or interpretive purposes. What do we do? Dualistic thinking would incline us to junk it and plump for the both/and. But a moment's reflection reveals that you can't have one without the other: there must be an either/or, two terms, in order that there be a both/and, a third. And what that third will turn out to be is contingent on the interaction in the either/or.

The third is no answer. It's just a moment in a process in which new possibilities are generated (Rorty, 1989, p. 108). Creating new tensions, it calls for new resolution, because it becomes an either/or to yet another term. Dialectics, viewed this way, is an ongoing process that in principle, as Ogden (1998) suggests, never stops, even if, at any given moment, closure seems to have been reached. In actuality, psychoanalyses end: the patient terminates, carrying the analysis away, one hopes, in an idiosyncratic, personal fashion. Whether one can say the same of the dialectics of social life is another question, and the results are not in. In the dialectics of psychic life, however, going from the either/or to the both/and is a voyage made repeatedly.

Irony and Patient Care. My work blushes with a slightly embarrassing tension: the contrast between an earnest, do-gooder wish to solve problems—to help my patients, make the world better—and an ironic sensibility. The sincere wish to make things better comes across as a mite naïve, in comparison with the world-weary, sophisticated recognition that things are rarely what they seem. I seem unable to resolve this tension (this dualism of my own). Indeed, my difficulty in eliminating it may explain the literary forms—the third—I have chosen. Notes, fragments, dual and multiple voices (Merleau-Ponty, 1961), these heteroglossic (Bakhtin, 1934–35) forms permit a certain provisionality. A unified thesis is hard to change, but you can always add another note. This flexibility is a good thing, since different languages, unveiling different features of reality, are differently useful (Rorty, 1989).

Certainly, "Perversion Is Us? Eight Notes" reveals the contradiction between earnestness and irony in a provisionally resolved form. Its format demonstrates, I find myself hoping, that the only way to help Dr. MH is by cleaving to postmodernist ironies. Here, perhaps, Rorty's (1989) cooler understanding of irony helps: the "opposite of common sense," irony means an awareness that one's language (he calls it "vocabulary") is contingent and fragile, that the terms with which one describes oneself "are subject to change" (p. 74). Call it skepticism: I hope, in other words, that, in telling by showing, I negotiate the Scylla of cynicism and the Charybdis of Babbitry. And, in all earnestness, I do want to report that, as of this writing, shifts are taking place in Dr. MH's treatment, especially in his engagement of the analytic relationship. The analytic third has begun quietly, perhaps provisionally, to enter the work, even as his literal and psychic struggle to get there endures.

Borders. But you never know, be it about a clinical approach or a way of writing or a life. Perhaps what I have been doing to resolve the tension is choosing not to resolve it. And maybe that paradoxical choice is yet another provisional resolution of dualism. Both/and. In contemporary psychoanalysis, the relation between dialectical method and paradox is not so clear. Nor is it any no longer so clear in social life; could it be that there never was going to be, as so many believe and believed, a single, universal solution to economic injustice? For psychoanalysis, at any rate, paradox may be how we currently understand contradiction (Benjamin, 1992), and out of that understanding emerges contingency—possibilities for multiple answers to old questions, varied solutions for varied problems on psychic and social fronts alike.

Why, anyway, should we have to choose? Earnestly recognizing that problems exist and invite solution, we might also keep in mind that solutions come and go. We could ironically reflect that, as poet Norman Fischer said at his installation as co-abbot of San Francisco Zen Center, "There's no end to trouble." Or, with the late Stephen Mitchell (1989), we might borrow Nietzsche's metaphor of the sand-castle you build at the shore—we know that the wave will knock it down, but we build and rebuild it anyway. The triple crossroads of psychoanalysis, feminism, and social theory at which my work plays is only the most recent way of asking time-honored questions about sexuality, intimacy, and power that are nigh universal in the West.

According to the late social theorist Pierre Bourdieu (1977), each culture generates two kinds of question. On one hand, there are the questions that may be asked, those within the "doxa" or orthodox systems of knowledge. On the other, there are the questions that are commonly thought to be unaskable (and therefore not usually asked), those pertaining to "paradoxic" regions of knowledge. In any discipline, work can proceed within the received paradigm, to switch to Thomas Kuhn's (1962) instantly classic, but also unfortunately instantly clichéd, characterization of Western science. Or, struggling to make the paradoxic intelligible, it can break through to the "heterodox" frontier, asking unconventional questions about the paradigm's odds and ends, which themselves furnish the raw material for new knowledge and new paradigms. Owen Lattimore (1951) held that cultural change tends to occur at cultural borders, the regions of Otherness where diverse ways of being, doing, and thinking meet, clash, mix, and change. In my work, I have been journeying toward and along that border and recording how I got there and what I found. Welcome to the border, to the heterodox frontier, where you think the unthinkable, speak the unspeakable, and ask whatever you want.

References

Bakhtin, M. M. (1934–1935), Discourse of the novel. In: *The Dialogic Imagination: Four Essays by M. M. Bakhtin*, ed. M. Holquist (trans. C. Emerson & M. Holquist). Austin: University of Texas Press, 1981, pp. 259–420.

Benjamin, J. (1992), Discussion of Judith Jordan's "The Relational Self: A New Perspective for Understanding Women's Development." *Contemp. Psychother. Rev.*, 7:82–96.

Bourdieu, P. (1977), *Outline of a Theory of Practice*, trans. R. Nice. New York: Cambridge University Press.

Dean, T. (2001). *Beyond Sexuality*. Chicago: University of Chicago Press.

Dimen, M. (2003), *Sexuality, Intimacy, Power*. Hillsdale, NJ: The Analytic Press.

——— (2005), "Sexuality and suffering, or the Eew! Factor," *Studies in Gender and Sexuality* 6:1–8.

Ferenczi, S. (1933), The confusion of tongues between adults and children. *Contemp. Psychoanal.*, 24:196–206, 1988.

Ghent, E. (1989), Credo: The dialectics of one-person and two-person psychologies. *Contemp. Psychoanal.*, 25:169–211.

Greenberg, J. & Mitchell, S. A. (1983), *Object Relations in Psychoanalytic Theory*. Cambridge, MA: Harvard University Press.

Hoffman, I. Z. (1998), *Ritual and Spontaneity in the Psychoanalytic Process: A Dialectical-Constructivist View*. Hillsdale, NJ: The Analytic Press.

Kuhn, T. (1972), *The Structure of Scientific Revolutions*. Chicago: University of Chicago Press.

Lattimore, O. (1951), *Inner Asian Frontiers of China*. Irvington-on-Hudson, NY: Capitol.

Merleau-Ponty, M. (1962), *The Phenomenology of Perception*, trans. C. Smith. New York: Routledge.

Mitchell, S. A. (1986), The wings of Icarus. In: *Relational Psychoanalysis*, ed. S. A. Mitchell & L. Aron. Hillsdale, NJ: The Analytic Press, 1999, pp. 153–179.

Ogden, T. (1994), *Subjects of Analysis*. Northvale, NJ: Aronson.

Rorty, R. (1989), *Contingency, Irony, Solidarity*. New York: Cambridge University Press.

Scheman, N. (1993), *Engenderings*. New York: Routledge.

Race, Self-Disclosure, and "Forbidden Talk": Race and Ethnicity in Contemporary Psychoanalytic Practice

(1997)

Kimberlyn Leary

❦   ❦   ❦   ❦   ❦

Editors' Introduction

Kimberlyn Leary has been at the leading edge of contemporary psychoanalytic work on race and racialized subjectivities for over a decade. Because her work has been concentrated on the understanding and psychodynamic processes with subjects in psychoanalytic work (very marginalized), she is in the unique but not entirely easy position of making theory; working out implications for practice; becoming an interdisciplinary master of studies of race, racism, and racialized identities; and educating her colleagues. In these respects, Leary's work has been conducted under many of the same conditions that feminists 20 years ago and queer theorists 10 years ago faced while making inroads into the hegemonic practices of psychoanalysis. Yet, as Leary would be the first to note, this groundbreaking and necessary work still is being undertaken by a very few practitioners.

Like many relationalists, Leary came from somewhere to find something of use and interest to her. It is perhaps important that this article originally was published in a classically inflected journal but includes a wide range of references across psychoanalytic approaches and social and cultural theories and embeds her work in an intriguing though sparse history of analytic writing on race. Her trajectory of publications shows a very unusual movement from critique to encounter to deconstruction and reconstruction. Like many relationalists, from the beginning, she has worked within a paradigm of theoretical fluidity, drawing on classical roots, social constructionist models, and relational perspectives. Of course, to say that race as an aspect of identity, as an aspect of social formations, and as a cultural phenomenon is a social construction is already to break new ground.

In this article, Leary notes the value of traditional psychoanalytic modes of understanding race and its dynamics through the use of projective mechanisms as a way of understanding racism and stereotyping. But from the outset she argues that race (and she likens this to work on gender) is always personal and political, social and intrapsychic, the province of psychoanalysis and of social theory. Within this essay, turning a psychoanalytic lens on the field itself, she notes that race, arguably the most pressing social problem of the past 200 years, is often a silenced presence in clinical dyads with mixed race and in the writing of the field at large. As analysts, we must appreciate immediately the meanings potentiated in the silences Leary notices. Her clinical vignette shows the careful, difficult work of making voice where silence prevails. The vignette also illuminates the power of voicing hidden fantasies and meaning for many areas of psychic functioning.

Finally, notice in her Afterword that Leary is thinking about writing. Any essay is both a progress report of the writer's thinking and another turn in a conversation that becomes more and more complex and interesting. It is certainly a very relational way to be thinking about writing. And this is a way of thinking also grounded in the particular kind of American pragmatism. Meaning and validity are adjudicated in a process of respectful and engaged conversation, addressed to the past surely but more crucially to the present and to future interlocutors.

Race, Self-Disclosure, and "Forbidden Talk": Race and Ethnicity in Contemporary Psychoanalytic Practice*

▼   ▼   ▼   ▼   ▼

In an interview with uncommon relevance for the present day, Ralph Greenson and Ellis Toney (Greenson, Toney, Lim & Romero, 1982), shared their thoughts about the impact of race on their analytic work. Toney's training analysis—conducted by Greenson from 1948 through 1954—was one of the first interracial analyses to involve a black and white analytic dyad. Greenson reflecting on the analysis commented on his realization that "we lived in two different worlds and we were try-ing to understand each other's. It took an unusual amount of courage on Toney's part and on my part to admit that we were millions of miles apart in certain ways of thinking, values and so forth" (p. 186). Toney, in reply, delineated trust as one of the most difficult areas in black-white relationships: "Blacks, practically every black individual today, has been traumatized, in some way by the white person. If blacks have not been traumatized directly by whites, then through talk and hearsay, they have incorporated experiences that were traumatic" (p. 188). This interview—remarkable for its candor and willingness to consider analytic interac-tions with respect to race (including by having an analyst and analysand engage in open dialogue about their shared work)—stands out as an effort to open up a psychoanalytic discussion on race, culture and the analytic process.

The aim of this paper is to extend psychoanalytic conversation about race and ethnicity further. This paper will discuss the impact of race and culture on psychoanalytic treatment. I will first consider the way in which race and ethnicity—and the social milieu in which they come to have meaning—explicitly and subtly influence the frame of psychoana-lytic work. Through a clinical illustration, I will then present material from an interracial treatment dyad in which interactions around race played a focal role in deepening the clinical process. This will be fol-lowed by a discussion of the psychoanalytic literature on race. I will sug-gest that contemporary psychoanalytic formulations and multicultural perspectives from outside of psychoanalysis can together define a new site for psychoanalytically meaningful conceptualizations of race.

* Originally published in *Psychoanalytic Quarterly*, 66:163–189. © 1997 The Psychoanalytic Quarterly, Inc. Reprinted by permission.

Some forty years after Greenson's analysis of Toney, race remains one of the most pressing problems of contemporary social life in the United States. In recent years, the popular imagination of this country has been captivated by public events in which race figured prominently. Race and racial resentments, never far from center stage, are again at the apex of social consciousness through events like the Clarence Thomas hearings, the acquittal in the police beating of Rodney King and in the open debate over Herrnstein and Murphy's *The Bell Curve* (1994). Nowhere was this more evident than in the aftermath of the O.J. Simpson trial and in the differing reactions of many blacks and whites to the verdict of not guilty. At the instant that many whites recoiled in stunned silence, many African-Americans cheered either because it seemed entirely plausible that Simpson had been framed by a police department long recognized as racist or because Simpson—guilty or innocent—was one of few black men in history who could marshal the resources necessary to use the legal system to his full advantage, making his success an ironic affirmation of social progress.

If nothing else, these reactions to the Simpson verdict confirm a post-modern social reality: In significant ways, most blacks and whites construct and are constructed by vastly different social worlds. At the same time, when these multiple realities interpenetrate, the result is far from the postmodern ideal of the co-existence of contradictory points-of-view. Dialogue about race in this country is instead tense and constrained. The clash of opposing realities often generates violence of one kind or another. As examples, just as whites feared blacks rioting in Los Angeles following the Rodney King verdict, many African-Americans expect that whites will exact their revenge for Simpson in the legislature and court room by further undermining affirmative action and other social programs.

At the *fin de siècle*, we remain a country that is obsessed with the problem of race and its multiple realities even as we are often paralyzed with respect to how we may respond effectively to them. As one columnist recently put it, "nothing is more important in America than what blacks and whites do in the name of race, to themselves or each other" (Rosenthal, 1995). In this respect, we have moved from the notion of a melting pot to the recognition that the pot is boiling over. How then does the racial divide of our culture affect the culture of the consulting room?

When I open the door to the waiting room to greet a new patient, that I am obviously a person of color constitutes an implicit and important self-disclosure. While one might argue that any of the particularities of us as people (e.g. age, gender or the way that we furnish our offices) also represent disclosures, I believe that they are of a different order in the climate of the present racial divide. At the present moment in time, racial similarity or difference in the consulting room immediately implicates us into a cultural conversation and one about which it is difficult to talk openly.

When I work with patients of color, most directly reference our shared racial background and/or shared status as members of minority groups. Many have elected to see me because I am a person of color. By contrast, most of the white patients I have worked with do not explicitly mention our racial difference though their metaphors, allusions and other derivatives suggest to me that it is very much on their minds (e.g. a patient in consultation who repeatedly states his "ability to get along with everybody—I mean everybody" when ostensibly this is not a part of the difficulties he trying to communicate to me).

With most patients, if racial similarity or, more typically, racial difference is not mentioned at some point during an evaluation or during the first month of a treatment, I typically comment on the fact that the patient hasn't mentioned it directly. I might, for example, acknowledge the social climate surrounding open talk about race in this country and then wonder with the patient as to whether thoughts about, for example, his ability to get along with all people has been his way of speaking about something he did not feel he could approach more directly. In this way, I am offering the patient an opportunity to consider the expanded possibilities for communication offered in treatment.

At the same time, I am also responding to the social milieu in which we practice: In contemporary America, race carries profound meaning. While it is undoubtedly true that my observation that the patient has avoided mention of our racial difference selectively focuses attention on only one aspect of the interactive field, it seems to me that clinical silence about race is equally directive. Failing to acknowledge racial difference is not neutral. We might consider what is conveyed when the clinician does not speak to, for example, her blackness or when his whiteness is assumed to speak for itself. Clinical silence about race may be perceived—and with some justification—as a commentary on the analyst's effort to stay out of the fray and opt out of the tension that comes with open talk about race. Ambiguity of this sort can close off the clinical encounter in ways that are at odds from what we ideally wish to offer our patients. Most of the time, opening a discussion about race by pointing out that neither the patient nor I have yet talked about the fact that she is white (or Japanese, or Latina, etc.) and I am African-American, does not prevent exploration of the patient's racial meanings or obviate fantasy. If anything, it facilities the admission of fantasy to the treatment relationship and sets a tone for the exploration to follow (cf. Greenberg, 1995) as that which was excluded from conversation is invited to assume a voice in the consulting room. If the invitation can not be accepted, understanding the reasons for this over time defines an equally important analytic exploration.

When previously unmentioned racial difference is acknowledged, my experience has been that white patients respond nearly universally by saying the difference is "not a problem," although this is usually then followed by a statement of exactly the problem the patient expects will complicate the treatment, namely the fear of saying something that would be perceived as racist or discriminatory. Holmes (1992) has commented on the regularly occurring fear for the patient in a cross-race treatment dyad that s/he will express aggressive urges in racist attitudes and the equally familiar wish that race will not come up in the patient's associations or if it does, that it will not be interpreted. Simpson (1993) suggests that therapists also fear that their counter-transference will be coded in racial terms. He further notes that it is "strange that those of us who are prepared to accept our murderous wishes, for example, towards members of our families cannot, or will not, accept that we might have 'racist' thoughts or feelings" (p. 291).

It seems inevitable that all of us—patients and analysts—will have racial thoughts and feelings that are libidinally and aggressively tinged. Just as the analyst may become aware of the patient's explicit and subtle immersion in cultural and personally idiosyncratic dialogues about race, it is also quite likely that the patient will, in time, catch the analyst in some unintended racial reflections of his or her own. Speaking to the patient's concerns about racist content and the sociocultural realities of race can become a way of understanding the patient's relationship to his/her own mind, including the patient's relationship to ideas, feelings and behaviors that evoke anxiety and vulnerability. I believe that a parallel process occurs with respect to the analyst's racial countertransference. In the case material which follows, I will describe how clinical interactions concerning race facilitated a patient's ability to articulate her own internal experience and deepen her involvement in a treatment process.

Clinical Illustration

Mrs. C. was a 30-year-old, white woman who entered treatment in an effort to cope with the divided loyalties she felt between progressing in her career and staying at home to raise her two young sons. She felt trapped by either option—critical of women who "abandoned" their children to daycare to fulfill their personal ambitions and unhappy with the prospect of being a "fifties housewife with no brain" dependent on her husband for financial security. At the same time, Mrs. C. wanted very much to be a good mother and worried that she was not. She felt continually angry with her husband whom she believed was free of comparable soul searching and was extremely critical of him in ways that dismayed both of them.

Mrs. C. spoke of her uncertainty about what she really wanted for herself and felt guilty that she was in the privileged position of even being able to make such a choice. She expected that whatever option she chose would expose her to punitive self-criticism and scrutiny from others. In sessions, Mrs. C. responded to me a kind of wary friendliness although it often seemed to me that she was also braced for our interactions to deteriorate into animosity. In an earlier phase of the work, we had talked about aspects of her history which seemed to relate to this problem, including Mrs. C.'s "adolescent rebellion" which had lasted well into her twenties and resulted in frequent clashes between Mrs. C. and her mother. Mother and daughter argued violently for years until a rapprochement before Mrs. C.'s marriage, purchased in part via the patient's defensive idealization of her mother.

Early in the treatment, Mrs. C. acknowledged that upon our first meeting she had been surprised to learn that I was black. The thought that she might be referred to a clinician who was a person of color had simply not occurred to her though she was quick to reassure us that she didn't expect "a problem." At the same time, Mrs. C. worried openly that she might say something that would be problematic, imagining that she might unthinkingly say something that would prove offensive to me or otherwise strain our ability to develop a relationship. This same concern was echoed in her relationship to non-racial material as well: Though she wished to speak freely, Mrs. C. felt worried about what her treatment would reveal about her and feared exposure.

During one session, Mrs. C. greeted me in the waiting room by noticing that I was wearing an engagement ring. As she walked into the office, she asked excitedly: "Is that an engagement ring?" Settling into the hour, she pressed further, repeating her question and appeared crestfallen when instead of answering, I asked for her thoughts. She reasoned that while it certainly *looked* like an engagement ring, she couldn't be sure. Perhaps the ring was for some other purpose. She obliged with a series of associations, offered in a lackluster manner. My efforts to wonder with Mrs. C. as to what interfered with her efforts to decide that the ring was an engagement ring did not meet with success.

When I thought about this session, I realized that Mrs. C. and I had engaged in something of a ritualized encounter. On the surface, each of us was doing as we were supposed to but nothing had happened. I was aware that Mrs. C.'s question about my engagement ring was a request that we interact more personally. Although I had in effect introduced my personal life into the session by wearing the ring in the first place, I believe that my retreat into stereotyped technique constituted my reluctance to engage with my patient more fully.

In the next hour, I acknowledged that I had not answered Mrs. C.'s question and told her that my ring was indeed an engagement ring. Mrs. C. became animated. She had been sure that it was an engagement ring but wasn't sure why she needed me to tell her so. This time, however, her associations about my engagement were more productive and included expression of her ambivalence about marriage and motherhood, including a joke about what I was getting myself into. Interspersed in her associations were thoughts about a recent news program in which blacks and whites discussed racial problems in some of the city's neighborhoods. Although I did not understand this particular shift at this particular time, responses of this sort were also typical for Mrs. C.: she talked often about political and community affairs. Mrs. C. had noticed that since beginning treatment with me, her interest in stories that concerned blacks and whites had increased.

Over the next several weeks, this same sequence was repeated: Mrs. C. would raise a question about a piece of information which she in fact already knew about me and present it for my confirmation. When I did so, her thoughts would soon encompass some piece of racial content—usually a reflection of some event from the media or with some reference to the fact that she was white and I black—not connected with the previous content in any way that I could discern.

After I became aware of this sequence, I noted it with Mrs. C. and we pieced together the following understanding: From her perspective, we were engaging in forbidden talk. She said that although she liked the idea that I answered her questions, from what she understood about therapy she believed that I was violating the rules by directly responding. Both of us were doing something we shouldn't. I wondered if that was the reason why her questions and my answers were followed by her talking about black issues or black-white problems. I said I thought that her thoughts about blacks and whites felt like a risky thing to discuss, especially as a topic between us. Mrs. C. agreed that this was not often done: Though she had known and worked with African-Americans, she had had few intimate contacts with blacks and in those they had not talked about racial issues with each other though she had wanted this. When reading the newspaper or watching television news, Mrs. C. felt worried about the state of racial relations in the United States. She was concerned about crime in urban areas (that were usually black) and troubled by how little contact she had with blacks (apart from me) and how little personal involvement blacks had with whites. At the same time, she felt that people needed to be "careful" around this topic because something problematic could emerge (e.g. something racist) and the situation would only get worse.

Mrs. C. and I discussed—in general terms at first—the sensitivities that blacks and whites have with respect to each other: Whites fear being labeled racist and blacks fear present and future mistreatment based on past history. Mrs. C. mentioned the likely possibility that were I or another black person to drive through her neighborhood, we would be assumed to be enroute to work rather than to our residence. Similarly, she wondered how welcome she would be in my (black) community.

As this interaction shows, my willingness to answer my patient's questions established a tacit negotiation: To the extent that I engaged in talk she considered to be forbidden (confirming her questions), she would too (by virtue of mentioning racial issues). Mrs. C., however, seemed to express her thoughts more freely following this discussion—talking with more feeling about the problems of her adolescence and the strife with her mother. She was attentive to the similarities and differences between us as women. She could, for example, now acknowledge feeling competitive with me (over my career), superior (because she had a new baby son) and was, to a limited extent, also able to express feelings of disappointment with me (because I had neither child rearing advice nor a prescription for the cessation of her conflicts). At the same time, her approach to me also remained somewhat idealized and her talk in the sessions, sanitized and polite.

My willingness to answer questions for which she already knew the answer prompted Mrs. C. to raise the stakes as she floated more involved questions. These questions were more personal and now concerned some aspect of me as an African-American woman (e.g. What were my plans on the upcoming Martin Luther King Day holiday? What kind of [racial] setting had I grown up in? Was my husband black?). I answered whatever she asked and as directly as I could although sometimes a given question remained between us for several sessions. The result usually involved a lessening of her constraint and an increase in her ability to be affectively expressive. I did not experience Mrs. C.'s questions as superficial or mainly voyeuristic. She confined many other of her thoughts about me (e.g. more specific curiosities about my sexual life) to her associations alone and did not ask questions of me about them. It was my impression—shared with the patient—that she was trying to get a fix on me as an African-American woman against whom she could reference herself. Her questions seemed designed to assess my racial self in terms of my difference and similarity to her.

Our interactions around the questions were also important. Mrs. C.'s caution and care was paralleled by my own. Mrs. C.'s relief with respect to my responsiveness to her questions alternated with ambivalence. On my side, I felt as if my answers were a kind of talking out of school, and as someone at the start of my career, I felt some concern about what colleagues would think were they to hear of my interactions with this patient. Mrs. C. and I talked together about this discomfort and several times assessed whether talking in this way was helpful to her. On this point, she was unequivocal, saying, "It makes me feel like we're both here." Admitting my racial self into the consulting room in a way that could not fail to implicate me personally seemed to permit Mrs. C. to grapple with hers and to expand what she could convey about herself.

As a typical example, now rather than only note a racial content in a film or news story, Mrs. C. began to describe her reactions in greater detail, aware that her attention reflected her interest in me and what went on in my mind. Mrs. C. spent the better part of another session captivated by the film *Pulp Fiction*, especially the relationship between the characters played by Samuel L. Jackson and John Travolta—both of whom enjoyed a casual relationship with one another even as they were involved in a considerable amount of violence. She thought that the characters—a black and white pair—spent their time together each getting into the other's head. This reminded her of some of the experiences she'd had with me. I also understood it as a commentary on her view of the interactive relationship between us, making us outlaws and outside of usual conventions.

Mrs. C. was disturbed (and fascinated) by the racial epithets used in the film by both blacks and whites. In her discussion, she hesitated to use the word "nigger"—the term used in the film—in her discussion and talked about the fact that while blacks could use this term between them with impunity, whites could not. When I pointed out that whites certainly had in the film, Mrs. C. wondered what blacks really thought about whites. I pointed out that this of course also raised the issue of what whites really thought about blacks as well. This became elaborated in more personal terms—and is still in play in treatment—as to what I as a black thought about her as a white and what she as a white thought about me as a black.

Mrs. C. became preoccupied for a time with thoughts about racialized violence—between blacks and whites as well as black-on-black crime. Consciously, she recognized she could also think about white-on-white violence as well but this "didn't mean anything" to her. In this way, Mrs. C. talked about the way in which her own racial identity as a Euro-American mainly acquired its meaning to her in relationship to someone of color. Talking about violence in black communities, she puzzled about how people "in the same group and the same community" could do this to each other. Her associations led her to discuss unacceptable impulses in herself, relating to the trouble she was having as a mother to her young sons. The struggles between Mrs. C. and her boys reminded her of her adolescent rebellion with her mother. Mrs. C. actively feared that her children were deliberately provoking her as she had her mother. She was frightened of her angry response, which was more extreme than she had previously been able to disclose, and she felt much less in control than she had been able to let on. Until this point, Mrs. C. had been struggling with her feelings of rage painfully, guiltily and alone.

It is clear that Mrs. C.'s selective focus on violence in African-American communities (a selectivity echoed in our culture at large) was a means to contend with aggressive impulses from which she struggled to distance herself. On later occasions, Mrs. C.'s racial reflections had a more libidinal cast and included expression of longings previously warded off. Her associations about black cultural life included envy of the familiarity and close connections she observed between many blacks. By virtue of my blackness I could belong and have access to an involvement from which she felt excluded. Reading an article on black feminism in the aftermath of the O.J. Simpson trial, Mrs. C. became interested in the question of whether African-American women would side with Simpson because he is black or withhold support because of his history of domestic violence. Were African-American women more committed to racial solidarity than their connections to other women? This echoed concerns Mrs. C. had in her relationship with me.

Expecting the article to confirm her ideas about race (namely that commitments to race superseded all else), Mrs. C. was surprised to read that younger African-American women, in particular, self-consciously differed from their mothers in permitting themselves more latitude, especially to find connections in their relationships with other women important. She also responded with some excitement to a phrase in the article which indicated that some younger African-American women declared that being black did not mitigate their attachments to whites ("some of whom we love"). Now Mrs. C. felt that there might be room for her in my world. That this might also include an erotic bond was ushered in through her articulation of the fantasy that I was biracial, a product of a sexual tie between black and white.

It remains my sense that the talk about race and racial difference between Mrs. C. and myself—once a forbidden topic—ushered in her ability to approach other materials that felt risky to her. This new material about her present life and history could then be admitted to the session for our joint consideration although it remained under the rubric of "forbidden talk" for some time.

Race, Ethnicity, and Culture in Psychoanalytic Treatment

As Goldstein (1994) notes, self-disclosures can take many forms: Disclosing information requested by the patient (e.g. Epstein, 1995); of the countertransference (Ehrenberg, 1995); the analyst's own difficulties in the analysis (cf. Miletec, 1996) as well as the analyst's difficulties in his/her own life (Abend, 1995; Dewald, 1982) all of which may require the patient to accommodate to the analyst's subjectivity. Similarly, analysts write that while they disclose for a variety of intended and unintended purposes, the motivation is often either to create room in the treatment space or repair a breach. In this way, the therapist's interactive availability and presence constitute the building materials and mortar of dyadic transactions. In the same way that two houses can have a different design and layout and so require different plans for effective maintenance, clinical work requires the flexibility of employing different tools at different times.

This clinical illustration concerned two types of disclosure: An implicit self-disclosure occasioned by the therapist being a person of color and a series of explicit answers in response to questions asked by the patient about the therapist's racialized experience. The therapist confirmed a reality (that the ring she was wearing was indeed an engagement ring) following a mild rupture occasioned by the therapist's use of stereotyped technique and a rebuff of the patient's interest in a more personal response. Thereafter, however, disclosures were employed in the context of clinical interactions directed at assisting the patient to say what was on her mind (Kris, 1990). My initial willingness to answer questions about information already known to the patient did occasion her desire to know more and led the patient to formulate a more specific and personal inquiry of my life circumstances and attitudes. The patient did not, in my view, become "insatiable" (cf. Freud, 1912) though her involvement in her treatment did deepen. As was evident here, patients' and analysts' talk about race can enliven a psychoanalytic dialogue. In some treatments, in fact, the talk about race may be the only way to enter into a psychoanalytic encounter so great are the social challenges of race in contemporary society.

Psychoanalytic clinicians have convincingly argued that clinical attention be directed at racial issues and racial stereotypes, especially where they overlap with conflicted affects and desires in the transference (cf.

Holmes, 1992; Schacter & Butts, 1968). Race and ethnicity are understood to be the context for expression of the patient's personal psychology and deployed to serve psychodynamically relevant agendas. Holmes (1992) offers one example of this approach, describing how her patient's attack of the analyst's race and gender as inferior served the protective function of warding off recognition of the patient's own feelings of self-loathing and rage. In this way, race comes to be treated as a psychoanalytic matter.

Although clinically valuable, this perspective may have the unintended consequence of obscuring the way in which race is both a psychoanalytic and a cultural experience. Talk about race becomes a vehicle for a psychoanalytic conversation and recedes as a matter of importance in and of itself. There is a tendency for race to become something to get past rather than something to live within. Race becomes something that is only "skin deep," rather than an intimate and enduring aspect of personal social identity. As a further illustration of this point, while psychoanalytic gender theory has a richly complicated and contested theory of gender and sexual identity, we have no comparable body of psychoanalytic work with respect to racial and cultural identity.

Even when race and ethnicity are considered more broadly they are also often treated as qualities that pertain only to patients or analysts of color. There is little in our literature, for instance, about the meaning that a shared racial background has in an analysis when both members of the analytic dyad are white. Frankenberg (1993) suggests that whiteness is an unnoticed aspect of identity for most Americans. In recognition of this, Chodorow (1995) notes that her work with Euro-American women has not typically "problematized their whiteness and its contribution to their sense of gender and sexuality" (footnote, p. 526).[1]

From its inception, psychoanalysis has had an ambivalent stake in racial discourse. Freud's recurring effort to forestall psychoanalysis from becoming "a Jewish science" (Blanton, 1971) is a potent reminder that anti-semitism was the definitive racial discourse in Europe in his day.

---

[1] Implicating whiteness into Euro-American identity is itself a problematic cultural affair. Berke Breathed, the creator of the comic strip "Bloom County," offers us one perspective on the difficulty in a piece he published in the late 1980s: Oliver, an African-American youngster, walks into the local drugstore to secure a copy of *Ebony* magazine. When the clerk asks him what *Ebony* is about, Oliver tells him "black persons, written for black persons, with exclusively black persons in the ads" then cheerfully purchases the latest issue. Moments later, Binkley, a white youngster, enters the same store inquiring about *Ivory* magazine whereupon the clerk anxiously shoos him out, saying "I run a progressive newsstand here."

Gilman (1992) writes that the last *fin de siècle*, Jews and perverts were almost interchangeable categories. Just as skin color functions as one of the most visible markers of difference in our time, racial difference in Freud's was also inscribed on the body through the male Jew's circumcision (Gilman, 1992). Even in this country, as few as thirty years ago, the legacy of anti-semitism differentiated those who were white from those who were Jewish. The long time psychoanalytic emphasis on the alienated other within has also been read by some as an echo of the fact that psychoanalysis was born in a culture hostile to the race of its creator and many of its practitioners (Hatcher, 1995; Bloom, 1991).

In a great many ways, psychoanalysis has maintained a contradictory relationship to culture even as contemporary re-readings of psychoanalytic thinking emphasize that the psychoanalytic theories of mind, development, and dysfunction are almost entirely the product of culture. Our psychoanalytic models are based nearly exclusively on the protections and pathologies afforded by the Western nuclear family, itself a cultural entity. In this way, psychoanalysis is cut from the very fabric of culture, albeit a very selective cloth. Although psychoanalysis resonates in this way with the Western culture in which it is chiefly practiced, for much of its history it has also considered itself to stand outside to offer a universal scientific rendering of human experience. With increasing recognition that science is itself a culture (cf. Keller, 1992; Mayer, 1996), psychoanalysis has begun its project of the next century of re-inventing itself as a contemporary discourse.

In a recent paper, Elliott and Spezzano (1996) argue that psychoanalysis is no more impervious to its cultural surround than was modern thought to the imprimatur of psychoanalysis. As a number of recent theorists have noted (e.g. Mitchell, 1993), during the last fifteen years, cultural shifts in how human beings understand themselves and the very nature of reality have occasioned major changes in the clinical theory of psychoanalysis. The technical emphasis on the analyst's anonymity and abstinence share the stage with models attending to the facilitative utility of the analyst's presence, self-disclosure and therapeutic provision (e.g. Bader, 1995; Lindon, 1994; Renik, 1994). Postmodern critiques are now increasingly imported into contemporary psychoanalytic practices

---

¹ *(cont'd)* For many Americans, the notion of white identity is synonymous with the idea of white supremicism. The hidden narrative is that whiteness can only mean one thing—a self-conscious violently-inclined superiority—that must be kept under wraps. Ironically, this hidden idea remains protected when whiteness is not assumed be a meaningful marker of identity for Euro-Americans and is not deconstructed psychoanalytically or culturally.

(e.g., Barratt, 1993) though these are not without their pitfalls (cf. Dunn, 1995; Leary, 1994; Glass, 1993).

At the same time, as Elliott and Spezzano indicate, it is also clear that psychoanalysis contributes to and is moved by cultural change of all kinds. Renik (1990) suggests, for example, that the oedipal constellation—sexual rivalry in the context of love—is an important psychic organizer because of the prevalence of nuclear families and the way that relationships are structured within them. He goes on to note that "future social changes may alter the shape of normative psychosexual development" (p. 201). It seems likely, for example, that ongoing revisions to the psychoanalytic theories of development and mind will be required as psychoanalysis takes seriously the extended family structure of African-, Hispanic- and Asian-Americans, families headed by gay partners as well as the new reproductive technologies currently reshaping the contemporary definition of "family."

Contemporary Psychoanalytic Practice and Multicultural Perspectives

There is now agreement across psychoanalytic models that psychoanalysis occupies an interactive landscape (cf. Mitchell, 1995). Critiques of the analyst's authoritative rendering of the analysand's subjectivity have given way to attention to the psychology of the analyst at work. Neither surgeon nor a technical instrument, the analyst is assumed to be a quite real counterforce in the treatment with a subjectivity of his/her own. As a result, psychoanalytic treatment has been increasingly recast as involving negotiated (e.g. Goldberg, 1987; Pizer, 1992; Hatcher, 1993) and intersubjective processes (e.g. Stolorow & Atwood, 1992).

The cultural landscape with respect to race and ethnicity has also shifted—a fact that is not yet represented in the psychoanalytic literature on race. Although race is treated as a carrier of cultural meaning which can be employed to serve any number of transference or defensive purposes, race usually carries only a limited number of cultural meanings. In the analytic literature, it most often symbolizes devalued, repudiated or pathological contents. As an example, Myers (1977) writes that in the black patients with whom he has worked most extensively ". . . many problems of early ego development as well as early and later conflicts in the psychosexual sphere, have been unconsciously organized in accord with meanings ascribed by the contrasting colors black and white." As a result, what is usually under discussion in most psychoanalytic writing is less about race per se than it is about racism and racial status. In consequence, much of the existing psychoanalytic literature is better appreciated for illustrating the psychodynamics of racism rather than offering a commentary on race or cultural identity.[2]

By contrast, new models of ethno-centric identity and psychotherapy (e.g. Greene & Comas-Diaz, 1994), emphasize that race may have a greater array of meanings culturally and psychologically than those occasioned by racism. Consider the following examples: Despite discriminatory practices, the United States is also home to a stable African-American middle and professional class whose considerable earning power has not gone unnoticed, as evidenced by advertising campaigns focused at people of color. Although at least four African-Americans have considered or attempted to run for the US presidency, there was widespread speculation that Colin Powell might have been able to win. Furthermore, "identity politics" (cf. Sampson, 1993) offers an another choice for the cultural life of people of color by endorsing, for example, an Afro-centric cultural ideal of racial solidarity which can include an affirmative separatism. Whether or not one agrees with these approaches, they do now represent alternatives to the devalued representations of people of color implicit in stereotypes. Race can and does mean more, at least to some people, than a devalued content. As such, we would expect that these new cultural meanings have their own agendas even as they also enter the psychoanalytic consulting room to be used to serve psychodynamically relevant agendas as well . In order to do so, this expanded array of racial meanings must also become recognizable to psychoanalysts so as to enter into the psychoanalytic lexicon.

Culturally sensitive treatment perspectives, including an emerging model of culturally sensitive psychoanalysis (e.g. Akhtar, 1995), begin with the assumption that culture plays a significant role in the development and maintenance of the self. Comas-Diaz & Greene (1994) also

---

[2] Psychoanalysis does offer several useful models with which to articulate the psychic reality of racism. The racially different other becomes a container for projected wishes that the majority repudiates in themselves. Other theorists concerned with the narcissistic dimension of human experience suggest that racism is a response to the pain attending difference: To notice distinction is to become cognizant that another mind, person or group possesses something that one does not. In consequence, the racially different other disturbs the sense of self-sufficiency and so evokes desire (Young-Bruehl, 1992). In either case, the group in power makes the other the repository of concerns that reflect their own preoccupations and effects a false sense of containing their disturbance by marginalizing the other. This becomes one means by which individual and group dynamics become translated into social policy with the result that psychic and social life become intertwined (cf. Kaplan, 1993).

note that people in majority and minority cultures in the United States also have multiple sources of identity which clash, leading to interpersonal and intrapsychic conflict. Employing the construct of projective identification as articulated by Burke and Tansey (1985), Comas-Diaz & Jacobsen (1987) has, for example, suggested that patients attribute ethnocultural characteristics to their therapists that relate to conflicts in their own ethnocultural identities.

While most models of culturally specific treatment recognize that the racial self is multiply determined, they also argue that the current and historical social climate of the United States means that racism remains a powerful and significant commonality for people of color (e.g. Greene, 1993) even as the terms in which racism is expressed may have been revised. While de facto exclusion and marginalization is apparent and widespread particularly in our urban cities, contemporary racism also shows itself in institutional practices, "glass ceilings" and environmental attitudes. Furthermore, while this form of racism is maddeningly evident to people of color and experienced as an inescapable aspect of American social life (Smith, 1993), it is often unacknowledged and dismissed by many in the majority culture.

From this perspective, while race is a social construction and specific racial meanings are socially determined, the fact of a racialized body also puts constraints on the psychological experience of African-Americans. For this reason, Comas-Diaz and Minrath (1985) have suggested that therapeutic work in an interethnic/racial patient/therapist dyad can only progress if both the manifest and the symbolic meanings of race and ethnicity are carefully worked through and *if* the reality of societal discrimination is acknowledged (including the possibility that discrimination exists in ways that the therapist can not herself yet apprehend).

Cultural change as well as changes in contemporary psychoanalytic practice and the emergence of alternative formulations of race in treatment models largely outside of psychoanalysis suggest the need to define a new site for psychoanalytically useful conceptualizations of race. In the first instance, race functions as a kind of positivistic fact. It is undoubtedly real and references real world history. In the second, it operates within the realm of postmodern possibility. Particular racial meanings represent social constructions that are elastic and shaped in accord with specific prerogatives, personally (as was the case for Mrs. C.) and culturally (as evidenced by enduring stereotypes).

I believe that a psychoanalytically meaningful approach to race for contemporary practice is situated in the conceptual space in between these perspectives. Race, in this sense, can not be taken-for-granted as a material entity and does not speak for itself. Neither is it only a socially-constructed harbinger of multiple re-readings. At the level of the culture and, more importantly, at the level of the individual it exists in the tension in between. A psychoanalytically productive conceptualization of race is as a result dynamic and context dependent even as race remains something that is "really real" (cf. Greene, 1993).[3] As a result, the conceptual and clinical space in which racial experience may be apprehended is fragile. It inheres in creative tension rather than settling for one perspective or another alone.

The approach to race that I am developing has much in common with Chodorow's (1995) recent theorizing with respect to gender. She argues that while psychoanalysts need to recognize the inextricable cultural and linguistic contributions to psychological gender experience, gender is also "not entirely culturally or politically constructed" (p. 517). Gender, she argues, is given psychic life via a universal process of subjectivity, namely the human capacity to endow experience with nonverbal emotion and unconscious fantasy meanings. This shared quality of subjectivity, however, does not give rise to universal or stable contents. Gender is psychologically personal and particular to the individual. Like race, gender is worn and lived similarly *and* differently by each of us. The analysis of gendered experience in analysis is a "product of interaction between therapist and patient as they work to create a consensual account of what is initially (and throughout) emotional, partially unconscious [and] fragmentary" (Chodorow, 1995, p. 525). Though Chodorow does not herself put it in these terms, her formulations suggest that gender flourishes in the tension between universal and unique experience.

Issues of race are sensitive in our multi-cultural, multi-ethnic and multi-racial society, just as sexuality was in Freud's day and continues to be in our own. As recent events like the Simpson verdict show it is usually difficult to discuss the unspoken beliefs, assumptions and textures of our different world views. It is clear that we as a country have considerable difficulty negotiating the racial divide. I'm not sure that we fare that much better in the consulting room.

To the extent that one endorses the view that race exists in the tension between lived actualities and constructed possibilities, the psychoanalytic clinician requires a clinical stance that admits both poles of the tension into the treatment encounter. Revisions to the clinical theory of psychoanalysis may offer one means to meet this challenge. Contem-

---

[3] Kaplan (1993) articulates a similar position: "Race and gender are constructs that produce material effects, material oppressions, even as one battles against such constructions and argues that they *are* alterable" (p. 510).

porary clinical theory now recognizes that features of the analyst's self are always at play, influencing the treatment interaction. This has led to a new interest in how the analyst may best make use of herself in order to further the goals of the treatment, namely the patient's capacity to better understand his or her own psychological experience.

Renik (1995) has offered a cogent critique of the notion of the anonymous analyst, noting that the principle of anonymity, rather than clearing the field, instead promotes active idealization of the analyst by assuming that if the analyst's ideas were known, the patient would no longer be in a position to think for him or herself. He offers the technical prescription that the analyst articulate everything that in the analyst's view will help the patient to understand where the analyst is coming from and where he wants to go with the patient. This may, as Renik notes, require the analyst to depart from his or her preferred ways of proceeding and bear a measure of discomfort just as the patient is asked to do. The analyst's understanding is also always open to a counter-critique by the patient.[4] As in the preceding discussion of race and gender, disclosures may be said to acquire their meaning in the tension ensuing between the principles by which the analyst is guided in offering them (Renik, 1995) and by their treatment effects as evaluated by both patients and analysts.

I believe the interactive process between Mrs. C. and myself facilitated the clinical work because of the particular way in which race was discussed. Race and racial difference were sustained within a dynamic tension: Mrs. C. and I worked within a context in which race was treated as a lived actuality and a sociocultural fact even as it was also available for the patient's idiosyncratic scripting of it to serve dynamic agendas. In this case, the shared acknowledgment and open dialogue about the difficulty of speaking openly about race actualized a sociocultural reality and was real life between us. My disclosures and the resultant open discussion about race and racial difference permitted the patient to access the reality of me as a racialized subject. This in turn permitted race and racial difference to exist between Mrs. C. and myself

---

[4] It is also the case that once the analyst discloses something to the patient, or analyst and patient highlight an implicit disclosure as being important, its status changes in the clinical encounter. Simply put, it becomes "for real." It can not be retrieved or "taken back" even as analyst and patient may agree or disagree about the meaning of what was conveyed. Furthermore, as Greenberg (1995) notes "if it is true that everything we do reveals something, it is equally true that everything we do conceals something else" (p. 195). Disclosures alone do not resolve the problem of the analyst's anonymity.

as something that implicated each of us personally, enabling the racial divide to also become a bridge to more meaningful clinical process (Margolis, 1996). Although this occurred in the context of a tacit negotiation that emerged as an enactment—engaging in forbidden talk—it also allowed the patient to enter more fully into her own subjectivity, including the ability to allow previously warded off material into her therapy.

It is clear that race and ethnicity exist as a potent force in the social milieu in which psychoanalysis and psychoanalytic psychotherapy are situated. It makes sense to assume that it operates as a powerful and pervasive influence on the treatment process in ways that clinical psychoanalysis has not been in a position to appreciate before. Increasing attention to cultural issues at large is drawing attention to the culture of the consulting room. This, in turn, may point to the utility of critiquing not only the anonymous analyst, but the racially anonymous one as well.

References

Abend, S. (1995), Discussion of Jay Greenberg's paper on self-disclosure. *Contemp. Psychoanal.*, 31 (2), 207–211.

Akhtar, S. (1995), Paper presented at the University of Michigan, unpublished.

Bader, M. (1995), Authenticity and the psychology of choice in the analyst. *Psychoanal. Q.*, 64 (2), 282–305.

Barratt, B. (1993), *Psychoanalysis and the postmodern impulse: Knowing and being since Freud's psychology.* Baltimore: Johns Hopkins Press.

Blanton, S. (1971), *Diary of my analysis with Sigmund Freud.* New York: Hawthorn Books.

Bloom, H. (1991), Freud: Frontier concepts, Jewishness and interpretation. *American Imago*, 1, 135–152.

Burke, W. & Tansey, M. (1983), Projective identification and countertransference turmoil: Disruptions in the empathic process. *Contemp. Psychoanal.*, 21 (3), 372–402.

Chodorow, N. (1995), Gender as a personal and cultural construction. *Signs*, 20 (31), 516–544.

Comas-Diaz, L. & Greene, B. (1994), Overview: Gender and ethnicity in the healing process. In B. Greene & L. Comas-Diaz (Eds.). *Women of color.* New York: Guilford.

Comas-Diaz, L. & Jacobsen, F. (1987), Ethnocultural identification in psychotherapy. *Psychiatry*, 50 (3), 232–241.

Comas-Diaz, L. & Minrath, M. (1985), Psychotherapy with ethnic minority borderline clients. *Psychotherapy*, 22 (supplement), 418–426.

Dewald, P. (1982), Serious illness in the analyst: Transference, counter-transference and reality responses. *J. Amer. Psychoanal. Assn.*, 30, 347–364.

Dunn, J. (1995), Intersubjectivity in psychoanalysis: A critical review. *Int. J. Psychoanal.*, 76, 723–738.

Ehrenberg, D. (1995), Self-disclosure: Therapeutic tool or indulgence? *Contem. Psychoanal.*, 31 (2), 213–228.

Ehrenberg, D. (1993), *The intimate edge.* New York: W.W. Norton.

Elliott, A. & Spezzano, C. (1996), Psychoanalysis at its limits: Navigating the post-modern turn. *Psychoanal. Q.*, in press.

Epstein, L. (1995), Self-disclosure and analytic space. *Contem. Psychoanal.*, 31 (2), 229–236.

Frankenberg, R.(1993), *White women, race matters: The social construction of whiteness.* Minneapolis: University of Minnesota Press.

Freud, S. (1912), Recommendations to physicians practicing psychoanalysis. *SE*, 12.

Gilman, S. (1992), Freud, race and gender. *American Imago*, 49 (2), 155–183.

Glass, J. (1993), *Shattered selves: Multiple personality in a postmodern world.* Ithaca, NY: Cornell University Press.

Goldberg, A. (1988), Psychoanalysis and negotiation. *Psychoanal. Q.*, 56, 109–129.

Goldstein, E. (1994), Self-disclosure in treatment: What therapists do and don't talk about. *Clinical Social Work Journal*, 22 (4), 417–433.

Greene, B. (1994), African-American women. In L. Comas-Diaz & B. Greene (Eds.) *Women of color.* New York: Guilford.

Greene, B. (1993), Psychotherapy with African-American Women: Integrating feminist and psychodynamic models. *Journal of Training and Practice in Professional Practice*, 7 (1), 49–66.

Greene, B. & Comas-Diaz, L. (1994), *Women of color.* New York: Guilford.

Greenberg, J. (1995), Self-disclosure: Is it psychoanalytic? *Contem. Psychoanal.*, 31 (2), 193–205.

Greenson, R., Toney, E., Lim, P. & Romero, A. (1982), Transference and counter-interracial psychotherapy. In B. Bass, G. Wyatt & G. Powell (Eds.), *The Afro-American family: Assessment, treatment and research issues.* New York: Grune & Stratton, 183–203.

Hatcher, R. (1995), Personal communication.

Hatcher, R. (1992), Negotiation between the patient and the therapist in the psychotherapy hour. Paper presented at the spring meeting of the American Psychological Association's Division 39, Philadelphia, PA.

Herrnstein, R. & Murphy, C. (1994), *The Bell Curve.* New York: The Free Press.

Hoffman, I. (1983), The patient as the interpreter of the analyst's experience. *Contem. Psychoanal.*, 19, 389–422.

Holmes, D. (1992), Race and transference in psychoanalysis and psychotherapy. *Int. J. Psychoanal.*, 73 (1), 1–12.

Kaplan, A. (1993), The couch affair: Gender and race in Hollywood transference. *American Imago*, 50 (4), 481–514.

Keller, E. (1992), *Secrets of life, secrets of death: Essays on language, gender and science.* New York: Routledge.

Kris, A. (1990). The analyst's stance and the method of free association. *Psychoanal. Study Child*, 45, 25–41.

Leary, K. (1994), Psychoanalytic "problems" and postmodern "solutions." *Psychoanal. Q.*, 63, 433–465.

Lindon, J. (1994), Gratification and provision in psychoanalysis: Should we get rid of "the rule of abstinence?" *Psychoanal. Dialogues*, 4 (4), 549–582.

Margolis. M. (1996), Personal communication.

Mayer, E. (1996), Changes in science and changing ideas about knowledge and authority in psychoanalysis. *Psychoanal. Q.*, 65:158–200.

Miletec, M. (1996), Practical aspects of self-disclosure. Paper presented at the spring meeting of the American Psychological Association's Division 39, New York, N.Y.

Mitchell, C. (1993), "Multiculturalism": The coded redescription of race in contemporary educational discourse. *Black Scholar*, 23 (3 & 4), 71–74.

Mitchell, S. (1995), Interaction in the Kleinian and interpersonal traditions. *Contemp. Psychoanal.*, 65–91.

Mitchell, S. (1993), *Hope and Dread in Psychoanalysis*. New York: Basic Books.

Myers, W. (1977), The significance of the colors black and white in the dreams of white and black patients. *J. Amer. Psychoanal. Assn.*, 25, 163–181.

Pizer, S. (1992), The negotiation of paradox in the analytic process. *Psychoanal. Dialogues*, 2 (2), 215–240.

Renik, O. (1995), The ideal of the anonymous analyst and the problem of self-disclosure. *Psychoanal. Q.*, 64 (3), 466–495.

Renik, O. (1990), The concept of the transference neurosis and psychoanalytic methodology. *Int. J. Psychoanal.*, 71 (2), 197–204.

Rosenthal, R. (1995), Upwardly mobile bigotry. *New York Times, A11*. October 13, 1995.

Sampson, E. (1993), Identity politics. *American Psychologist*, 48 (12), 1210–1218.

Schacter, J. & Butts, H. (1968), Transference and countertransference. *J. Am. Psychoanal. Assn.*, 16, 792–808.

Simpson, I. (1993), Discussion of a paper by Farhad N. Dalal. *Group Analysis*, 26 (3), 290–293.

Smith, D. (1993), Let our people go. *Black Scholar*, 23 (3 & 4), 74–76.

Stolorow, R. & Atwood, G. (1992), *Contexts of being: The intersubjective foundations of psychological life*. Hillsdale, NJ: The Analytic Press.

Young-Bruehl, E. (1992), Discriminations. *Transitions*, 60, 53–69.

Afterword

An experience I had some years ago stands out in my decision to write within our profession. I had recently read Jerome Bruner's (1983) autobiography, *In Search of Mind*. The book had a tremendous effect on me. I was drawn to Bruner's passion for ideas and his willingness to follow his nose in the direction of the things about which he was most curious. While attending my first American Psychological Association meeting, I chanced upon Bruner in the hallway as he was en route to give a paper. I caught up to him and blurted out "Professor Bruner. I loved your book. It really made me think." Bruner, always the teacher, boomed out, "And that is why one writes."

Looking back on this paper—now some seven years since it was published—I can appreciate how it served as a transitional work in my development toward the psychoanalyst I would become. My first exposure to psychoanalysis was to the ego psychology and contemporary Freudian perspectives I learned in my graduate training in clinical psychology at the University of Michigan. In an earlier paper on psychoanalytic problems and postmodern solutions (Leary, 1994), I used those models and others to critique formulations from relational psychoanalysis. A useful process ensued: that paper was itself debated and heavily critiqued. With those discussions, I found myself part of a conversation about contemporary clinical process. This, in turn, made me think. I examined anew the assumptions I had previously taken for granted about the goals and methods of psychoanalytic exploration. Now I found myself drawn back to relational perspectives and intersubjective formulations. I was deeply curious about what I might learn from the analysts whose approach to clinical work was so distinctly different from that I had encountered during my graduate training.

As an African-American woman, I had been interested for some time in how race shaped the personal and cultural experiences I had growing up, in school, with colleagues, and now in my consulting room. The psychoanalysis I knew best offered a way to think about race that was only partially satisfactory. The basic model—disavowed impulses were projected onto racially different others—made sense. It accounted for some aspects of the psychology of racism. Most important, this model allowed psychoanalysts to put racial experience within the purview of psychoanalysis. At the same time, I could not help but find the prevailing psychoanalytic accounts of race extremely limiting. They were also at some considerable distance from the multicultural perspectives that were then emerging in clinical psychology and different, as well as from the affirmative way that I was able to experience my own identity as a person of color.

Relational psychoanalysis, with its attention to socially constructed accounts of gender and its awareness of the clinical encounter as a social relationship, offered the possibility of a different conversation. I wondered if thinking relationally about race might enable new points of access to the subjectivity of racial experience as it is lived differently by different people. The topic of race as self-disclosure enabled me to explore ideas from within relational psychoanalysis that intrigued me and also to consider how those ideas might inform, expand, or interrogate my understandings about how race worked in the United States. It seemed to me that such an endeavor might enable us to rethink our ideas about race in the consulting room, especially by recognizing that race is not something "out there," but something that is always "in here," inflecting clinical practice, including when analyst and analysand are of similar racial backgrounds and traditions.

By writing this paper, I hoped to add to the efforts of those who came before me. I wanted to put psychoanalysis in dialogue with multicultural perspectives that I thought might enable our profession to consider more culturally responsive forms of practice and theory. For me, it was the starting point of an inquiry that I have continued in subsequent papers by considering the challenges that exist for the analytic couple when racial enactments take place; by examining what is psychically at stake for blacks and for whites when racial passing occurs and by looking at the intersection of identities that are both raced and gendered.

I have learned from the sharp challenges I have sometimes received when I have had occasion to present this work. Those comments have helped me to focus my arguments. I am also appreciative of the feedback I have received from colleagues, and especially from students, who have found my papers facilitative to their own thinking and clinical work. Writing, for me, has always been a matter of participating in the larger conversations going on in our profession about what psychoanalysis is and what it ought to be. To paraphrase Bruner, this is why I write and why I have encouraged others to do the same.

References

Bruner, J. (1983), *In Search of Mind: Essays in Autobiography*. New York: HarperCollins.
Leary, K. (1994), Psychoanalytic "problems" and postmodern "solutions." *Psychoanal. Quart.*, 63:433–465.

More Life:
Centrality and Marginality in
Human Development

(2001)

Ken Corbett

Editors' Introduction

Ken Corbett, by virtue of his training and his current theoretical interests, embodies a certain kind of conceptual multiplicity, a comfort with border jumping and interdisciplinary work. Trained both in clinical and in developmental psychology, working with children and with adults, Corbett has addressed topics that are both highly specific—work on masculinity, on homosexuality in men, on homophobia, on children's use of phallic potential—and highly metatheoretical. Interested in developmental theory and in critiques of stage theory, in this essay he introduces a variety of axioms as new ways to configure matters of development.

This work, indebted to nonlinear dynamic systems, to queer theory, and to relational approaches to intersubjectivity and emergent coconstruction, challenges the standard-issue developmental account with its linearity, its stage reifications, and its focus on single lines and separate spheres of psychological process. His model emphasizes process over structure and, as one of the strengths of both postmodernism and queer theory, he keeps a watchful eye on the complex interfaces of culture and person.

More Life:
Centrality and Marginality in
Human Development*

▼   ▼   ▼   ▼   ▼

In the concluding scene of Tony Kushner's (1992) drama, *Angels in America*, Prior Alter turns to the audience and offers a benediction: "You are are all fabulous creatures, each and every one. And I bless you. More Life" (p. 146).

I begin with Prior's parting wish because of the way in which his beneficence captures the utopian liberality and generosity of a postmodern queer ethic, which is perhaps best captured in his description of us "each and every one" as "fabulous"—a veritable shibboleth of the queer lexicon, a seemingly ever-expansive qualifier that can apply to states of attire and states of desire as well as encapsulate states of being. Is it possible that "fabulous" enunciates the entirety of postmodernism? In the throes of the postmodern passion for an excess of subjectivity and subversion, for "countering the contradictions of experience by endlessly complicating the interpretations that experience can have" (Canguilhem, 1994, p. 71), we might hear Prior to be saying: You are all manifold and multiple, excessive and extravagant, fabled, fabricated, and fictional. You are all a lie—a lie that lies the truth.

In keeping with such postmodern rapacity, Prior then ices his fabulous cake with the wish for "More Life." In so wishing, he makes a moral demand. Pursuing the queer quest to expand the volume of mental freedom, and heeding the postmodern imperative, as Phillips (1995) put it, to create "a society without margins and therefore without humiliation" (p. 186), the voluptuary Prior licks the icing spatula and elbows the margin with his demand for "More Life." His emphatic demand exemplifies the postmodern call for greater sovereignty, for the opportunity that all persons be granted the possibility of self-respect and relief from suffering, and for the particular dignity of self-determination—a wish for a democracy of the multiple, underscored by a nonnormative ethic of difference as liberty.

So here we are at the margin of yet another century, and here we have yet another homosexual at the margin. I refer to the manner in which Freud's *fin-de-siècle* "invert" also occupied the margin. Following

---

* Originally published in *Psychoanalytic Dialogues*, 11:313–335. © 2001 The Analytic Press, Inc.

on late 19th-century sexological nomenclature, Freud (1905) used the term *invert* (interchangeably with *homosexual*) to describe what he felt to be homosexuals' constitutional reversal of sex roles. This so-called sex-role reversal placed the invert in opposition to what was considered the natural and normative heterosexual sex-role arrangement. Turned around and out of step, the homosexual was seen as a twisted other who turned away from nature, reality, and cultural coherence.

A century hence, it is precisely this cultural incoherence and aberrance on which the queer twists. "Queer" is a late-20th-century reappropriation of a pejorative term for homosexuality. Such reappropriation represents the efforts of theorists and activists to assume and empower a marginal position. The aim of vigorously occupying the margin, and boldly being out of step, is to shift the homosexual from the object who is known (the investigated invert) to the subject who knows (the interrogating queer). The queer is held forward as the eccentric subject whose knowledge and capacity for critique derive from his privileged position at the margin. Following such queer reasoning, one would argue that, in the course of the 20th century, privilege has migrated from the center to the margin.

Both the late-19th-century invert and the late-20th-century queer serve as exemplars of an aberrant other—the other by whom the normative heterosexual is contrasted. As other, the invert and the queer provide the margin for the normative, central, ideal citizen who is encoded as heterosexual and who, in turn, constitutes ideal cultural standards. Included in these standards are overarching injunctions as to the composition of mental freedom—ideals regarding the characteristics of a mind open to experiences of expansion and revision.

But, unlike the invert, the queer talks back. The queer not only illuminates normative logic, he critiques it. Postmodern theorists, following largely on Foucault, have in relatively short order ennobled the queer as the ideal nonnormative, noncentral citizen, who is generally, though not exclusively, encoded as homosexual, and who articulates his own set of cultural imperatives and injunctions, including his own brand of mental freedom.[1]

---

[1] Along these lines, consider Foucault's observation (as quoted in and translated by Halperin, 1995): "Homosexuality is a historic opportunity to open up new relational and affective potentialities [virtualities], not in virtue of qualities intrinsic to the homosexual, but because the position of the homosexual 'off-center,' somehow, together with the diagonal lines which the homosexual can draw through the social fabric, makes it possible to bring to light these potentialities" (p. 67).

At both ends of the century, a border between the aberrant-marginal them and the ideal-central us has been constructed around and through the homosexual subject. It is at this border that this essay embarks. I turn toward the homosexual at this border, so that we may learn more, not only about homosexuality, but also about mental freedom and the ways in which it infuses human development. I focus on the insufficient way in which mental freedom has been characterized as either marginal or central, along with the further insufficiency of linking centrality with heterosexuality and marginality with homosexuality. Through such critique, I argue for a conception of human development and mental freedom that promotes an interplay between centrality and marginality.

Regarding the expression "mental freedom," I am following on Benjamin (1998), who followed, in turn, Freud's (1915) description of "that extra piece of mental freedom that distinguishes conscious mental activity" (p. 170). In using this expression, Freud was attempting to clarify his view that freedom followed overcoming the pleasure principle through consciousness. As Benjamin (1998) pointed out, this belief corresponds with one of Freud's two implicit antithetical theories of mental freedom:

1. The *associative mode* is the mode in which freedom is gained by and through association, and one is freed of the unconscious as resistance is lifted.
2. The *reality mode* rests on being freed from the unconscious through the organizing authority of the reality principle.

I show how Freud's concept of the invert reflects the reality mode whereas the associative mode reflects today's queer. I link the invert with Freud's reality model of mental freedom, which might also be characterized as Freud's model of centrality; this mode exclusively informs Freudian developmental theory. Then I examine the "more life" life of the queer, who seems to have fallen heir to Freud's associative mode of mental freedom, which might also be characterized as his model of marginality.

Neither the reality mode nor the associative mode sufficiently problematizes mental freedom, or development—in the same way that neither the invert nor the queer sufficiently problematizes homosexual subjectivity. In particular, traditional developmental models are dominated by the normative logic of centrality, with limited accounting for the developmental phenomenon and necessity of marginality, whereas postmodern theories of subjectivity overvalue the potential of the margin and fail to account for the significance of similarity and coherence in human relations. I then use that criticism as a platform for proposing five quasi-axioms toward a new developmental model. Central to this new model is the interplay of centrality and marginality—the inter-implication of reality and association—in any given life. In imagining such a model, I employ constructs derived from chaos and systems theories in order to advance an idea of human development that is open to the perplexity and the complexity that are embodied in the simple certainty that no two humans are the same.

The Invert, Reality, Centrality, and Determinism

To be sure, the concept and possibility of mental freedom have an elaborate history both inside and outside the psychoanalytic canon. Philosophers and poets have long referred to the conflict humans face between the construction of a just and shared reality and the desire for liberation from reality's control, including the quest for an independent mind free of restrictions and obligations. This conflict is noted as early as Plato's recognition of the pull between justice and happiness. It is perhaps the Romantics, though, who best described the tension between reality and liberty. Taylor (1992) linked the quest for mental freedom with the Romantic philosophers of the late 18th century and credited the German philosopher Herder with putting forward the idea that each of us has an original way of being human. However, it was Rousseau, the philosopher most often identified with this belief in originality, who linked mental freedom with the liberty and expansion needed for growth.

Indeed, it was the Romantics to whom Freud (1900) turned in his first ruminations on mental freedom in *The Interpretation of Dreams*. As Benjamin (1998) detailed, Freud (1900), in pondering the surrender of reason to imagination, invoked Schiller, the 18th-century Romantic poet and philosopher. Freud (1900) (on Rank's suggestion) quotes from Schiller's reflections on the relationship between creativity and reason: "Where there is a creative mind, Reason relaxes its watch upon the gates, and ideas rush in pell-mell" (p. 103). By recasting Schiller's observations linking reason with censorship and imagination with wish, Freud began to construct his first model of mental freedom: freedom is gained as one is relieved of reason/reality, and resistance to association is thereby lifted. His second theory of mental freedom, wherein freedom rests on the authority of reality, emerged through his later discussions of sexual development (Freud, 1905) and more directly through his discussion of transference (Freud, 1915).

In "Three Essays on the Theory of Sexuality," Freud (1905) undertook to set forth a developmental account of mental freedom. Uncharacteristically, Freud returned to this text (between 1905 and 1920) and tried repeatedly to elaborate and refine his developmental theory. As is often remarked, the repeated reworking of the essays invests them with a unique vigor equal to the significance of the ideas developed therein. Dimen (1999), for example, observed that there is a particularly energetic and instructive rhythm created between Freud's two modes of mental freedom as they dance an intricate pas de deux, shadowing each other between the text and the margin of the essays. Quite literally, the hierarchy of text and margin mirrors the hierarchy established between the centrality of reality (the body of the text) and the marginality of the associative mode (the margin of the text).

Freud (1905) began to construct his second model of mental freedom—the reality mode—through his developmental theory of psychosexual stages. In the course of his "Three Essays on the Theory of Sexuality," Freud tethered mental freedom to a particular form of developmental hierarchy—an order of things (a specific intrapsychic organization) that, according to Freud, reflects the organizing authority of reality. The reality of cultural imperatives slowly commingles with biologically scheduled stages, reflecting and reproducing a progressive human evolution. The invert stands outside this evolution, and via negativa provides the margin for this model of developmental hierarchy. The invert never ascends to a position of maturity—never grabs the brass ring of mature desire. Instead, he remains a haunted and haunting object who occupies the margin, from which he can never fully desire or love as a mature subject but only in an act of displaced heterosexuality.

The invert also illustrates the manner in which psychosexual evolution could, on the level of the individual, be altered by personal events that lead to unique developmental stories. Such stories are absent from "Three Essays," although Freud did present developmental narratives within the case studies that he was writing during the same period. Within these case studies, Freud brought to life the developmental explanatory concepts he outlined in "Three Essays," including repression, maturation, fixation, and identification (arguably the linchpin of Freudian developmental theory). In reading about Dora, Little Hans, and Leonardo, one certainly gains a sense of each of these individuals as unique. Clearly and often gloriously, Freud reached toward describing each subject as a web of contingent associations and relations—an ever-expansive relay of wishes and reconstructions that move unhindered through past, present, and future.

Yet the pragmatic effect of these progress narratives is one whereby the development of each subject is yoked to a stage theory that is at once linear and unwavering in its deterministic predictability. In an effort to capture the forward movement of development, Freud brought a kind of Newtonian determinism to bear on this problem of developmental hierarchy.[2] In accord with Newtonian axioms, Freud assumed that, given an approximate knowledge of a system's initial conditions and an understanding of natural law, one could calculate the approximate behavior of the system. Working with what he believed to be the naturalism of the reproduction of matrimonial relations, Freud proposed a theory of serial initial conditions and behaviors (his libidinal stages) that become reorganized at successively more complex hierarchical levels. This developmental stairway culminates in a heterosexual object choice and in subordination of the sexual instinct to the reproductive function. The reproduction of reproduction melds into a "naturalized" notion of the hierarchical reorganization of psychic structure. This manner of "natural" development (reorganization and structure) is then held forward as both the product and progenitor of mental freedom.

The Queer, Association, Marginality, and Complexity

But deterministic predictability and the stage have seen their day. Even the simplest systems are now seen to create extraordinarily difficult problems of predictability. Developmental psychologists and psychoanalysts reflecting on the complex intersubjective field within which any individual develops have begun to point out that stage theories and linear conceptions of development do not adequately capture the complexity of what Kennedy (1997, p. 553) called "subjective organizations" (Mitchell, 1993; Bromberg, 1994, 1996; Ogden, 1994; Thelan and Smith, 1994; Chodorow, 1996; Davies, 1996, 1998; Harris, 1996, 1999; Wolff, 1996; Coates, 1997; Fajardo, 1998). Linear conceptions of development also tidy up the complexity of mental freedom—linearity has a way of confusing the minimalism of order with freedom.

On a parallel track, feminist and queer theorists have been arguing for some time now that a theory of developmental hierarchy that rests on the reproduction of matrimonial relations does not adequately account for the variety that characterizes human existence (Foucault, 1978; Butler, 1990; Sedgwick, 1990; Goldner, 1991; Harris, 1991; Flax, 1993; Schwartz, 1993; Warner, 1993; Dimen, 1995; Lesser, 1995). In an

---

[2] Reisner (2001) made what might be thought of as the opposite argument—for the prescient elasticity and antifoundationalism that can be found in Freudian thought. Although I largely concur with Reisner, I maintain that there is a difference between Freud's antifoundational thinking and the pragmatic effect of his developmentalism—most especially as it is represented in his psychosexual stage theory.

effort to capture this human variance and to illuminate the nonnormative margin, postmodern theorists have set out to deconstruct naturalism, disarticulate identification, and relativize normativity. Postmodern theorists force us to question the degree to which we promote a life wedded to maintaining and generating a normative order of existence. We are confronted with our commitments to the construction of new cultural forms—along with our allegiance to fellow citizens who refuse or possibly even renounce the reproduction of matrimonial relations, who are reinventing reproduction, who may embrace the alterity of so-called primitive or perverse acts for their disruptive potential, and who may even defy tribal ethics in favor of the mental freedom born of individual self-determination. Such contemporaries are now called "queer." Nonredemptive and verily Rousseauian, the queer reaches toward individual autonomy, passionately warning against the idea of prevailing social realities and the force of such realities to promote conformity to depersonalizing customs.

"Queer" obtains its very meaning and energy through its oppositional relation to normal social realities. As Halperin (1995) explained, "Queer is by definition *whatever* is at odds with the normal, the legitimate, the dominant. *There is nothing in particular to which it necessarily refers*. It is an identity without an essence" (p. 62). The queer maintains his edge through endless mutations and associations. Freedom is not gained in accord with reality principles; rather, freedom is gained by dismantling reality's resistance. So-called reality is challenged, or queered, through the freedom of association—the liberty to realign and reconfigure associative links and thereby deconstruct established meanings. Examples of such queering maneuvers include reappropriation and resignification of pejorative labels such as queer; employment of camp theatrics such as drag to highlight the possibility and pleasure of extreme fantasies that are liberated from moral relevance, duty, and seriousness (Sontag, 1964); and persistent exposure of hierarchies (e.g., heterosexual privilege and presumption), which leads to overturning the positions of the center and the margin.

An especially amusing and obviously parodic example of such queer exhortation can be found in John Waters's (1974) *Female Trouble*, a film I am sure Kushner's Prior would have seen, likely more than once. In the film, Aunt Ida explains to her nephew, Gator, that she would "be so happy if [he] turned Nellie." Gator objects, and maintains that he is straight. But Aunt Ida persists, exclaiming, "But you could change. Queers are just better. I'd be so proud if you was a fag and had a nice beautician boyfriend—I'd never have to worry . . . that you'd work in an office, have children, celebrate wedding anniversaries. The world of a heterosexual is a sick and boring life!"

Through this parodic retaliatory tweak, Waters reverses the manner in which homosexuals have often been implored to change their identities and desires, and thereby illuminates the way in which such interdiction creates a them–us border. Waters also manages to call our attention to the absurdity of creating an aberrant-marginal them and an ideal-central us. Posting the homosexual at the margin invites a discourse based on how different they are, how much better or worse they are, how much more or less imaginative or reasoned they are, and who would change them, or who they would change—when, alas, the homosexual is not much better, or much worse, is not less reasoned, or more fabulous, and alack, the homosexual's experience of difference coexists, as does all experience of difference, with experience of similarity. Moreover, this dialogic movement of similarity and difference may or may not drive one in the quest for self-determination to resist the regulatory force of normativity.

Queer theorists have had much to say about the oppression of regulatory force and the dulling consequences of normativity. But what of the strain of living outside the regular, the reliable, the customary? What does it cost to be always and already fabulous? What of the subjective strain of living "without an essence"? What might be the consequences of an illusory subjectivity built on a chain of constantly shifting associations? And how might the forces of nonregulation regulate? Might the illusory queer underestimate the potential of living in reliable relations with others as opposed to always living through opposition to others? Queer transcendence is largely configured through opposition, thereby ignoring the possibilities of transformation through relation. Another possible consequence is the construction of evacuating associating subjects who have limited capacities for self reflection or relational reverie. Although queer theorists may have succeeded in moving the homosexual from a Freudian couch, do they now leave the homosexual to squirm in a heap of relationally unbounded free associations on a "Foucauldian couch" (Boyarin's, 1995, phrase, p. 137)?

The construction of the invert resulted in the projection of the other as aberrant and outside. The construction of the queer results in the projection of similitude as negligible and outside—similarity is often postmodernly constructed as some manner of autistic white or banalizing narcissistic beige. Each case points to the failure of both the Freudian and the postmodern efforts to sufficiently heed the complex interimplication of centrality and marginality—of similitude and difference. We are in need of a model of mental freedom—along with a way to account for the developmental phenomenon of psychic reorganization—that is not dominated by the notion of ego coherence, social cohesion, and maturity ceded to the center. At the same time, such a model should not be governed by an overestimation of the liberty and deliverance born of the vivacity and veracity that are currently attributed to the margin.

From Three Essays to Five Quasi-Axioms

In what follows, I outline five quasi-axioms toward a new model of development. I qualify these axioms as "quasi," because I want to emphasize my wish that they be heard as an effort toward improved self-description as opposed to a set of foundations. In qualifying these axioms as "quasi," I am working a contradiction, for, indeed, a quasi-axiom is an oxymoron. Through this oxymoronic coupling, I am attempting to capture my dual commitment to the contingency of subjective repertoire and the possibility of a developmental vocabulary (Corbett, 1996, 1997). I am not suggesting that this developmental vocabulary can "hold all the sides of our life in a single vision" (Rorty, 1989, p. xvi) or provide a single lexicon for all human lives; rather I envision this developmental vocabulary as one possible form of redescription, one possible way to build a narrative amid present, past, and future.

1. The first quasi-axiom of my theory of development is that it be a *theory of process rather than state*, of position rather than stage, of becoming rather than being.

Recognizing that learning and relational contingencies produce indeterminacy and disturbance and that perplexity and complexity are ingrained by-products of process reorients our theorizing about human development from compositional (or substantialist) stage models to relational (or ecological) position models. As Fajardo (1998) pointed out, "The questions posed no longer concern invariant causal sequences but instead concern regularities in the patterns of organization and synchrony among elements" (p. 195).

How we imagine growth is pivotal to this model shift. Positions afford a conceptualization of growth that not only emphasizes regularity but pattern, coherence, complexity, and movement between developmental periods. Positions offer a degree of perplexity that is missing from stage theories that emphasize movement through developmental periods guided by unvarying sequence, order, and cause. Developmental narratives framed by the idea of positions also become more complex—moving from causal stage narratives that tend to promote telic constitutive explanations toward dynamic analyses of subjective phenomenologies. Developmental stories are pursued not only with an eye toward pattern, but also with an eye toward the ways in which patterns are modified by the contingent and often paradoxical structure of subjectivity. Patterns, tropes, and regularities may be gleaned from these phenomenologies, but they are always subject to the vicissitudes of variance and context.

Variability and multiplicity are emphasized, and follow increased attention to the long-known (but less often observed) principles of multiple function and overdetermination. This emphasis on variance stimulates and resonates with a corresponding reexamination of linear time and context specificity. Just as increased attention to variability calls deterministic predictability into question, increased attention to the vicissitudes of time and context discredits the idea of a determining telos.

As Chodorow (1996) demonstrated, deconstructing deterministic predictability has particular relevance with regard to the predictive authority we grant to the past and with regard to the manner in which we establish so-called developmental determinants that culminate in producing developmental stages. Although recognizing the ways in which the human child remains sensitive to initial conditions, less explanatory value is acceded to childhood, developmental tasks, and initial conditions. Freud (1930) metaphorically captures this dilemma regarding predictive authority, when he wrote, "In the marrow-bones of the grown man I can, it is true, trace the outline of the child's bone, but it itself has disappeared, having lengthened and thickened until it has attained its definitive form" (p. 71).

Childhood must now be reconceived as a resonant yet emergent process, open to oscillation and transformation within the multiple relational worlds constructed throughout a life. Central to childhood's reconception will be an effort to locate children within an intrasubjective and intersubjective "relational matrix" (Mitchell, 1988) of multiple relations, spaces, times, and selves. This matrix formation bespeaks the ways in which neither time (past/present/future) nor relationships (one/two/multiple) are conceived as veridical, but rather as fabulous, combined, and perpetually dynamic (Mitchell, 1993; Ogden, 1994; Aron, 1996; Bromberg, 1996; Chodorow, 1996; Harris, 1996; Davies, 1998). In other words, not only is the past a palimpsest, so is the present—experience is always being rewritten or overwritten. The act of living a life constructs or changes the supposed determinants (during both childhood and beyond); a constant importance cannot always be assigned to initial conditions (even as they are under way).

Similarly, a constant and determining importance cannot always be assigned to the fit between any given subject and global regularities. As Thelan and Smith (1994) observed, global regularities may be reliably predicted and observed. Yet, "local variability, complexity, and context-specificity" (p. vxiii) lead to the perpetual dynamism of subjectivity (even within the so-called normal subject). The postmodern attunement to contingency has shown us that, though norms and global regularities capture what is most conspicuous about human development, they do not capture what is perhaps most interesting about human development—the way in which the repetition of patterns or averages is never exact, the way in which it can occur only with variance.[3]

Considering the interplay of variance, context, time, and chance in determining our fates also changes our quest to find causal origins and to provide constitutive explanations. As Freud (1910) suggested by paraphrasing Da Vinci, "[life] is full of countless causes that never enter experience" (p. 137). Asking why someone is homosexual, for example, leads to an unprofitable quest. In the Nietzschean sense, we may wish to track our sexuality home—we may wish to discover the causes of our being what we are. But in so doing, we must recognize that we will find and create multiple, contingent, and indeterminate causes and homes.

Along these lines, I cannot recall a treatment with a contemporary gay patient in which the question of the origin of homosexuality was relevant to the movement of the patient's anxiety. The overwhelming majority of my gay patients approach their sexuality with a certain inevitability that does not brook questions of specific origin or legitimization. Through this assertion, I do not mean to imply that I do not set out with my patients to understand—to the degree that we can—in what manner their sexuality has developed. But our efforts in this regard are guided by the question "How homosexuality?" (With what meaning and to what effect?) as opposed to what I consider to be the ill-conceived etiologic project of "Why homosexuality?" (For what reason, cause, motive, or purpose?). With this interrogative shift in mind, we

---

[3] In like manner, although the material reality of the body and the brain exerts a certain influence over development—including the ways in which, as Kandel (1998) summarized, the material reality of "genes and their protein products are important determinants of the pattern of interconnections between neurons in the brain"—these bodily and neurologic exertions do not by themselves explain all the variance of human development (p. 460). The material reality of the body and brain is polygenic and in a state of perpetual dynamic equilibrium. As Birch (1992) explained, "What a gene is depends upon neighbouring genes on the same and on different chromosomes and upon other aspects of its environment in the cell. The gene (DNA) makes nothing by itself" (p. 395). Genetic expression is further dependent on and entangled with the relational excess of human life. For example, it is now well known that, through learning and social contingencies, gene expression is open to alterations that in turn modify synaptic connections and produce structural changes between nerve cells of the brain (Vaughn, 1997; Kandel, 1998).

then attempt to address the meanings and possible causes of specific aspects of a patient's desires and object relations; however, those meanings and causes are always overdetermined and often contradicted.

2. The second quasi-axiom calls for a theory that *accounts for the dialogic movement of chaos and coherence.*

This condition follows in recognition of the manner in which the disturbance of process generates richly organized patterns. These patterns emerge between the chaos of contingency and the coherence of integrative need. They develop out of relations with external and internal objects and result in "persisting inner regulations" (Schafer, 1964, p. 14) and motivating fantasies. Davies (1998) captured the way in which these patterns are "kaleidoscop[ic], . . . multitudinous yet finite organizations of substructures, always shifting, yet always moving in relationship to one another; patterns, at first novel, [that become] identifiable over time with repeated exposure" (p. 195). The regulatory persistence of these patterns, however, is not the product of a simple unity; such patterns are not simple maps or simply a matter of hierarchical layering. They are, instead, variegated pathways open to the tension of integration and unintegration (Ogden, 1994).

An intriguing example of this chaotic–coherent pattern organization and regulation can be found in the mysterious and seemingly contradictory manner in which sexuality, liable as it is to multiplicity, is notoriously transitory—yet equally notorious for its stability. As postmodern theorists are fond of pointing out, multiple identifications within the same subject can rival one another, overthrow one another, or even revive, following their apparent demise (Fuss, 1995). Identities composed as they are of multiple identifications (including disidentifications) and confounded as they are by the vicissitudes of other forms of internalization (including incorporation and introjection) are never brought to full closure.

Identities and desires can and do change, but they also persist and, through their relative coherence, resist change. This phenomenon is perhaps best recognized through varying conceptions of self-sameness (consider, e.g., Bollas's construct of the "human idiom"). Self-sameness and the persistence of identity have also been observed relative to the ways in which change in sexual orientation or even in what Person (1980) referred to as the "sex print" or "an individual's erotic signature" (p. 620) is achieved only with great difficulty and generally not at all. For example, Robert had multiple lovers throughout the course of his six-year psychotherapy. Although Robert's lovers were outwardly quite dissimilar (distinguished by class, age, race, and, on two occasions, gender), his relationships were marked by the similarity in his mode of sexual desire and lack of satisfaction. Robert referred to himself as a "bottom-top" and explained, "I like to be seduced, but then I run the show." Rarely, it seemed, could he find a compatible sexual partner who would surrender to his desire. Often these relations ended abruptly, with limited understanding on Robert's part as to his partner's anger and confusion. In accord with the assumption of overdetermination, we approached Robert's relations from a variety of directions. An important byway of our analysis centered on his conflicted identification with a generally passive though easily provoked and aggressive father. As Robert said of his father, "He could turn the table." Gradually, Robert was able to take stock of the relational dynamics of his desire. He was able to appreciate the manner in which his sexual excitement hinged on his partner's confusion. Further, he began to grasp the ways in which he projected his own confusion (his own contradictory experience of excitement and fear) onto his partners. This awareness allowed us to pursue another byway of analysis regarding Robert's defense against his own desire for surrender, and the conflicts he faced in wishing for a trustworthy other who could "run the show." It was especially important to examine this particular wish and anxiety within the transference. With time, Robert's relations became less rigid, and compatibility and reciprocity were enhanced with his partners. He developed greater flexibility with regard to sexual satisfaction. He even formed a relationship wherein he described himself as a "switch," as opposed to either a "top" or a "bottom." Yet, his "bottom-top" identity—one that he could now better communicate and negotiate—continued to color his experience of sexual passion and excitement, and this identity was most typically expressed within the more stable relationship he formed near the end of his treatment.

In the same way that identity is confounded by multiplicity, it is also founded on multiplicity or, as Schafer (1964) described, "multiplication of minds within minds" (p. 62). It is through the chaotic and dialogic repetition of identification, negation, disidentification, incorporation, and introjection that inner regulations, mental representations, and characteristic motivations are internalized. The regulatory structure of internalization and the force of identity persistence have often been overlooked when postmodern theorists turn to theories of identification—as Fuss (1995) aptly pointed out—in order to pity them as "painful and poignant meditations on the possibility of identification's own impossibility" (p. 39).

But, by reading the impossibility of identification's multiplicity as the redundant dead end within a closed system, postmodern theorists circumvent the ways in which identification's impossibility could be read as part and parcel of the complex and chaotic workings of an open nonlinear system—a system wherein identifications stimulate intricate feed-back loops forming patterns of exchange and transfer. It is through the flow, feedback, and repetition of such patterns that structure and regulation emerge. As Rapaport (1967) suggested, "Structures are processes of a slow rate of change" (p. 787). And as chaos and complexity theorists have found, complexity is characteristic not of objects but of events (e.g., identification) through which structures emerge (Gleick, 1987; Waldrop, 1992; Gell-Mann, 1994; Holland, 1995). Identity is an ongoing "event," not a discrete endpoint. And the structure that emerges is in motion—imagine a building the walls of which are aquiver with atomic movement.

Another way to imagine the structuring quality of identification is to consider that the repeated consequences of internalization are as much a verb as they are a noun. Like the present participle verb form "-ing," identifications flow. In turn, this flow produces inflections and connections that bind internalizations and build structures; these flowing structures then function as feedback systems. As the expressed action of the present participle suggests, these structures are always in the process of becoming, and they are never complete; they are transforming and revising but always postponing resolution. Moreover, in league with the plastic quality of a verb, these systems are intrinsically "coadaptive" (Gell-Mann, 1994); just as verbs rely on a subject to make a sentence, so too does internalization rely on the back-and-forth correspondence between psychic representations and the actual world to structure an identification.

3.   The third quasi-axiom calls for the representation of developmental hierarchy as a multidimensional topology. Following this axiom entails rethinking our basic developmental metaphors—especially the metaphors of developmental line and developmental core.

In a recent critique of the construct of developmental line, Coates (1997) suggested we think of development as more like "complex multiple spirals." I wish to build on Coates's spirals by suggesting that we imagine them made of a weblike substance, imagine a spiral web or tissue that can be stretched, twisted, elongated, folded in on itself—and that springs back . . . but is never quite the same. I imagine these webs as being like taffy but each having a different tensile strength (some spirals are more flexible than others).

Further, I envision these webs moving in a manner like that described by the poet August Kleinzahler (1998),

the way parallelograms move
across computer screens, cooling the points

as they turn through themselves
driven by an algorithm
into new shapes that bend and dissolve
only to reappear and move on
to the next set of coordinates [p. 38].

Kleinzahler's moving parallelograms and Davies's kaleidoscopic patterns are metaphors reaching for the same idea—the perpetual dynamism of pattern repetition. If we then consider the lingering effect of such dynamism—when the pattern itself is past or invisible, the evidence or residue of the pattern remains—we come to my idea of the web. We can also begin to consider the ways in which chaos builds structure. The lacework of a web articulates the confluence and coadaptive dependence of the interlacing on the context; it is not a Newtonian a priori structure, or a fixed form, but rather a structure that is never fixed and always in transition, always moving in accord with the atmosphere.

I offer this metaphor of the web as a substitute for the idea of the core. In place of the core, which implies a hard, static nucleus that is formed, unified, self-contained, and whole, the web represents a woven network that contains and interconnects in intricate patterns, some of which may be tightly woven (or well integrated), others less so, still others subject to dropped stitches (leading to unintegration). Construction of a core also implies hierarchically layered stages, whereas the open-weave construction of a web suggests the synchronic quality of positions. Further, a web seems a more apt metaphor for internalization within an intersubjective frame. We can envision a web as a link between subjects. We can imagine a weaving, linking, mutually created intersubjectivity, as opposed to a core that is completely centered and created within the self.

4.   The fourth quasi-axiom calls for a theory that accounts for a *culture's need to read pattern, as well as a culture's need for individuals who reach beyond patterns.*

I find much to be admired in the postmodern explanation of the ways in which power and norms shape our subjectivities. Yet I remain troubled by the prospect that, through our incessant deconstruction of patterns of enculturation, we run the risk of undervaluing our needs to be recognized by others. I do not mean to overlook that such recognition often comes with the oppressive and repressive cost of social regulation, including submission and subordination (Flax, 1993; Butler, 1997). And I do not wish to overlook the potentialities born of resisting social regulation—the will to surpass one's self, to transform, to create the future.

For example, the queer (a curious amalgamation of Blake's exuberance and Genet's abjection) is always reaching for the future. This heroic temptation and effort toward futurity are manifestations of a utopian quest. As Halperin (1995) explained, "Utopian vision is an experiment we perform on ourselves so as to discover our otherness to ourselves in the experience of our own futurity" (p. 106). Otherness produces the rupture that creates room for new cultural forms, new social bonds, and new futures.

Some might respond to this heroic temptation by critiquing its omnipotence, or by questioning its flirtation with outright sentimentality. Still and all, we could stand to be less wary of transforming hope and confident expectation. My concern lies with the manner in which a utopian quest is always and forever oriented toward the future. Despite the postmodern critique of linearity, queer theory's utopianism is exquisitely linear. Through its linear futurity, utopianism skims over the manner in which subjectivity is nourished by the unencumbered movement among past, present, and future. Subjects and relations are constructed not only by reaching together toward a future, but also by resting together in the relationality of customs, traditions, and norms. There could be an appreciation of approximation, recognition, convergence, and, dare I say, beauty. There could be room for an imperfectly structured structure. Harmonies and relations are to be discovered.

I find the postmodern insistence on the sheer contingency of individual existence to be too limiting. Are we only to recognize contingency and difference? Indeed, how do we understand difference apart from similarity? Are we forever captive to contingency? Or might we acknowledge and appropriate contingency as we explore the liminal and liberatory possibility of transformation? In his estimable fashion, Proust (1928) circled around the tension between our near constant efforts to reach beyond ourselves (to transform) and the circumscription of such efforts when he suggested:

> Even if we have the sensation of being always enveloped in, surrounded by our own soul, still it does not seem a fixed and immovable prison; rather do we seem to be borne away with it, and perpetually struggling to transcend it. To break out into the world, with a perpetual discouragement as we hear endlessly all around us that unvarying sound which is not an echo from without, but the resonance of a vibration from within [p. 119].

Contrary to their frequent employment of rhetorical strategies that rely on imagination, postmodern theorists rather consistently fail to recognize our fantasmatic desires and imaginative efforts to reach through normativity toward recognition and to reach beyond normativity toward transformation. We are in need of a theory of mental freedom that not only allows for the utopian rupture of normativity but also heeds the quotidian rhythm of regularity and the structuring potential of relational reverie.

5. The fifth quasi-axiom promotes *interplay between Freud's two modes of mental freedom*. Neither the associative mode nor the reality mode holds a privileged position in relation to the other—they coexist in a mutually preserving and negating relationship.

Distinct from Freud's implicit proposition that mental freedom is divided into antithetical modes (reality vs. associative), I am proposing a mutuality of reality and association. One vantage point on this mutuality is the way in which analysts have reoriented their focus toward the action of free association within the analytic dyad. Through the modern reappraisal of psychoanalytic technique, with its emphasis on enactment, intersubjectivity, and mutuality, we can no longer view free association as occurring simply through words, and we can no longer assume, as Greenberg (1996) argued that "we understand the meaning of the act of free-associating just from the fact of its occurrence" (p. 202). The meaning of free association can be gleaned only from a deeper understanding of the relation created through the patient's action. Meaning can be understood only between the patient and the analyst and, more specifically, between the patient's associations and the analyst's associations, which are in turn fed by the mutuality of the transference and countertransference relationship(s) (Aron, 1996). These associations then interact with the realities (both psychic and material) of the analytic situation. Neither association nor reality stands alone.

Daniel, a bright and energetic young academic, entered a period in his analysis wherein he set about to "free-associate." He would lapse into lengthy periods of near "word-salad" and pointedly ignore my attempts to understand the action of his efforts. He was most reluctant to examine his effort as anything other than the act of free-associating and doing the work of an exemplary "analysand." He was equally angered by my struggle to turn our attention to the ways in which he was utilizing so-called free-associating to create a relationship with me. I was aware that Daniel's turn toward this manner of free-associating followed a period in the analysis wherein he had begun to become more freely aware of long repressed erotic desires, and had begun to act on some of those desires within two short-lived affairs. I was also aware of a move toward schizoid withdrawal—an old retreat that often took the form of shrouding his mind in a marijuana haze. My countertransference response was to feel cut-off, bored, deadened, and, yet, anxiously confused.

One day during this period, Daniel ended an analytic session by exclaiming with a mix of vexation and awe, "Damn, sexuality is so disordered." I noted my feeling of optimism in response. During this hour, he reported a dream in which he was playing with a little boy in a backyard. In the dream, he was anxiously aware that the play was colored by a kind of sexual tension ("not exactly like being turned on, just a sort of 'freesion'"). His anxiety was heightened when he was made aware that a woman was also in the yard, and he thought she was looking over his shoulder as he played with the boy. Something about this dream seemed to allow Daniel to break with his pattern of word association, and he allowed the convoluted interplay of association and reality to emerge. He ventured forth with associations to the dream that ranged from homosexual pederastic impulses to repressed heterosexual fantasies—fantasies that he feared might contradict both his identity as an adult and as a homosexual. But whence or with whom did the excitement arise, the boy or the woman? He was especially aware of his feeling of being watched while in a state of near arousal. He then wondered if I would react as the "gay police." I asked if he meant, "Would I police his homosexual excitement?" "No," he replied, "Will you police my heterosexual fantasies?" He went on to say he felt that that was not likely, yet he had been aware of holding back. He then detailed a recurring daydream of holding a woman from behind while fondling her. I wondered if he thought that being homosexual meant having to hold back his heterosexuality. He responded with multiple associations to policing: Did one of the figures in the dream represent his policing mother? Was she more comfortable when he did not deal with his heterosexuality? Had he found her in me? Had she adequately held back her own incestuous (heterosexual) wishes? How did that relate to his fears where I was concerned? He then remembered that the woman in the dream was looking over his shoulder. Or was he also looking over my shoulder? Was he policing his own fantasies regarding my life and sexuality as a way to fend off what he felt to be the threat of a growing closeness?

At that point, I asked if he might fear a growing "freesion," what seemed to be his curious blend of *free*, *frisson*, and *association*. What kind of excitement might occur if he allowed himself to relate and associate in my backyard? We both laughed, for at that moment we both became aware that my office literally looks out on a backyard. Ah, I thought, we were now at the welcome edge of chaos. Along this fabulous border, where complex systems can remain open and nonlinear, networks of exchange and transfer can occur (Gell-Mann, 1994). Neither patient nor analyst is autonomous—the convolution transpires within both the material and the psychic realities of the analytic situation.

Associations and reality are constantly reconstructed in and through their complex interactions. It is through this kind of mutual reconstruction that the "radically poetic character" of a patient's life conjoins the "poetic foundations" of the analytic dyad, and the poetry ("freesion") of psychoanalysis occurs (Rorty, 1989, p. 67). And it is through the revision and expansion of these fabulous borders that perceptions shift, thought is transformed, and more life circulates.

References

Aron, L. (1996), *A Meeting of Minds: Mutuality in Psychoanalysis*. Hillsdale, NJ: The Analytic Press.

Benjamin, J. (1998), *Shadow of the Other*. New York: Routledge.

Birch, C. (1992), The postmodern challenge to biology. In: *The Post-Modern Reader*, ed. C. Jencks. New York: St. Martin's Press, pp. 392–398.

Boyarin, D. (1995), Freud's baby, Fliess's maybe: Homophobia, anti-Semitism, and the invention of Oedipus. *GLQ*, 2:115–147.

Bromberg, P. (1994), "Speak that I may see you": Some reflections on dissociation, reality, and psychoanalytic listening. *Psychoanal. Dial.*, 4:517–547.

———— (1996), Standing in the spaces: The multiplicity of self and the psychoanalytic relationship, *Contemp. Psychoanal.*, 32:509–535.

Butler, J. (1990), *Gender Trouble*. New York: Routledge.

———— (1997), Response to Lynne Layton's "The doer behind the deed: Tensions and intersections between Butler's vision of performativity and relational psychoanalysis." *Gender Psychoanal*, 2:515–520.

Canguilhem, G. (1994), The death of man, or exhaustion of the cogito. In: *The Cambridge Companion to Foucault*, ed. G. Gutting. Cambridge, England: Cambridge University Press.

Chodorow, N. (1996), Reflections on the authority of the past in psychoanalytic thinking. *Psychoanal. Quart.*, 65:32–51.

Coates, S. (1997), Is it time to jettison the concept of developmental lines? Commentary on deMarneffe's paper "Bodies and words." *Gender Psychoanal.*, 2:35–54.

Corbett, K. (1996), Homosexual boyhood: Notes on girlyboys. *Gender Psychoanal.*, 1:429–462.

———— (1997), Speaking queer. *Gender Psychoanal.*, 2:495–514.

Davies, J. (1996), Linking the "pre-analytic" and the postclassical: Integration, dissociation, and the multiplicity of unconscious process. *Contemp. Psychoanal.*, 32:553–576.

———— (1998), Multiple perspectives on multiplicity. *Psychoanal. Dial.*, 8:195–206.

Dimen, M. (1995), On "our nature": Prolegomenon to a relational theory of sexuality. In: *Disorienting Sexuality*, ed. T. Domenici & R. Lesser. New York: Routledge, pp. 129–152.

———— (1999), Between lust and libido: Sex, psychoanalysis, and the moment before. *Psychoanal. Dial.*, 9:415–440.

Fajardo, B. (1998), A new view of developmental research for psychoanalysts. *J. Amer. Psychoanal. Assn.*, 46:185–207.

Flax, J. (1993), *Disputed Subjects: Essays on Psychoanalysis, Politics, and Philosophy*. New York: Routledge.

Foucault, M. (1978), *The History of Sexuality*. New York: Random House.

Freud, S. (1900), The interpretation of dreams. *Standard Edition*, 4 & 5. London: Hogarth Press, 1953.

———— (1905), Three essays on the theory of sexuality. *Standard Edition*, 7:130–243. London: Hogarth Press, 1953.

———— (1910), Leonardo Da Vinci and a memory of his childhood. *Standard Edition*, 11:63–137. London: Hogarth Press, 1957.

———— (1915), Observations on transference-love. *Standard Edition*, 12:157–171. London: Hogarth Press, 1958.

———— (1930), Civilization and its discontents. *Standard Edition*, 21:64–145. London: Hogarth Press, 1961.

Fuss, D. (1995), *Identification Papers*. New York: Routledge.

Gell-Mann, M. (1994), *The Quark and the Jaguar: Adventures in the Simple and the Complex*. New York: Freeman.

Gleick, J. (1987), *Chaos: Making a New Science*. New York: Penguin Books.

Goldner, V. (1991), Toward a critical relational theory of gender. *Psychoanal. Dial.*, 1:243–248.

Greenberg, J. (1996), Psychoanalytic words and psychoanalytic acts: A brief history. *Contemp. Psychoanal.*, 32:195–214.

Halperin, D. (1995), *Saint-Foucault*. New York: Oxford University Press.

Harris, A. (1991), Gender as contradiction. *Psychoanal. Dial.*, 1:197–224.

———— (1996), The conceptual power of multiplicity. *Contemp. Psychoanal.*, 32:537–552.

———— (1999), Making genders: Commentary on paper by Irene Fast. *Psychoanal. Dial.*, 9:663–674.

Holland, J. (1995), *Hidden Order: How Adaptation Builds Complexity*. New York: Addison-Wesley.

Kandel, E. (1998), A new intellectual framework for psychiatry. *Amer. J. Psychiat.*, 155:457–469.

Kennedy, R. (1997), On subjective organizations: Toward a theory of subject relations. *Psychoanal. Dial.*, 7:553–582.

Kleinzahler, A. (1998), *Green Sees Things in Waves*. New York: Farrar, Straus & Giroux.

Kushner, T. (1992), *Angels in America, Part Two: Perestroika*. New York: Theatre Communication Group.

Lesser, R. (1995), Objectivity as masquerade. In: *Disorienting Sexuality*, ed. T. Domenici & R. Lesser. New York: Routledge, pp. 83–96.

Mitchell, S. (1988), *Relational Concepts in Psychoanalysis*. Cambridge, MA: Harvard University Press.

———— (1993), *Hope and Dread in Psychoanalysis*. New York: Basic Books.

Ogden, T. (1994), *Subjects of Analysis*. Northvale, NJ: Aronson.

Person, E. (1980), Sexuality as the mainstay of identity: Psychoanalytic perspectives. *Signs: Women in Culture Society*, 5:605–630.

Phillips, A. (1995), Keeping it moving: Commentary on Judith Butler's "Melancholy gender—refused identification. *Psychoanal. Dial.*, 5:181–188.

Proust, M. (1928), *In Search of Lost Time, Vol. 1. Swann's Way*. New York: Modern Library.

Rapaport, D. (1967), *The Collected Papers of David Rapaport*, ed. M. Gill. New York: Basic Books.

Reisner, S. (2001), Freud and developmental theory: A 21st century look at the origin myth of psychoanalysis. *Stud. Gender. Sexual.*, 2:97–128.

Rorty, R. (1989), *Contingency, Irony, and Solidarity*. Cambridge, England: Cambridge University Press.

Schafer, R. (1964), *Aspects of Internalization*. New York: International Universities Press.

Schwartz, D. (1993), Heterophilia—The love that dare not speak its aim. *Psychoanal. Dial.*, 3:643–652.

Sedgwick, E. (1990), *The Epistemology of the Closet*. Berkeley: University of California Press.

Sontag, S. (1964), *A Susan Sontag Reader*. New York: Farrar, Straus & Giroux.

Taylor, C. (1992), *Multiculturalism and "The Politics of Recognition."* Princeton, NJ: Princeton University Press.

Thelan, E. & Smith, L. (1994), *A Dynamic Systems Approach to the Development of Cognition and Action*. Cambridge, MA: MIT Press.

Vaughn, S. (1997), *Talking Cure: The Science Behind Psychotherapy*. New York: Putman.

Waldrop, M. M. (1992), *Complexity: The Emerging Science at the Edge of Order and Chaos*. New York: Simon & Schuster.

Warner, M. (1993), *Fear of a Queer Planet*. Minneapolis: University of Minnesota Press.

Waters, J., Dir. (1974), *Female Trouble* [film]. New Line Cinema.

Wolff, P. (1996), Infant observation and psychoanalysis. *J. Amer. Psychoanal. Assn.*, 44:369–392.

Afterword

Looking back at this essay, I elaborate on two themes that intertwine with current questions regarding psychoanalytic technique: the developmental action of affinity, and the function of developmental models as tools.

Affinity and Development

I think it likely correct to assert that within the psychoanalytic literature more has been written about the fear of similarity (and suscep-
tibility) and the defense of affection than about the capacity and
positive action of affinity. Apart from discussion of early parent–child
relations (what used to be referred to as the anaclitic relationship),
the psychoanalytic discourse on growth privileges experiences of difference and loss. When the experience of sameness is approached,
it is often folded into discussions of identification (blended, as it were,
with the conflicts of desire), and there is little or no consideration of
what Phillips (2001) in a discussion of "More Life" so aptly referred
to as "noncollusive sameness" (p. 337).[1]

If we turn to discussions about psychoanalytic technique, we can note
a similar trend. Beyond standard introductory nods toward the establishment of a therapeutic alliance there has been limited discussion
of the positive psychotherapeutic action of affinity. Affinity in the consulting room has most often been handled through avoidance. There
are, of course, exceptions to this general "rule" (Ferenczi and Kohut
to name but two). Nevertheless, I think I am correct to assert that our
literature on the kindred undertaking, the noncollusive sameness, and
the reliable relatedness of a psychoanalytic treatment is remarkably
spare and insufficiently problematized.

Can one, we might ask, speak of anything noncollusive and sustain a
psychoanalytic line of inquiry? In the current climate of *vive la différ-
ence*, especially as it informs contemporary Continental perspectives
on psychic life (French neo-Freudian, Lacanian, neo-Bionian), one
cannot approach the idea of noncollusive sameness unaware of the
looming critique that such consideration is insufficiently reflective and
nonpsychoanalytic. This critique is often coupled with a chastening
emphasis on the power of the unconscious and the foundational
experience of sexual difference (see, for example, Green, 1995; Dyess
and Dean, 2000). In particular, American analysts are portrayed as
too involved in relating while too little involved with unconscious
process. Too much ego, too little id.

This critique has proven to be both constructive and corrective.
Consider, for example, recent relational retheorizing of the body that
answers, in part, such critiques (see Dimen, 1998; Harris, 1998,

---

[1] Benjamin's (1995) efforts to examine the forces of liking and loving, as
well as her critique of the classical split between identification and desire, represent an interesting departure from this traditional discourse.

2000). That said, it is important to note that this relational retheo-rizing succeeds in a manner that is distinct from the splitting of rela-tional and unconscious experience that so often informs Continental discussions of American relational theory. Dimen (1998) and Harris (1998, 2000) pursue a view of psychic life that knits relational experience into a perplexing network of unconscious processes. I too have set out a similarly perplexing course, and at this stage in my career I find that I am often taken up by two central issues or questions that inform my pursuit: (1) the relationship between affection and desire—is desire always and already privileged? (2) the relationship of sameness to dif-ference (or affinity to conflict)—is difference (is conflict) always and already privileged?

Thinking about the distinction between affection and desire, I was led back to the distinction that Winnicott (1958) drew between what he termed ego-relatedness and the id-impulse. He embedded his dis-cussion of ego-relatedness within the larger framework of his ideas about ego-integration and psychic equilibrium. For Winnicott, suc-cessful ego-integration rests on successful ego support. Ego support, in turn, rests to a certain degree on affinity. Affinity, in its turn, is established through a certain daily-ness, in particular; for Winnicott, mother–child daily-ness.

Winnicott (1958) was careful to distinguish but not separate related-ness, the ego, and the id: "In a frame of ego-relatedness, id-rela-tionships occur and strengthen rather than disrupt the immature ego" (p. 36). He also considered that relatedness, the ego, and the id could come together in varying titrations. For example, he proposed a realm of ego-relatedness that is colored by a different "quality as well as quantity of id" (p. 35). He illustrated this idea by referring to what he called the "happy play" of children: "The so-called normal child is able to play, to get excited while playing, and to feel *satisfied with the game*, without feeling threatened by a physical orgasm of local excitement" (p. 35). Similarly, he referred to the experience of an adult at a concert or the experience of friendship as evidence of happy play. He even went so far as to suggest that such experiences may result in "ecstasy" or an "ego orgasm"—"a climax that may occur in satisfactory ego-relatedness" (p. 35).

Clearly, psychoanalytic treatments are most often focused on conflict. Life, sadly, is also often absorbed in conflict. As Freud (1930) so aptly reminded us, "Life as we know it is too hard for us" (p. 75). Still and all, we could stand to be less wary of those moments of equilibrium when life temporarily halts or exalts in ecstasy. Or when life rests in ego-relatedness.

Winnicott (1958) attached great importance to the potentialities of ego-relatedness and argued that it "may turn out to be the *matrix of transference*" (p. 33). It is precisely this manner of affinity, coupled with the daily-ness of the psychoanalytic relationship, that is missing from (and mystifying within) much of the current Continental discussion of clinical practice. This is not to say that the Continental emphasis on the restlessness of the unconscious is without merit. Hardly. But I am suggesting that much of human development and much of psychotherapeutic action unfolds in daily ego-related ways that are not always informed by the same quality or quantity of restless unconscious action. Some even occur in the course of happy play.

Herein lies the challenge of more life: to live through (and theorize through) daily ego-relatedness without collapsing the paradox of the multiple valences of psychic life. How else? Living as we do between difference and similarity. Living as we do between the wish for more and the fear of too much. Living as we do between effort and desire.[2] Living as we do through memory and the succession of years superimposed one upon another. Living as we do through aspects of life that are more or less episodic, familiar, and daily while simultaneously living through those currents of life that are marked by vicissitude, the unheeding unknown, and difference.

---

[2] Here I would like to respond to Dyess and Dean's (2000) misreading of my proposition (following Ricoeur) that any account of psychic life must speak to the relationship between effort and desire, including accounts of that which falls out of psychic awareness. As I indicated in my discussion of their essay, I concur with Dyess and Dean that we are in need of a way to theorize a dimension of subjectivity that cannot be superseded as well as a way to speak about that which falls out of psychic awareness. Unlike Dyess and Dean, however, I do not privilege this dimension of impossibility over relational effort. Effort need not, as they incorrectly assume, morph the impossible into the possible. Nor do I privilege effort, as Dyess and Dean incorrectly assume. Effort often fails, and most certainly fails in light of that which falls out of psychic awareness. But an account of psychic life, as presented by Dyess and Dean, that constructs the relationship between effort and the impossible only as oppositional is inadequate. It reduces effort to some doomed and naïve manifestation of will. It is too linear and constructs internal processes as too correspondent. Effort and impossibility are always at hand (with a host of other psychic forces), and we would do better to begin entertaining these forces in a less static interimplicated relationship that moves beyond overly simplified opposition toward the possibility of relations that are perplexing, complexing, and paradoxical.

Developmental Models as Tools

Even though psychoanalysis challenges flat-footed psychologies and trips them up with unconscious process, it is nonetheless still a psychology. As such, psychoanalysis is charged with the responsibility to present a multifaceted view of psychic life—one that imagines and theorizes psychic reality as it knits and is knit into the material reality of daily life.

Psychologists, myself included, have often turned to models in their effort to map the intricacies of psychic life. I am speaking to the dicey and often confusing tension inherent in my effort to employ the antifoundational thinking of postmodernism while at the same time upholding the necessity to think about foundations that is inherent in developmentalism. A similar tension imbues my relationship to developmental models. I wish to resist the standard bearing brutishness of models, yet I continue to desire their service.

Fuss (2001) in a discussion of "More Life," referred to the "stranglehold of models" (p. 346), a phrase that has a particular resonance for me. Models do strangle. They do ignore the pain of others. Yet models also hold. They store perceptions through which foundations emerge. I suggest, however, that we lessen a model's stranglehold by reconsidering and reinvigorating our conceptions regarding foundations. We can get a more complex purchase on development by imagining foundations whose joists and joints are always in motion, or as Rapaport (1967) might have it, foundations that are "processes of a slow rate of change" (p. 787).

It might also be helpful to parse—to the degree that one can (hence, the fly in the ointment)—a model's modeling function or its use as a prototype from its function as a way to know (a struggle toward perception, conception, and construction). Models are built, and, more important, rebuilt (foundations are built and constantly rebuilt), in an effort to capture that developmental hierarchy.

This assertion, however, does not answer whether model building is the best way to engage this project. I do not feel prepared at this juncture to answer either in the affirmative or negative. Yet I can say that I desire the possibility of construction that models imply and provide. I am reminded here of the pleasure I used to take as a boy in building models, the intricate and painstaking effort to master plastic, glue, and representation. Once they were built, though, I had little to no use for these models. They would gradually move from desk to shelf to closet. Whence I'm not sure where they ended up. Perhaps this association illustrates the gap between the dynamism of model building and the static quality of a model built.

It is precisely this static quality of developmental models that has been much criticized in our modern reconsideration of development. It is a critique that I largely support and one to which I have also contributed. Yet I find that such a critique rests too heavily on the action of deconstruction. This does not mean that I approach developmental model building naïve to the postmodern deconstruction of the unity and stability of human subjectivity. Nor do I undertake such a course in opposition to postmodern theories. But I do contend that a complex appreciation of human subjectivity rests not only on the reversing force of deconstruction, but also on an equal and opposite forwarding force of construction.

Developmental models are constructed and employed through the clinical psychoanalyst's effort to grasp the forwarding force of development. Models provide a useable way to consider what might be called the ontogenetic significance of certain features of development. In this regard models function as tools. Like any tool, they do not function simply; they function as history, as description, as diagnosis. They are used and abused. Consequently, those of us who are eager to diminish cruelty can only *self-consciously* rely on developmental models. We can use them only knowing they are not true—not true, insofar as they do not have a privileged relationship to the truth, nor do they offer any metaphysical guarantees.

I propose that we follow Rorty (cited in Rorty, Nystrom, and Puckett, 1998) (who, in turn, was following Wittgenstein) by suggesting that "we view our ways of describing and explaining the world as 'tools' which help us get along in that world, rather than as representations of that world which could be said to be more or less correct" (p. viii). Key to this strategy is the element of self-consciousness—the degree of reflection and tension that elevates description and redescription over representation. That elevates model building and rebuilding over static representation. This manner of self-consciousness is key, in turn, to More Life—a strategy that rests on the constant reconstruction of association and reality and the perpetually perplexed circulation of revision and expansion.

References

Benjamin, J. (1995), Sameness and difference: An "overinclusive" view of gender constitution. In: *Like Subjects, Love Objects*. New Haven, CT: Yale University Press.

Dimen, M. (1998), Polyglot bodies: Thinking through the relational. In: *Relational Perspectives on the Body*, ed. L. Aron & F. S. Anderson. Hillsdale, NJ: The Analytic Press, pp. 65–93.

Dyess, C. & Dean, T. (2000), Gender: The impossibility of meaning. *Psychoanal. Dial.*, 10:735–756.

Freud, S. (1930), Civilization and its discontents. *Standard Edition*, 21:64–145. London: Hogarth Press, 1961.

Fuss, D. (2001), More metaphor: Commentary on paper by Ken Corbett. *Psychoanal. Dial.*, 11:343–346.

Green, A. (1995), Has sexuality anything to do with psychoanalysis? *Internat. J. Psycho-Anal.*, 76:871–884.

Harris, A. (1998), Psychic envelopes and sonorous baths: Siting the body in relational theory and clinical practice. In: *Relational Perspectives on the Body*, ed. L. Aron & F. S. Anderson. Hillsdale, NJ: The Analytic Press, pp. 39–64.

———— (2000), Gender as soft assembly: Tomboys' stories. *Psychoanal. Dial.*, 1:223–250.

Phillips, A. (2001), More or less life: Commentary on paper by Ken Corbett. *Psychoanal. Dial.*, 11:337–342.

Rapaport, D. (1967), *The Collected Papers of David Rapaport*, ed. M. Gill. New York: Basic Books.

Rorty, R., Nystrom, D. & Puckett, K. (1998), *Against Bosses, Against Oligarchies: A Conversation with Richard Rorty*. Charlottesville, VA: Prickly Pear Pamphlets.

Winnicott, D. W. (1958), The capacity to be alone. In: *The Maturational Processes and the Facilitating Environment*. New York: International Universities Press, 1965, pp. 29–36.

Author Index

Author Index

collusion(s) *(continued)*
  "coherent," 320
  open, 318
  unconscious, 126
conduct disorders, 265–266
conflict (in analytic relationship),
    107. *See also under* analyst(s),
    identity of; negotiation;
    supervisory situation
  and deception. *See also* cases,
    Edward, Nancy, Tanya
  how analytic situation heightens
    the experience of, 86–88,
    91–92, 100–102, 111–117
  as essential constituent of relating,
    77–82
"confusion of interest(s)," 78n, 92.
constructivism, 57, 66, 312–313. *See
    also* enactive (relational)
    representation(s)
constructivist view of defenses, 327
containing function, criticism related
    to, 129
containment. *See also* holding
  contributors to the concept of, 31n
  of mental states, 260, 261
contingencies, 213
continuity-contiguity moment, 6
control, 131. *See also* overcontrolled
    patients
  of analyst, 136
  over the other, 14, 21–23
  sense of losing emotional
    equated with losing control of
      behavior and boundaries, 129
    fear of, 129, 136
control systems, unique features of
    relational, 336–338
control systems model of mind, 328–332
"core" of personality, 79–80
corrective emotional experience, 341–
    343. *See also* new experience
countertransference, 147–148,
    177–181, 384. *See also*
    analyst(s), affective responses
    and expression; enactments;
    self-disclosure; supervision
  cannot be relegated to candidate's
    analysis, 148–150

concordant and complementary
    identifications, 154
disclosure and open discussion of,
    149–150, 179–180. *See also*
    self-disclosure
  dangers of not disclosing, 139, 140
  as multiply determined, 177
  "objective," 79
  patient's perception of, 180–181
  racial, 422. *See also* cases, Mrs.
    C.; race
cultural context of psychoanalysis,
    353–354, 357–358, 414. *See
    also* perversion; psychoanalytic
    treatment, and the urban
    poor; race
cultural factors in development,
    432–433
cultures, need to read patterns and
    for individuals to read beyond
    patterns, 456–458

D
deceptive potentials in analytic frame,
    111. *See also* conflict (in analytic
    relationship), and deception
defenses, 325–328
defensiveness, 22–23
dependence and holding, 33
depression, 289. *See also* cases,
    Edward
derailment, 215
desire *vs.* affection, 464
determinism. *See under* homosexuality
development. *See also* affect
    development; cognitive-
    developmental theory; enactive
    relational procedures
  affinity and, 462–465
  cultural factors in, 432–433
  and dialogic movement of chaos
    and coherence, 453–455
  as process *vs.* state, 450–453
  quasi-axioms of new model of,
    450–458
developmental and psychoanalytic
    change. *See also* enactive
    (relational) representation(s),
    and change process

Printed and bound by CPI Group (UK) Ltd, Croydon, CR0 4YY

17/10/2024

01775687-0011